Anti-Obesity Drug Discovery and Development
(Volume 2)

Editor

Atta-ur-Rahman, *FRS*

Kings College
University of Cambridge
Cambridge
UK

&

M. Iqbal Choudhary

H.E.J. Research Institute of Chemistry
International Center for Chemical and Biological Sciences
University of Karachi
Karachi
Pakistan

CONTENTS

PREFACE

Obesity is a disease which leads to several chronic illnesses and reduces the life expectancy. It is a complex health problem, caused by a number of factors, such as excessive food intake, lack of physical activity, genetic predisposition, endocrine disorders, use of certain medications, and psychiatric illnesses. More recently a linkage between infection with Adenovirus 36 and obesity has also been investigated. Obesity has been identified as the leading preventable cause of mortality and morbidity, and substantial research has been conducted to identify the molecular targets for pharmacological interventions. Extensive studies on nutritional aspects and life style changes have also been carried out to prevent the on-set of obesity. Prevalence of obesity in both developing and developed world has reached to an epidemic proportion. In response to this, efforts to control and treat obesity have also been vigorously pursued, ranging from raising awareness about lifestyle modifications to the discovery and development of safe and effective anti-obesity drugs.

"*Anti-Obesity Drug Discovery and Development*" focuses on this important area of healthcare research. The second volume of this eBook series is a compilation of five well written reviews on the state-of-the-art developments in obesity research.

This volume begins with a review of Sabán-Ruíz *et al.,* explaining the relationship between obesity and cardiometabolic syndrome. This comprehensive review covers basic research and epidemiology about obesity, metabolic syndrome and cardiac diseases, as well as old and new drugs used to treat obesity and hypertension. The problem with such drugs that were approved for prescription, was they are effective in the short-term but that they often exhibit several adverse side effects. These include newer drugs, such as sibutramine, rimonabant and orlistart. This has been an ongoing concern in anti-obesity drug development. The researchers have also mentioned progress in the new drug development and combined therapies in clinical trials. The chapter concludes with a discussion of anti-obesity therapy using Topiramate, a drug used to treat psychological disorders and the implications of such drugs for the treatment of cardiovascular disorders.

Obesity is also be regarded as a consequence of homeostatic imbalance within the body. Homeostatic balance is influenced by hormone levels, food intake, epigenetics, immunological factors, and others. Suba, in chapter 2, explores the hypothesis of estrogen as an anti-obesity agent. The author suggests that estrogen has positive regulatory effects on the lipid distribution in the body as well as resistance to insulin. Research also suggests that insulin helps to promote pancreatic insulin secretion and controls the inflammatory response of adipocytes. Hormonal therapy, such as estrogen administration to patients - postmenopausal women in particular - has shown positive outcomes with respect to curbing fat deposition in the body.

In chapter 3, Essam Abdel-Sattar and colleagues have reviewed the scientific works on herbal and microbial remedies of obesity. This review presents the mechanisms of action of active ingredients and contains a comprehensive list of herbs that can be used to treat obesity and associated disorders. The authors have also included illustrations of some of these herbs, many of which could be used to develop effective nutritional supplements.

Reyna and Banu have reviewed the work conducted on the capacity of natural extracts which can be used to interface with lipid metabolism. Natural products can provide a safe and cost effective OTC solution for the treatment of obesity. This review focuses on several types of plant extracts and also discusses some benefits of common dietary herbs, such as tea, lotus and certain oriental and eastern spices. The review also provides information about the anti-obesity mechanism of action of selected natural products.

Babenko has contributed a lucidly written review on the possibility of targeting sphingolipids metabolism in the quest for controlling obesity. Specifically, this can be achieved by targeting sphingomyelin hydrolysis and nucleotide synthesis pathways to limit the ceramide production in cells. Since an increased ceramide levels in obesity patients has been observed, it is believed that reducing the concentration of ceramides, by inhibiting the enzymes involve in its biosynthesis, can help in tackling the disease. The author discusses the results of inhibition of sphingolipids in mice as a first step towards drug development.

At the end we would like to express our deep gratitude to all the contributors for making this volume an excellent compilation of state-of-the-art knowledge on the molecular basis of obesity and its effective treatment. We also wish to express our thanks to Ms. Maria Baig (Manager Publications) and other members of the Bentham Science Publishers for their efforts in the timely completion of this volume. We are also most grateful to Mr. Mahmood Alam (Director Publications) for efficiently leading the Bentham team in this project.

Atta-ur-Rahman, FRS
Kings College
University of Cambridge
Cambridge
UK

&

M. Iqbal Choudhary
H.E.J. Research Institute of Chemistry
International Center for Chemical and Biological Sciences
University of Karachi
Karachi
Pakistan

List of Contributors

Alcira Andrés

Endothelium and Cardiometabolic Medicine Unit, Internal Medicine Service, Ramón y Cajal Hospital, Madrid, Spain

Ana Alonso-Pacho

Endothelium and Cardiometabolic Medicine Unit, Internal Medicine Service, Ramón y Cajal Hospital, Madrid, Spain

Asunción Guerri

Endothelium and Cardiometabolic Medicine Unit, Internal Medicine Service, Ramón y Cajal Hospital, Madrid, Spain

Cristina de la Puerta González-Quevedo

Endothelium and Cardiometabolic Medicine Unit, Internal Medicine Service, Ramón y Cajal Hospital, Madrid, Spain

Delia Barrio

Endothelium and Cardiometabolic Medicine Unit, Internal Medicine Service, Ramón y Cajal Hospital, Madrid, Spain

Essam Abdel-Sattar

Pharmacognosy Department, College of Pharmacy, Cairo University, 11562, Cairo, Egypt

Jameela Banu

Coordinated Program in Dietetics and Department of Biology, University of Texas-Pan American, 1201, W. University Dr., Edinburg, TX 78539-2999, USA

José Sabán-Ruíz

Endothelium and Cardiometabolic Medicine Unit, Internal Medicine Service, Ramón y Cajal Hospital, Madrid, Spain

Maha M. Salama

Pharmacognosy Department, College of Pharmacy, Cairo University, 11562, Cairo, Egypt

Martin Fabregate-Fuente

Endothelium and Cardiometabolic Medicine Unit, Internal Medicine Service, Ramón y Cajal Hospital, Madrid, Spain

Nataliya A. Babenko

Department of Physiology of Ontogenesis, Institute of Biology, Kharkov Karazin National University, 4 Svobody pl., 61077 Kharkov, Ukraine

Rosa Fabregate-Fuente

Endothelium and Cardiometabolic Medicine Unit, Internal Medicine Service, Ramón y Cajal Hospital, Madrid, Spain

Sara M. Reyna

Department of Medicine and Medical Research Division, Edinburg Regional Academic Health Center, University of Texas Health Science Center at San Antonio, 1214, W Schunior, Edinburg, TX 78541, USA

Soheir M. El Zalabani

Pharmacognosy Department, College of Pharmacy, Cairo University, 11562, Cairo, Egypt

Susana Tello Blasco

Endothelium and Cardiometabolic Medicine Unit, Internal Medicine Service, Ramón y Cajal Hospital, Madrid, Spain

Zsuzsanna Suba

National Institute of Oncology, Department of Surgical and Molecular Pathology, Budapest, Hungary

Send Orders for Reprints to reprints@benthamscience.net

Anti-Obesity Drug Discovery and Development, Vol. 2, 2014, 3-85

CHAPTER 1

An Approach to Obesity as a Cardiometabolic Disease: Potential Implications for Clinical Practice

José Sabán-Ruíz*, Martin Fabregate-Fuente, Rosa Fabregate-Fuente, Ana Alonso-Pacho, Cristina de la Puerta González-Quevedo, Susana Tello Blasco, Asunción Guerri, Alcira Andrés and Delia Barrio

Endothelium and Cardiometabolic Medicine Unit, Internal Medicine Service, Ramón y Cajal Hospital, Madrid, Spain

Abstract: Obesity is a multifactorial disease that is currently developing a threatening tendency towards becoming the main cause of chronic disease in the world. Obesity can induce type 2 diabetes mellitus, dyslipidemia, cardiovascular disease and other chronic disorders with high social and health costs. Obesity was firstly described in 2000 as a cardiometabolic disease, even before Metabolic Syndrome, type 2 diabetes mellitus and coronary disease were considered as such. In this chapter we recover this approach to obesity, which has remained almost forgotten for the last decade. In obese subjects, adipokines and miokines interact to promote reticulum stress, insulin resistance, metabolic inflexibility and endothelial dysfunction. These pathological processes are amplified when hyperglycemia is present, leading to an increased risk for atherosclerosis. A number of potential implications for clinical practice are derived from the cardiometabolic state underlying obesity and its comorbidities. The first step in the therapeutic strategy against obesity should be the correct diagnosis of its causes and the promotion of lifestyle changes including physical exercise and a healthy diet. In the usual case of failing to achieve results, we can still resort to the pharmacological therapy. While awaiting the release of new drugs, topiramate, alone or combined with phentermine, has been proposed as a novel anti-obesity drug, showing relevant effects not only on weight loss but also on cardiometabolic alterations and biomarkers, even though new studies should clarify the mechanisms of these findings. Finally, our own experience with topiramate is described, focusing on its effects upon weight loss and inflammatory markers.

Keywords: Adipokine, adiposity, adiposopathy endoplasmic reticulum stress, anti-obesity drugs, atherosclerosis, cardiometabolic disease, coronary heart disease, diet, endothelial dysfunction, inflammation, insulin resistance, lifestyle changes, metabolic inflexibility, miokine, obesity, physical activity, topiramate, weight loss.

---

*Address correspondence to José Sabán-Ruiz: Endothelium and Cardiometabolic Medicine Unit, Internal Medicine Service, Ramón y Cajal Hospital, Madrid, Spain; E-mail: psaban@gmail.com

INTRODUCTION

Obesity constitutes a multifactorial pathology whose acquired influences exceed genetic factors, and nowadays threatens to become the major cause of chronic disease in the world [1], with high social and health costs [2]. The medical expenditure related to the treatment of obesity in the USA was $147 billion in 2008, which has doubled in the course of the last ten years [3]. WHO definition [4] for obesity is a body mass index (BMI, weight/(height)^2) greater than or equal to 30, while overweight is defined as a BMI between 25 and 30 kg/m^2. Within obesity, different grades have been defined according to BMI: Grade 1 (BMI from 30 to less than 35), Grade 2 (35 to less than 40) and Grade 3 (40 or greater) [4].

According to WHO data [4], every year at least 2.8 million of deaths are caused by overweight and obesity, being the fifth leading risk for global deaths. Moreover, overweight and obesity account for 44% of the diabetes burden, 23% of the coronary heart disease and between 7% and 41% of certain types of cancer. The most recent data on obesity prevalence in the US show that more than one out of three adults and almost 17% of children and adolescents were obese in 2009-2010. With regard to sex, differences have diminished in the last years, with men reaching almost identical prevalence than women. A higher prevalence of obesity has been observed among older women compared with younger women, but there were no age-related differences by age among men [5]. In 2007-2010, 20% of US adults had Grade 1 obesity, 9% Grade 2 obesity, and 6% Grade 3 obesity, whereas 33.3% of adults over 20 years were overweight (and not obese) [6]. In European countries, the prevalence of overweight in 2008 was 58% among males and 51% among females, whereas the obesity prevalence was 20% in males and 23% in females. Worldwide data show that 34% of males and 35% of females had overweight, whereas the prevalence of obesity was 10% in males, 14% in females and 12% in both genders [7]. The Figs. **1** and **2** show the prevalence of overweight and obesity worldwide.

**Prevalence of overweight*, ages 20+, age standardized
Both sexes, 2008**

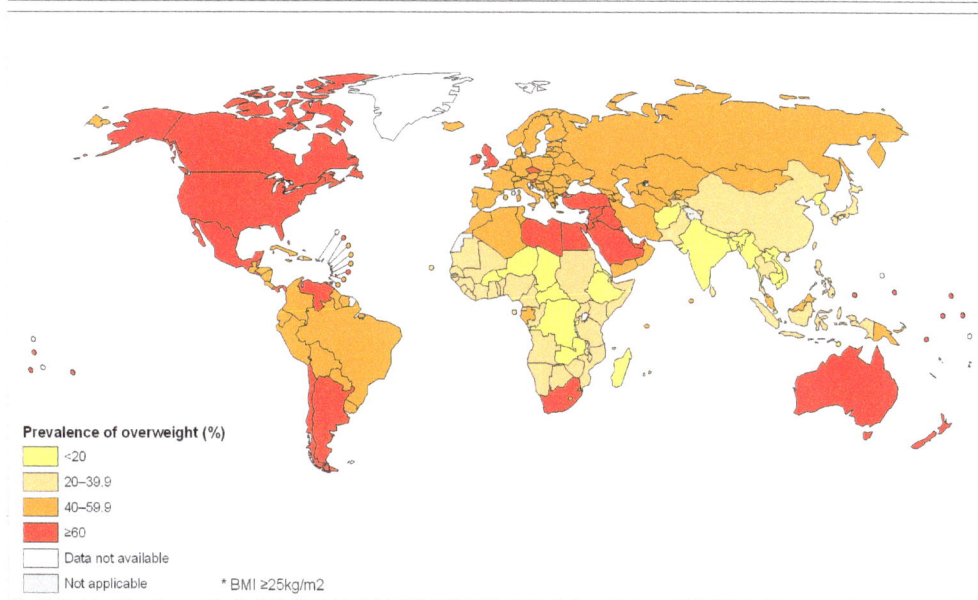

Figure 1: Prevalence of overweight. Source: World Health Organization.

**Prevalence of obesity*, ages 20+, age standardized
Both sexes, 2008**

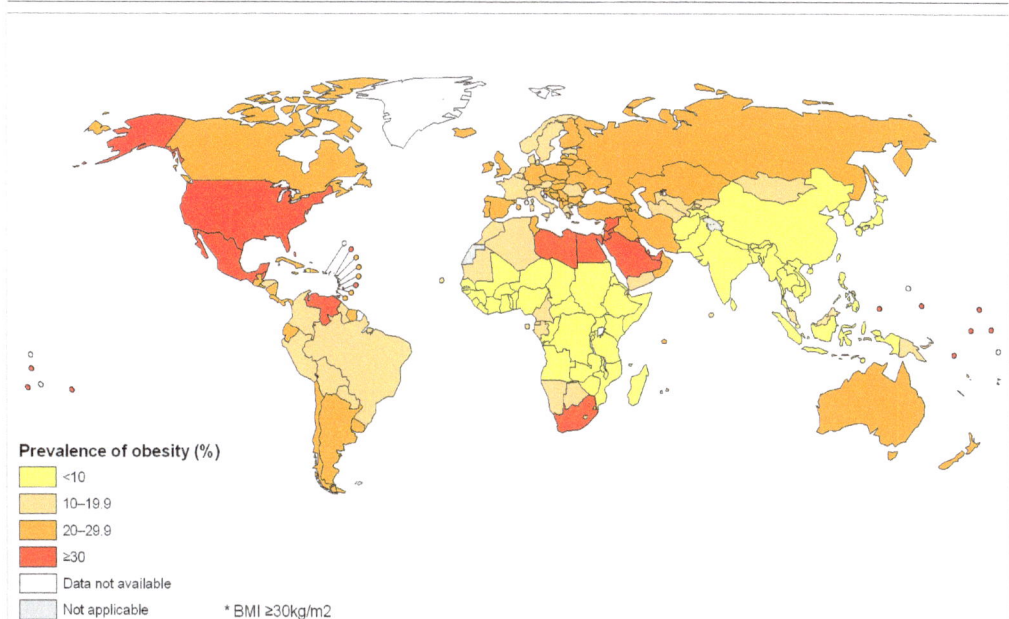

Figure 2: Prevalence of obesity. Source: World Health Organization.

In this scenario, a current strategy leading to improve six cardiovascular health metrics (weight, blood pressure, physical activity; diabetes, total cholesterol and smoking) could prevent 24-30% of the CHD deaths expected in 2020 [8]. Four of these items keep a direct relationship with obesity as a cardiometabolic disease (weight, sedentary lifestyle, blood pressure and diabetes). Future prevention of cardiovascular disease necessarily involves acting now energetically without further delay. A better understanding of the pathophysiology involved in obese will help us in this hard and arduous task.

At present, different prevention strategies against the worrying prevalence of obesity have been implemented, especially in the childhood period. But hitherto, these approaches have not shown results, so we have to act improving the compliance with conventional therapy. There is a triple obesity treatment objective: a) at short term, lowering weight; b) at medium term, reducing cardiovascular risk factors associated; c) at long term, stopping the cardiovascular events and the obesity comorbidities, such as arthrosis or obstructive sleep apnoea syndrome. Regarding weight reduction, several studies focused on obesity therapies have confirmed that a moderate reduction of initial body weight could have positive results such as significant improvements in blood pressure and/or serum lipid concentrations, increased insulin sensitivity or improved glycaemia [9-12]. The "Look AHEAD Study" has shown that a body weight reduction of 7% improves glycemic control and cardiovascular risk factors in subjects with type 2 diabetes [13].

Traditionally, therapies for weight loss have been based on lifestyle changes: mainly diet and exercise or a combination of both. This is still a useful tool for this purpose, but it faces a great disadvantage: compliance by obese or overweight subject is usually low [14]. Thus, when these measures fail, a fact that is very frequently verified in daily clinical practice, the pharmacological treatment of obesity constitutes an effective alternative which should not be postponed. In order to stop this epidemic, the American College of Physicians published in 2005 the first obesity guideline [15], which was based upon the results of two previous meta-analysis on recent therapies for weight loss [16, 17]. In this guideline, pharmacological treatment is presented as a useful alternative for patients who have failed with treatments based upon life-style changes such as diet and/or exercise, becoming "resistant" to these therapies. Drug therapy is considered to be suitable for subjects with BMI higher or equal to 27 Kg/m^2, especially for those (a very frequent circumstance in this range of BMI) who present obesity-related morbidities such as Type 2 diabetes mellitus or impaired glucose tolerance, dyslipidemia and/or high blood pressure.

The National Institutes of Health (NIH) also recommends that adults with a BMI > 35 Kg/m^2 with serious associated comorbidities such as sleep apnoea, obesity-related cardiomyopathy or severe joint disease may also be candidates for bariatric surgery [9]. However, the experts' opinion is to run out all treatment options before carrying out this surgery. The place of so the called "Metabolic Surgery" [18] for the treatment of type 2 diabetes exceeds the purpose of this chapter.

In the last years, several drugs have been used for the treatment of obesity: orlistat [19, 20], an inhibitor of gastric and pancreatic lipases; selective serotonin reuptake inhibitors (SSRIs) [21]; sibutramine, a serotonin-norepinephrine reuptake inhibitor which is structurally related to amphetamines [22, 23]; and rimonabant, a selective cannabinoid receptor antagonist (CB1) [24, 25]. However, all of these drugs produce severe side effects, especially sibutramine [26] and rimonabant [27, 28].

Human appetite is controlled by neurological networks in the Central Nervous System (CNS), more precisely by serotonergic, opioid, dopaminergic and cannabinoid systems, which are regulated in a very precise and complex way by intricate signalling pathways [29]. With regard to these neural pathways, despite the evident failure of current drugs (amphetamine derivatives, fenfluramine, sibutramine, rimonabant) [30], several additional gut hormone-based treatments for obesity are under investigation, with particular focus on leptin, ghrelin, peptide YY or pancreatic polypeptide [31], due to its participation together with the neural pathways involved in appetite.

While awaiting the release of new drugs, topiramate (TPM), an antiepileptic drug (AED), also approved as a treatment for migraine headaches, has been proposed as a novel anti-obesity drug. Furthermore, the combination of TPM plus phentermine, an appetite suppressant, has been recently approved for chronic weight management in overweight or obese adults [32].

The main purpose of this chapter is to position obesity as a cardiometabolic disease with an underlying vascular damage. In this sense, it is necessary to differentiate syndromes related to obesity such as Metabolic Syndrome (MetS), Cardiometabolic Syndrome (CMS) and Cardiometabolic Risk (CMR), and the role of overweigh in each other. It is also important to analyze the role of low-grade inflammation or metaflammation in fat tissue, as well as two new metabolic phenomena, Metabolic Inflexibility and Endoplasmic Reticulum Stress, and their interaction with the vascular triad (Endothelial Dysfunction, Oxidative Stress and Vascular Inflammation). In this context, new drugs should consider the mechanisms related to the physiopathology of obesity as a cardiometabolic disease, and not only in the weight loss in a narrow sense.

PATHOGENESIS OF OBESITY

The pathogenesis of obesity is influenced by interactions among several factors including inherited genetic features, a dysfunctional appetite regulation and the energy consumption. It is also influenced by behavioural, physical or psychological factors, cultural identity, education level, and socioeconomic status.

Genetic Factors

There is a genetic basis upon which environmental factors interact in the development of obesity [33]. Moreover, there are some forms of obesity transmitted by both recessive and dominant modes of inheritance. Amongst them, the Prader-Willi syndrome is the most common. Obesity, as many of the most prevalent diseases in human being, is thought to be polygenic, although there are some very rare types of monogenic obesity [34, 35].

Up to now, genetic variation in the FTO (Fat Mass and Obesity Associate) gene has the largest effect on BMI since Frayling and colleagues found a strong association between this gene and human obesity in 2007 [36]. Many others mutations associated with the nutrient intake and energy expenditure have been described, although they are beyond the purpose of this chapter.

In summary, as genetic disorders represent only a small fraction of the obese population, they cannot explain the magnitude of the obesity.

Energy Expenditure and Nutrient Imbalance

Obesity results from a chronic energy imbalance, as food intake over-matches the body's energy output. Increase in body weight and body fat with age cannot be associated with an increased caloric intake, but rather to a reduction in energy consumption, as energy requirements decline with age. Resting metabolism, defined as the total energy required by the body in a resting state, typically represents about 70% of total energy expenditure. It depends mainly on age, sex, body weight, drugs and genetics, and it is closely related to fat-free body mass as well as to body surface area because of its relationship to heat loss from the skin [37].

The other key player in obesity is appetite. It is regulated by specific molecular processes and neural pathways which are ultimately integrated at hypothalamus [38, 39], producing the expression of behavior and the associated subjective sensations [40]. Food intake is controlled by the complex integration of hormonal signals from the gut, pancreas, liver and fat.

Hunger and satiety are the psychological experiences regulating food intake behavior. Handling energy balance demands extensive coordination from the central nervous system (CNS), as the regions controlling energy homeostasis are accessible to numerous circulating hormones as well as the information from the sensory experience of eating and from peripheral receptors related to the ingestion and the utilization of food nutrients. These include signals from receptors in the gut and metabolic changes in the liver. Cholecystokinin (CCK), glucagon-like peptide-1 (GLP-1), peptide YY (PYY) and amylin are the chemical signals related to satiety [38], whereas ghrelin, a peptide hormone, is involved in the short-term regulation of appetite. Blood levels of ghrelin secreted by the stomach and duodenum are raised during fasting and decreased after food intake. In addition, these appetite pathways also involve other signals from receptors within the CNS detecting circulating levels of nutrients, their metabolites and other substances, such as glucose [39].

Daily food intake and eating behavior are not only related to appetite and satiety, but also respond to processes of energy storage and the status of the body's energy stores [41]. Lipostatic signals including leptin and insulin, or levels of cytokine signals, such as the IL-6 and TNF-α, may also be influenced by adipose tissue.

PATHOPHYSIOLOGY OF OBESITY AND ITS RELATIONSHIP WITH CARDIOMETABOLIC SYNDROME

The Importance of Type of Fat and Body Distribution

With regard to obesity in humans, a wide array of research has focused on white adipose tissue (WAT). Although brown adipose tissue (BAT) depots were thought to disappear shortly after the perinatal period, recently positron emission tomography (PET) imaging using the glucose analog F-deoxy-d-glucose (FDG) has shown the existence of functional BAT in adult humans. BAT is activated in response to cold stimulation, [42], as a energy-dissipating mechanism responsible for "adaptive thermogenesis" in adults during cold stress. In this context, adipocytes within WAT can be converted into multilocular adipocytes (known as "browning-WAT" or "beige" adipocytes) expressing UCP1, a mitochondrial protein capable of uncoupling the activity of the respiratory chain from ATP synthesis, which plays a key role in heat production. Whereas BAT has been extensively studied in rodent models [43], both *in vivo* and *in vitro*, there is still a lack of human models to assess critical factors involved in the induction of thermogenic response within adipocytes. Although even in subjects with relatively large depots, BAT accounts just for 20 kcal/day during moderate cold stress, recent discoveries on thermogenic BAT in human adults has opened a new field for innovative strategies in the fight against obesity and its associated diseases. Even so, further research is required in order to clarify the conversion and metabolism of white-to-brown converted adipocytes, which would enable the development of new therapeutic strategies targeting overweight/obesity [44].

The physiopathological effects of adipose tissue are related to the specific site where fat is stored [45-47], besides other factors such as genetic factors, gender, age, and physical exercise [48]. There is a clear functional distinction between visceral or intraperitoneal fat, extraperitoneal (peripancreatic and perirenal) and intrapelvic (gonadal/epididymal and urogenital) adipose tissues, all of them presenting a higher metabolic activity than subcutaneous peripheral adipose tissue [49].

Classically, obesity is classified into two types according to fat mass distribution. The "android type" obesity, also called central or abdominal obesity, and the "ginoid" or peripheral obesity. Central obesity, characterized by the storage of the excess of fat in the upper part of the body, is typically related to male individuals, although this fat distribution is also present in women, especially during the menopausal and post-menopausal period, as well as in elderly subjects, both men and women [50]. Although it is always present in Caucasian subjects with BMI higher than 30 kg/m^2, also subjects of medium or even low BMI may develop central obesity. Moreover, abdominal obesity is strongly associated with associated with Metabolic Syndrome (MetS), Cardiometabolic Risk and Cardiovascular Disease [51].

As explained in the introduction, obesity has been defined according to the Body Mass Index (BMI), although it leads to a not very accurate assessment of obesity, since it does not take into account differences in body composition and body fat distribution [52, 53]. However, despite its limitations, diagnosis of obesity and overweight in epidemiological studies is assessed according to BMI [54]. With regard to Cardiometabolic disease, a concept that includes essentially obesity, MetS, diabetes mellitus and atherosclerosis, several alternatives to BMI have been proposed to assess fat mass, such as waist circumference, skinfold thickness measurements (with calipers), underwater weighing, bioelectrical impedance, dual-energy X-ray absorptiometry (DXA) and computerized tomography. In clinical practice, waist circumference (WC), waist-to-hip ratio (WHR) and waist-to-height ratio (WHtR), are useful tools for assessing adiposity/obesity, providing a better approach to cardiometabolic risk than BMI [55, 56]

In addition to the abdominal fat, two locations of fat in obesity could take part in the active form of the disease that later we will name "adiposopathy": pericardial fat and fatty liver (Figs. **3** and **4**). Pericardial fat, also known as epicardial fat when assessed by echography [57], is strategically located next to coronary vessels. This ectopic fat depot has been recently correlated to BMI, visceral adipose tissue (VAT), metabolic risk factors, insulin resistance and coronary artery disease [58-61]. In a study by Rosito *et al.,* [62], VAT showed a stronger correlation to Cardiovascular Risk than pericardial fat, but these fat depots were associated with vascular calcification, which suggests that they may exert local toxic effects on the vasculature. According to this attractive cardiometabolic hypothesis, epicardial fat could contribute to the pathogenesis of coronary heart disease in a straightforward manner.

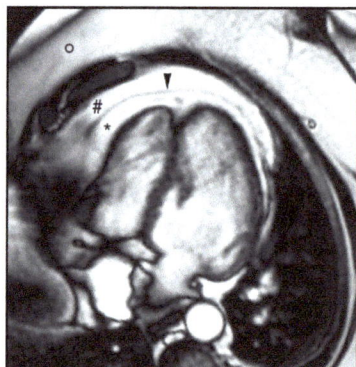

Figure 3: Pericardial fat.

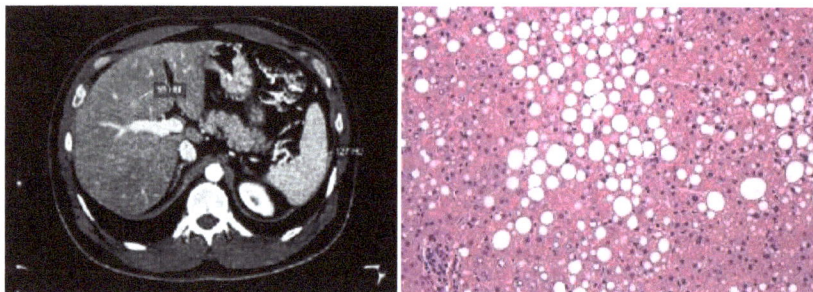

Figure 4: Hepatic steatosis.

On the other hand, nonalcoholic fatty liver disease (NAFLD) is the most important cause of chronic liver disease and it is considered the hepatic manifestation of the obesity, especially in subjects with Metabolic Syndrome and/or type 2 diabetes mellitus. The prevalence of NAFLD in the general population reaches 15-20%, whereas nonalcoholic steatohepatitis (NASH), an advanced stage of the disease, affects 3% of the population. NAFLD includes a wide range of liver damage, from simple steatosis or accumulation of triglycerides in the liver to inflammation (NASH), fibrosis and cirrhosis [63-65]. Subjects with steatosis and NASH present liver oxidative stress, which is a plausible mediator of cellular injury, inflammatory recruitment, and fibrogenesis. CYPs 2E1 and 4A, the microsomal oxidases involved in fatty acid oxidation, can reduce molecular oxygen to produce prooxidant species, increasing oxidative stress [66]. Both in obese and non-obese cohorts of non-alcoholic patients without hereditary hemochromatosis, high serum ferritin levels increase risk for steatosis [67]. The benefits of iron reduction are still unclear, and the final decision to treat such patients should be individualized [68].

INSULIN RESISTANCE (IR) AND ITS RELATIONSHIP WITH METABOLIC SYNDROME (METS) AND TYPE-2 DIABETES MELLITUS (T2DM)

Insulin resistance (IR) is a pathophysiological phenomenon that usually occurs along with weight gain. Moreover, weight increment and IR may be accompanied by a MetS. Around one third of obese subjects will develop T2DM, but if we take into account pre-diabetes, this figure raises over 50%, which is the percentage of patients with hyperglycemia. T2DM development requires not only IR but also a genetic susceptibility of β-cell in addition to others factor which take part in β cell dysfunction [69].

MetS history starts in 1921 when Eskyl Kylin, a Swiss physician, related for the first time the occurrence of high blood pressure to diabetes. This association was confirmed one year later by Gregorio Maranon, a Spanish physician, on the same medical publication (Zentralblatt für Innere Medizin). In 1923, Kylin [70] widened the concept, adding the diagnosis of hyperuricemia. Later in 1929 Samuel A. Levine [71] not only added new components to this concept, such as the presence of dyslipemia, but also underlined the importance of the cardiovascular risk associated to smoking, foreseeing 30 years in advance to what was much later demonstrated in the Framingham Study [72], thus laying the first stone of what today is denominated "Cardiometabolic Risk (CMR)".

In 1936, Harold Percival Himsworth, used the term Insulin Insensibility in those diabetic patients who were non-responders to that hormone [73]. In 1947 J. Vague [74], a French doctor, underlined the difference in body fat distribution between genders and later in 1956 related abdominal obesity to an increased risk of diabetes, atherosclerosis, gout and uric lithiasis [75]. The association between obesity, dyslipidemia and diabetes was named Plurimetabolic Syndrome by Avogadro and Crepaldi in 1967 [76], highlighting its relationship with coronary risk.

In 1979, De Fronzo *et al.,* [77], described IR, quantified by the clamp technique, as an essential element in the T2DM physiopathology. As IR was observed not only in diabetics but also in non-diabetic patients, a deficit in insulin secretion, later showed of multifactorial origin, was suggested as necessary for T2DM development.

MetS was dubbed as X Syndrome by Reaven [78] in the 1980s including hyperglycemia, high blood pressure, low HDL-cholesterol, high triglycerides and IR; and later by Kaplan as Deathly Quarter [79], adding central obesity with impaired glucose tolerance, hypertriglyceridemia and high blood pressure. However, the term Metabolic Syndrome, previously used by Hanefeld and Leonhardt [80], was later imposed on. In 1997 DeFronzo and Ferranini deepend in the IR concept, coining the Insulin Resistance Syndrome term [81] (Fig. **5**).

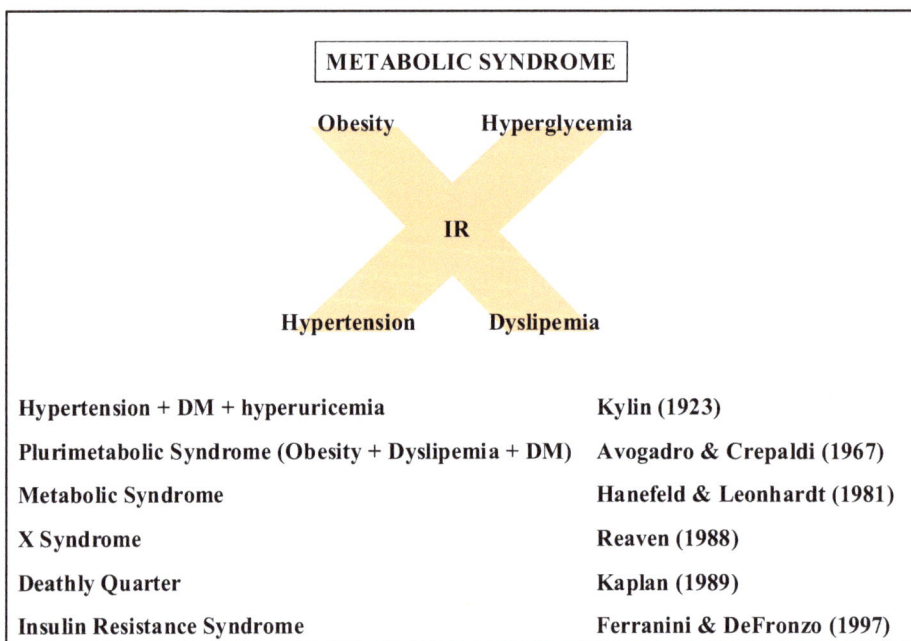

METABOLIC SYNDROME

Hypertension + DM + hyperuricemia	**Kylin (1923)**
Plurimetabolic Syndrome (Obesity + Dyslipemia + DM)	**Avogadro & Crepaldi (1967)**
Metabolic Syndrome	**Hanefeld & Leonhardt (1981)**
X Syndrome	**Reaven (1988)**
Deathly Quarter	**Kaplan (1989)**
Insulin Resistance Syndrome	**Ferranini & DeFronzo (1997)**

Figure 5: History evolution of the Metabolic Syndrome (MetS) concept.

Nowadays, MetS is considered to be between T2DM and cardiovascular disease, taking part in the development of both processes, but not simultaneously. Table **1** shows the ATP III-2005 criteria for MetS.

After reviewing the evolution of the Metabolic Syndrome concept and its relationship with IR, the following provides an in-depth revision of the physiological mechanisms involved in IR. The most important physiological action exerted by insulin is to allow the entrance of the plasma glucose into the cell. This is carried out through a biological phenomenon called activation of the trans-membrane transport for which two previous phases are necessary: the translocation of the glucose transporters (named GLUT) from the microsomes to the plasmatic membrane and their phosphorilation to convert them into "GLUT-P", which is the active form. The entrance of glucose into the cell also depends on the so called "mass action effect", which is independent of insulin, so that glycemic levels promote the uptake of glucose by a direct action upon GLUT. But this mechanism is impaired in both type 1 and type 2diabetes. This peculiar phenomenon was named "resistance to glucose" by Del Prato and De Fronzo [82]. However, it is necessary to clarify that the insulin receptor does not only allows glucose enter to the cells through the GLUT transporter, but also facilitates its metabolism, by activating particular enzymes which are key factors in its metabolic pathway, including storage and oxidative routes.

The first question we should ask ourselves is: in a normal cell, what mechanisms regulate the activation cascade of the insulin receptor? This cascade is activated by an enzyme called Rad, which is a GTP (Guanosine-5'-triphosphate) hydrolase related to PC-1, a plasmatic membrane protein. Both molecules are involved in the inhibition of the physiological actions of insulin. Some authors attribute to PC-1 a role in insulin resistance, when this membrane protein is over-expressed, as it is the case in the obesity [83].

IR is evidenced by the failure of endogenous insulin to hinder hepatic gluconeogenesis and to induce glucose peripheral uptake. Such dysfunction is compensated by increasing insulin levels (hyperinsulinemia) [84]. Peripheral insulin resistance emanates from interaction the interaction between liver, adipose tissue and skeletal muscles, when altered insulin signaling stems from altered insulin receptors and post-receptor defects. These alterations include an imbalance between the two insulin receptor isoforms, decreased insulin receptor affinity, improper insulin receptor kinase activity, decreased autophosphorylation and impaired glucose transporter translocation and activation [81].

Table 1: NCEP ATP III 2005: Metabolic Syndrome (MetS) criteria

Risk Factor	Defining Level
Abdominal obesity (waist circumference)	
Men	≥ 102 cm
Women	≥ 88 cm
HDL-cholesterol	
Men	< 40 mg/dl
Women	< 50 mg/dl
Triglycerides	≥ 150 mg/dl
Blood Pressure	≥ 130 mm Hg / ≥ 85 mm Hg
Fasting glucose	≥ 100 mg/dl
MetS diagnosis if ≥ 3 risk factors are present	

Hyperinsulinemia is classically defined as a basal level of insulin higher or equal to 16 mU/l, or more recently by a quite lower basal value (higher than or equal to 10.9 mU/l) [85], which constitutes a useful cut-off point for IR. Hyperinsulinemia is a constant in the MetS, but is not a required criterion for its diagnosis. It is possible to present a level of insulin 10-fold higher than the normal range with normal glucose plasma levels. However when both are elevated many other parameters such as triglycerides, HDL-cholesterol and blood pressure result in raised values. In particular, among obese normotensive patients hyperinsulinemia is more prevalent than insulin resistance (38% *vs.* 26%) [86], although the mechanisms causing hyperinsulinemia in absence of insulin resistance still remain unclear. Nevertheless, when hyperinsulinemia appears, insulin resistance becomes aggravated.

With regard to blood pressure, hyperinsulinemia is involved in four potential hypertensive mechanisms: the activation of the Sympathetic Nervous System (SNS), the hypertrophy of the smooth muscle cells, the renal sodium retention and the increase of intracellular levels of calcium [87]. Moreover, clinical trials as the

"San Antonio Heart Study" have confirmed that hyperinsulinemia is a key factor in the development of hypertension [88]. Both hypertensive and normotensive subjects showed a positive correlation between serum insulin concentrations and blood pressure.

Hyperinsulinemia also comes along with raised levels of PAI-1 (Plasminogen-Activator Inhibitor-1), a serine protease inhibitor. PAI-1 is the main inhibitor of tissue plasminogen activator (tPA) and urokinase (uPA), the activators of plasminogen and hence fibrinolysis, and it appears to be also associated with endothelial dysfunction, left ventricular hypertrophy and coronary disease [89].

According to data obtained from nondiabetic subjects in the Framingham Offspring Study, IR might not be the only precedent condition in MetS, but also other independent physiological processes may be involved [90]. Recently, IKKβ/NF-κB in the mediobasal hypothalamus, in particular in the hypothalamic POMC (proopiomelanocortin) neurons, has been proposed as a primary pathogenic link between obesity and hypertension [91]. In addition, subjects presenting insulin resistance are also at risk for developing other pathologies such as non-alcoholic fatty liver disease, polycystic ovary, and certain types of cancer, among others [92].

The genetic underpinning of the MetS and its individual risk factors is reflected in the substantial heritability observed in different ethnic groups for the individual syndrome components including the IR [93]. So, adiposity evaluated by BMI or WC has been found to be highly heritable, with estimates ranging from 0.52 to 0.80, IR and fasting insulin ranging from 0.24 to 0.61, fasting triglyceride and high-density lipoprotein cholesterol (HDL-C) ranging from 0.20 to 0.47 and 0.60 to 0.78, respectively (Table **2**) [93]. The range of heritability estimates for systolic, diastolic, and pulse blood pressures are 0.30 to 0.37, 0.24 to 0.37, and 0.21 to 0.63, respectively and were similar in White and Eastern African cohort studies. Although studies assessing the heritability of MetS itself, rather than its individual risk factors, are less common, a range from 0.13 to 0.42 has been reported in several studies [94-96].

Genetics is especially important in the development of diabetes mellitus, but it is not the only cause. The multiple causes involved in β-cell dysfunction are represented in Fig. **6** according to Unger [97] and LeRoith [98].

Table 2: Heritability of MetS components and MetS itself [93]

MetS Components	Heritability
Adiposity (BMI/WC)	0.52 - 0.80
IR & Fasting glucose	0.24 - 0.61
Fasting TG	0.20 - 0.47
High HDL-C	0.60 - 0.78
Systolic blood pressure	0.30 - 0.37
Diastolic blood pressure	0.24 - 0.37
Pulse	0.21 - 0.63
MetS	0.13 - 0.42

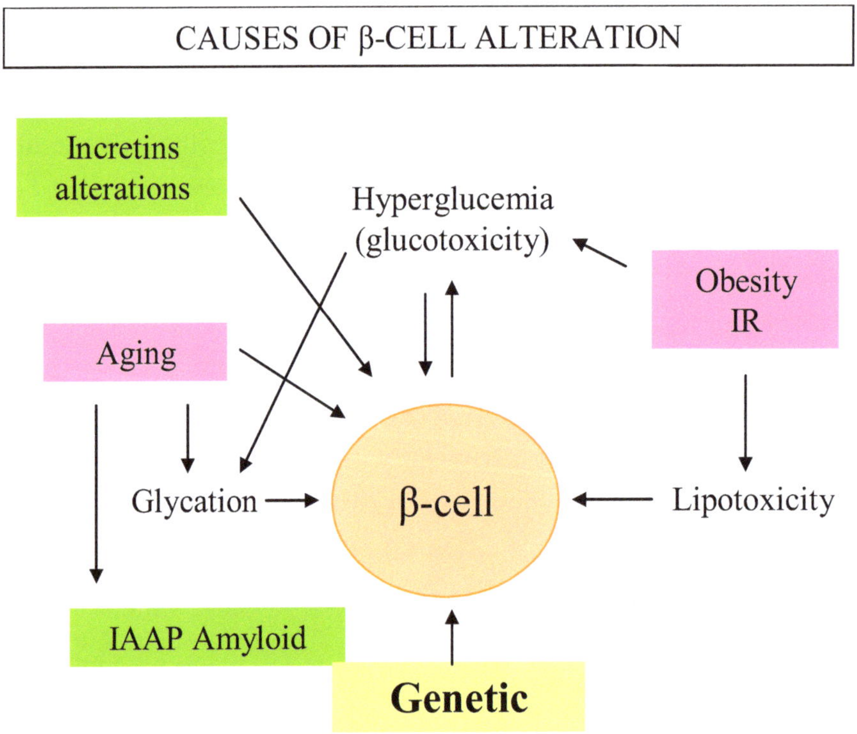

CAUSES OF β-CELL ALTERATION

Incretins alterations

Hyperglucemia (glucotoxicity)

Obesity IR

Aging

Glycation → β-cell ← Lipotoxicity

IAAP Amyloid

Genetic

Figure 6: Multiple causes involved in β-cell dysfunction. IR together with beta-cell alteration from multifactorial origin and genetic susceptibility lead to the development of diabetes. Abbreviations: IAAP: islet amyloid polypeptide; IR: Insulin Resistance.

FREE FATTY ACIDS, VICTIMS OR EXECUTIONERS IN THE OBESE SUBJECT? SYSTEMIC LIPOTOXICITY, INCLUDING B-CELL DAMAGE

In the context of obesity, circulating free fatty acids or non-esterified fatty acids (NEFA or FFA) are among the first victims of insulin resistance (IR), as the normal antilipolytic action of insulin is lost in the early stages of the IR. On the other hand, increased FFAs levels are of paramount concern in the pathogenesis of obesity-related diseases, becoming a very dangerous executioner in the obese patient. These actions are influenced by many factors, such as: i) patient situation regarding ingestion of food; if the subject is fasting or at postprandial state; ii) how active are other body organs (muscle, liver) in metabolizing free fatty acids; iii) the degree to which adipose tissue stores free fatty acids in the form of triglycerides.

With regard to FFAs, one of the key points is that the impaired ability of adipose tissue to suitably store free fatty acids results in increased levels of circulating FFAs, which may significantly contribute to the metabolic disease. As subcutaneous adipose tissue is the largest fat depot (making up 80% of body fat), it produces most of the FFAs [99]. Nevertheless, an increase in visceral adipocyte hypertrophy and/or visceral adipose tissue often increases FFAs delivery to the liver through its portal drainage, which may promote hepatic "lipotoxicity". This increased delivery of FFAs to the liver has been associated with the development of hepatic-mediated insulin resistance and dyslipidemia [100, 101]. This fact explains that although visceral adipose tissue is considered the main responsible for metabolic disease generation and/or aggravation, subcutaneous fat has pathogenic potential [102]. In addition, some patients present impaired ability to metabolize intramuscular fat [103], which may result in ectopic FFA storage in muscle and the accumulation of "toxic" intramyocellular lipids such as diacylglycerol, fatty acyl coenzyme A and ceramides [104]. This lipotoxicity promotes IR in the muscular tissue [105]. Moreover, FFAs may also damage pancreatic β-cell, and this pancreatic lipotoxicity may contribute to type-2 diabetes mellitus development in subjects genetically predisposed [106, 107]. The role of certain fatty acids in the beta-cell dysfunction through its interaction with GPR-40 receptors will be discussed later in this chapter.

Hypothalamic sensing of circulating lipids and modulation of hypothalamic endogenous fatty acid and lipid metabolism are proven mechanisms involved in body energy homeostasis [108, 109]. Enzymes such as AMP-activated protein kinase (AMPK) and fatty acid synthase (FAS) as well as intermediate metabolites as malonyl-CoA and long-chain fatty acids-CoA (LCFAs-CoA) play a key role in this neuronal network, pooling peripheral signals with neuropeptide-based mechanisms. Recent evidence have shown that impaired lipid metabolism and accumulation of specific lipid species in the hypothalamus leads to "hypothalamic lipotoxicity", resulting in adverse effects on hypothalamic neurons and causing endoplasmic reticulum (ER) stress in the hypothalamus [110], which contributes to the development of MetS [111].

Finally, of particular interest is "cardiac lipotoxicity". Excess lipid accumulation in the heart is associated with decreased cardiac function both in human and animal models [112]. The mechanisms are still unclear, but it may result from either toxic effects of intracellular lipids (acylcarnitines) or excessive fatty acid oxidation (FAO) [113, 114]. In subjects with MetS, both cardicac PPARγ overexpression and use of PPARγ agonists are associated with heart failure. A significant association between accumulation of long chain fatty acyl carnitines and poor cardiac function has been observed in subjects with coronary disease. These compounds may be associated with effects on sarcolemmal ion channels, resulting in cardiac arrhythmias [115], which are the main cause of death in heart failure patients. Future development of specific inhibitors of carnitine acyltransferase may be a promising therapeutic strategy to attenuate the incidence of severe arrhythmias associated with coronary heart disease.

ADIPOSE TISSUE AS AN ENDOCRINE ORGAN. FROM ADIPOSITY TO ADIPOSOPATHY

Adipose tissue is more than just the storage place for lipids, an energy reservoir. It is a highly active metabolic and endocrine organ secreting a range of peptides known as adipocytokines with both local and remote actions [116, 117]. These have been lately renamed as adipokines, since they are not only produced by the adipocytes. Some of these peptides can be more accurately termed adipose-derived hormones, among which leptin and adiponectin have a critical role in obesity-related processes.

Adipokines [118, 119], including IL-1-β, IL-6, IL-8, IL-10, TNF-α, TGF-β, acylation stimulating protein (ASP), visfatin, apelin and the acute-phase proteins (serum amyloid A, PAI-1), are involved in appetite, lipid metabolism, insulin sensitivity, vascular homeostasis (endothelium), blood pressure regulation, lipid and glucose metabolism and energy homeostasis [120, 121].

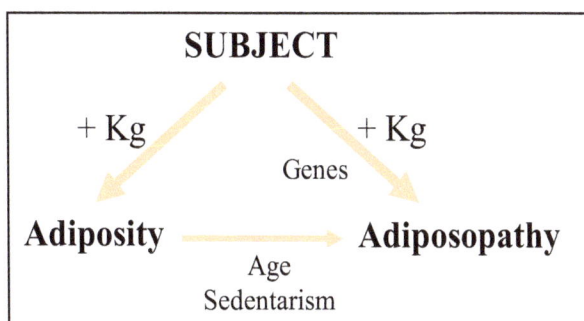

Figure 7: Adiposity *vs.* adiposopathy. Both are accompanied by overweight but the patient with adiposity is a "metabolically-healthy overweight subject" +Kg: Weight gain.

The term adiposity refers just to an excess of adipose tissue. However, when adiposity results in functional abnormalities, including endocrine and immune disorders, the term adiposopathy or "sick fat" [48] has been recently proposed to better describe this metabolic disease. Adiposopathy characterizes the pathogenic enlargement of fat cells and fat tissue leading to adverse clinical consequences including the most common metabolic diseases encountered in obese subjects in clinical practice such as type-2 diabetes mellitus (the most severe form of adiposopathy), prediabetes, high blood pressure, dyslipidemia and MetS [104, 122]. Moreover, some factors such as age or sedentary lifestyle may also convert adiposity into adiposopathy (Fig. **7**). In summary, adiposity and adiposopathy are both accompanied by overweight, but the patient with just adiposity is a "metabolically-healthy overweight subject" [123, 124].

Adiponectin

Adiponectin, or "adipocyte complement-related protein" is a 30 Kd protein secreted by the adipocyte, being the most abundant inflammatory mediator expressed in white adipose tissue (WAT). In healthy subjects, adiponectin levels are around 5-10 µg/ml [125]. This hormone exerts both metabolic and vascular actions. Metabolically, it is directly involved in hepatic and peripheral glucose metabolism. In the liver, adiponectin diminishes the hepatic production of glucose, while at a peripheral level, it improves insulin resistance. Decreased adiponectin plasma levels have been described in obese subjects and patients with T2DM. In addition, adiponectin regulates energy balance [126], reducing the triglyceride content of muscular and hepatic tissues as well circulating levels. With regard to vasculature, adiponectin modulates cell adhesion to the endothelium. Both metabolic and vascular actions are always opposite to those exerted by two other adipokines: TNF-α and resistin (Fig. **8**).

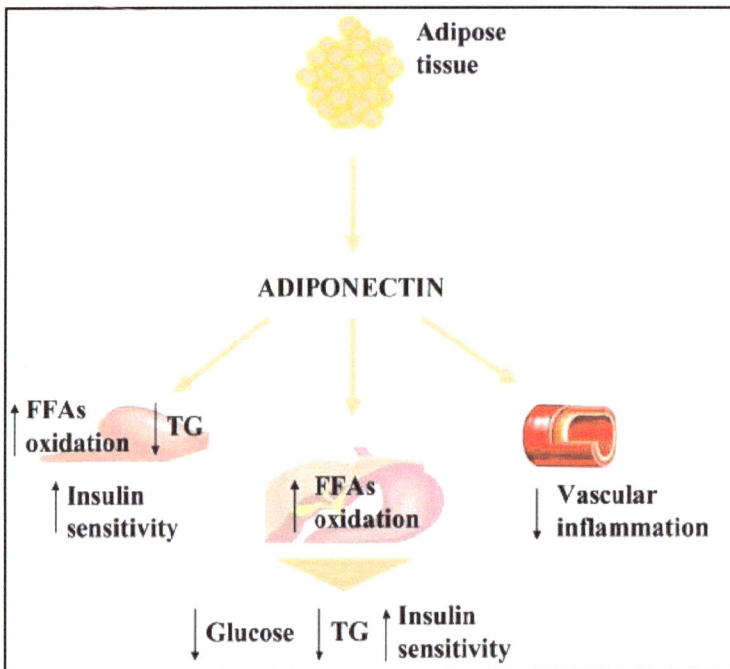

Figure 8: Adiponectin is released by adipose tissue, and promotes Metabolic and vascular actions on muscle tissue, liver and vasculature, such as increased FFAs oxidation and insulin sensitivity, as well as decreased triglycerides, glucose and vascular inflammation. FFAS: free-fatty acids. TG: triglycerides.

Adiponectin is responsible for the entire inhibition of VCAM-1(Vascular Adhesion Molecule-1) and inhibits partially ICAM-1 (Intercellular Adhesion Molecule-1), both induced by resistin. In addition, it has also been observed that adiponectin inhibits signaling from NF-kappaB [127] through cAMP (Ciclic Adenosin Monophosphate). On the other hand, adiponectin also exerts a beneficial action on nitric oxide (NO) released by the endothelial cells, which seems to be directly dependent on NOSe (Endothelial Nitric Oxide Synthetase) activation. Moreover, Iwashima *et al.,* [128] reported a direct relationship between lower levels of adiponectin and hypertension, independently of other components of MetS. This is a remarkable fact in the context of obesity and the MetS, as similar effects had been described with regard to other adipokine, leptin.

Resistin

Resistin is a cysteine-rich adipokine produced by the monocyte in humans and primates, and by the adipocyte in rodents [129]. Resitin levels are increased in obese [130] and smoking patients[131], but in spite of its name, resistin has a controversial role in IR [132]. Recently this adipokine has been related to advanced atherosclerosis [133] and heart failure [134]. Previously, *in vitro* studies had associated resistin with an increase in the mRNA expression of adhesion molecules VCAM-1 and ICAM-1 as well as in MCP-1 (Monocyte Chemotactic Protein-1) and Endothelin-1 (ET-1), a peptide produced by the endothelial cells [135]. However, the relationship between resistin and CRP has shown mixed results [130, 131]. In any case, while resistin being related to CV risk could be expected, its involvement in atopic dermatitis and asthma atopic in childhood [119], as well as to primary asthma in obese adults, even predicting the response to glucocorticoids, may be considered as surprising [136, 137]. It should be noted that leptin has been also associated with asthma [138].

Moreover, in the last years, the adiponectin/resistin ratio has been defined as a useful indicator for the assessment of obesity-related health problems [139].

6.3. Leptin

Another important factor to take into account in the context of obesity and inflammation is leptin. This molecule, involved in energy homeostasis, is the product of the so called "ob-gene" [121]. Leptin also regulates appetite, and its absence or deficiency has been demonstrated to cause obesity in animal models [140]. Accordingly, hypothalamus and the adipocyte itself are the targets for leptin. Leptin receptor belongs to the superfamily of receptors for cytokines class I, while STAT (Signal Transducer and Activator of Transcription) proteins serve as intracellular messengers, which become activated when their tyrosine residues are phosphorilated.

With regard to central nervous system, leptin regulates appetite in animals, acting in two different ways: both stimulating and inhibiting appetite [140]. Nevertheless, the role played in appetite regulation in humans is still unclear. Both in animals and humans leptin increases the sympathetic tone [141], which may be responsible for high blood pressure in MetS subjects. It has been suggested that these patients present resistance to the metabolic actions of leptin, regardless of its hypertensive effect [142]. Moreover, leptin has been proposed as a cardiovascular risk biomarker [143].

THE ROLE OF OBESITY IN CARDIOMETABOLIC SYNDROME AND CARDIOMETABOLIC RISK

Historical Perspective

In the last decade two new terms, "Cardiometabolic Syndrome" (CMS) and "Cardiometabolic Risk" (CMR), have emerged as an amplified evolution of Metabolic Syndrome (MetS) with different nuances. But even more interesting in our contexts, the term "cardiometabolic" appeared for the first time in a medical article related to obesity: Pescatello and Van-Heest in 2000 [144].

In 2001, Sowers, Epstein and Frölich, experts from the American Diabetes Association (ADA), coined the term CMS putting together the classic components of MetS, such as central obesity, hyperglycemia, hypertriglyceridemia, low-HDL-cholesterol, high blood pressure and IR, and IR-related new factors such as loss of the circadian rhythm of the blood pressure, hyperuricemia and microalbuminuria. Alongside these, they also included the "Pearson risk biomarkers", which are indicators of systemic inflammation, namely C-Reactive protein (CRP) levels, endothelial dysfunction, oxidative stress and hypercoagulability (Fig. **9**).

In 2005 Khan, Buse, Ferrannini and Stern, also ADA experts, used the term Cardiometabolic Risk (CMR) instead of MetS, but with a difference with respect to CMS: CMR complements the risk associated with MetS adding classic risk factors not related to IR, such as family history of cardiovascular disease, sedentary life-style, hypercholesterolemia and smoking (Fig. **10**).

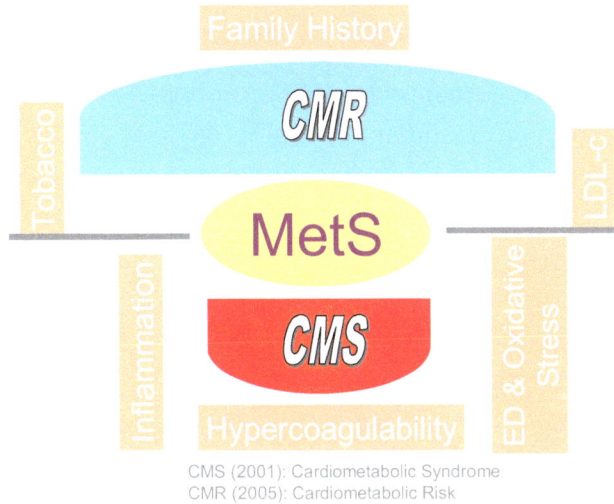

Figure 9: Relationship between Metabolic Syndrome (MetS), Cardiometabolic Syndrome (CMS) and Cardiometabolic Risk (CMR). Abbreviations: ED: endothelial dysfunction; LDL-c: LDL-cholesterol.

In fact, CMR and CMS are not different concepts, but complementary. While CMR defines a non-quantifiable clinical risk, unlike the classical cardiovascular risk scores, CMS is a pathophysiological concept, and thus it is a pivotal notion in this chapter. The differential key: if we include biomarkers of inflammation, oxidative stress, endothelial dysfunction and prothrombotic state, we should rather refer to CMS, otherwise CMR.

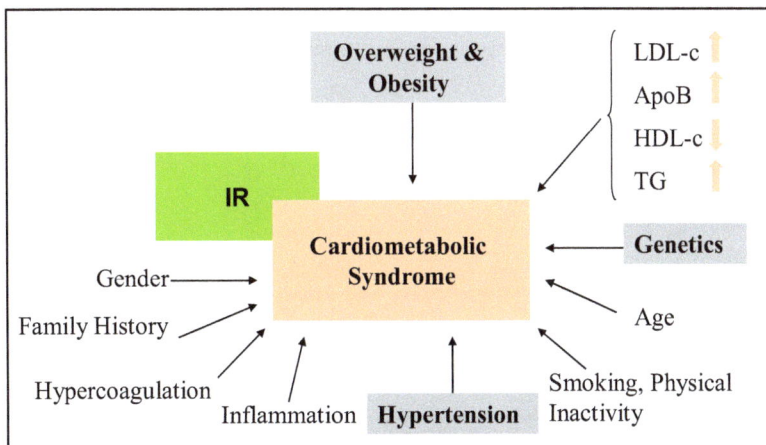

Figure 10: Cardiometabolic Syndrome. Abbreviations: LDL-C: LDL-cholesterol, ApoB: apolipoprotein B; HDL-c: HDL cholesterol; TG: triglycerides; IR: insulin resistance.

Obesity as a Low-Grade Inflammatory Disease: *Metaflammation*

The anatomical-functional base of obesity as a cardiometabolic disease is a chronic low-grade inflammation or "metaflammation" [145] that compromises the fat and the vascular stroma. So, it involves not only the adipocyte of WAT, but also the SVF (Stroma-Vascular Fraction), consisting of macrophages, endothelial cells, progenitor cells and leukocytes. As a result of inflammation, the obese patient presents increased levels of IL-6, TNF-α, resistin and leptin, along with reduced adiponectin [146]. In obese subjects WAT is infiltrated by macrophages, which at the same time constitute a great source of pro-inflammatory cytokines. The latter is consistent with the fact that weight loss is associated with a reduction in the rate of macrophage infiltration into WAT, and subsequently with a reduction in the levels of circulating inflammatory cytokines and interleukins [147, 148]. The molecules produced by immune cells and adipocytes, such as cytokines or reactive oxygen species (ROS), can activate important stress pathways and disrupt critical metabolic processes involved in obesity as the insulin signalling cascade and regulation of energy homeostasis [149]. Examples include their participation in lipid metabolism inhibiting lipoprotein lipase (LPL), and subsequently increasing the production of triglycerides in the liver, leading to hypertriglyceridemia, typical in the MetS.

Besides the inflammation-involved molecules already described, which are secreted by adipose tissue, there are many other key cells, such as pre-adipocytes, endothelial cells, fibroblasts, and immune cells [150], which are related to the health of the tissue involved in the pathogenesis of obesity.

WAT monocyte-macrophage system, besides releasing resistin, also produces two other factors involved in both inflammation and IR: CXC ligand 5 [151] and macrophage inflammatory protein (MIP)-1α [152]. In addition, granulocyte-macrophage colony-stimulating factor (GM-CSF), a proinflammatory cytokine that induces myeloid-lineage differentiation of hematopoietic stem cells, may also take part in obesity-related inflammation, involving central (hypothalamic neurons related to food intake) and peripheral (WAT increase) mechanisms [152, 153].

With regard to anti-obesity drugs, these may act on reducing inflammatory markers in a direct, indirect or mixed way. Those drugs achieving a double goal, weight loss and modulation or improvement of their underlying metabolic and immunological states, would be the best choice as anti-obesity drugs. Thus, reducing or at least modulating the inflammatory state associated with the excess of body fat through drugs whose molecular targets are implicated in the synthesis and release of pro-inflammatory mediators generated at the adipocyte, would result in effective therapies not only to treat obesity, but also, what is more important, its complications.

Many authors are drawing attention to the fact that weight loss is not only a matter of diminishing BMI below values of 30 or 25 kg/m^2. Obesity, when is linked to inflammation places obese subjects at moderate to severe cardiovascular risk [154].

Adipose Tissue Inflammation in the Origin of Insulin Resistance

According to recent data, plasma levels of inflammatory mediators, such as TNF-α and IL-6, are increased in obesity and type 2 diabetes, raising questions about the role played by these cytokines in the mechanisms underlying inflammation in insulin resistant states [155].

TNF-α, also called "caquectine", is secreted by adipocytes, macrophages and lymphocytes. This cytokine induces resistance to insulin when it is overproduced at skeletal muscle and/or adipocytes. The most likely explanation is that TNF-α interferes with the insulin signalling cascade. Thus, TNF-α would be over-expressed in the adipose tissue of subjects suffering from MetS, leading to a state of IR. According to Hube *et al.,* [156], this would constitute a "defensive mechanism" to avoid further fat accumulation in the obese subject. Such hypothesis was outlined for the first time by Eckel in 1992, suggesting that insulin resistance protects from gaining more weight [157].

In accordance with these theories linking TNF-α and IR, TNF-α would act by inhibiting glucose transport and facilitating lipolysis, and thus producing free fatty acids, which is just the opposite to insulin action. The inhibitory role played by TNF-α on the signalling cascade of insulin is not based on its lipolitic activity, but rather on the inhibition of the phosporilation cascade of insulin by activating protein kinase C (PKC) enzymes [158].

Meanwhile IL-6, produced in WAT by adipocytes, macrophages and stroma vascular fraction (SVF) cells [155, 159, 160], could be directly involved in the onset and/or development of metabolic states of IR and its associated health complications [161, 162]. This theory arises from the fact that IL-6 receptor belongs to the "cytokine class I receptor family" involving JAK/STATs (Janus kinases/signal transducers and activators of transcription) signal transduction pathway. Interplay between IL-6 and insulin signalling pathways results in decreased insulin action, and thus leading to a insulin resistant state [163, 164]. With regard to vascular damage, IL-6 induces CRP production in the liver by activating JAK/STATs mediators which enable the CRP gene expression [165].

Cross-Talk Between Inflammated Adipose Tissue and other Tissues

According to some authors [166], as visceral fat grows larger, the influence of monocytes in the insterstitial area between adipocytes also becomes greater, since they establish a sort of "dialogue". This theory has changed the way we used to conceive these biological phenomena. Accordingly, adipose tissue is not only composed of adipocytes, but also of Stroma-Vascular Fraction (SVF), including endothelial cells, stem-cells and leucocytes. Regarding the adipokines produced by adipose tissue, only adiponectin and leptin are produced by adipocytes, while it is not clear if resistin is synthesized and secreted by other types of cells also present in adipose tissue. The remaining hormones secreted by visceral WAT are released by the macrophage. These findings contribute to confirm the idea that we are speaking of an inflammatory state when dealing with obesity. Most of visceral WAT macrophages derive from bone marrow, while just a small proportion come from mitotic division.

MCP-1 (Monocyte Chemoacttratant Protein) is one of the molecules involved in the recruitment of macrophages from the bone marrow into the adipose tissue. It is synthesized by the adipocyte in collaboration with the endothelial cells from the SVF. The endothelial MCP-1 is stimulated by leptin, so that adipocyte has a double role in this process. On the other hand, MCP-1 activates the circulating monocyte, increasing the expression of CD11-b. Once the monocyte is "called", it leaves the vessel and enters into the adipose tissue. In order to remain within the WAT, the monocyte requires the presence of the macrophage inhibitory factor (MIF) and the macrophage colony-stimulating factor (M-CSF).

A dysfunctional or impaired adipose tissue does not cause metabolic disease on its own. Actually, what takes place is a sort of "dialogue" or "cross-talk" with other tissues and organs, what determines whether endocrine and immune responses from adipose tissue end up causing the metabolic disease [104]. The pathogenic responses during positive caloric balance are modulated by several organs [104]. One of the best described pathogenic responses of dysfunctional adipose tissue, which is an example of this dialogue, is the concept previously described as adiposopathy. In postprandial state, increased insulin secretion stimulates FFAs storage in adipose tissue and other body tissues, resulting in reduced circulating FFAs. In the hours following initial insulin release, FFAs levels gradually tend to increase again [167]. During positive caloric balance, fat gain can result in adipocyte hypertrophy and adipose tissue dysfunction, leading to impaired storage of FFAs within adipocytes and IR. Lack of balance between lipolysis and lipogenesis in adipose tissue increases both fasting and postprandial circulating FFAs in IR [168]. In such a situation, adverse metabolic consequences of increased FFAs, such as hepatic IR and dyslipidemia [103], depend on whether or not the liver is able to manage the pathogenic responses of adipose tissue. In this scenario, a negative caloric balance would be expected to improve adipose tissue function and FFA storage in adipose tissue, as well as reducing circulating FFAs and lipid delivery to skeletal muscle, and thus reducing lipid storage in skeletal muscle, which may improve insulin sensitivity [169]. Likewise, type 2 diabetes mellitus is often developed when obesity comes along with pathogenic endocrine and immune responses from the adipose tissue, including an increased release of FFAs. In this situation, a genetic limitation in the ability of β-pancreatic cells to release insulin would result in an even further impairment in insulin secretion [170]. Moreover, adipose tissue is also known to have important interactions with the immune system, heart, brain, endothelium, kidneys, endocrine glands or gastrointestinal tract, what potentially may lead to a number of metabolic alterations [104].

Recently, the importance of targeting adiposity dysfunctionalities when approaching to obesity treatments has been pointed out, since this therapeutic goal does not only lead to loss of excessive weight, but also improves patient general health. If the patient has an adiposopathy-induced metabolic disease (*e.g.*, Type 2 diabetes mellitus, dyslipidemia, and/or high blood pressure), then weight loss interventions may reduce adipocyte hypertrophy and visceral adiposity, and thus improve adipose tissue pathogenic endocrine and immune responses, and subsequently metabolic disease [171]. This paradigm is a key issue in the treatment of obesity.

Metabolic Inflexibility and Endoplasmic Reticulum Stress Underlying Obesity

In addition to IR, two concepts have been recently coined to "complete the picture" of a more accurate and comprehensive explanation of the physiological phenomena converging in obesity and its associated morbidities: the so called "Metabolic Inflexibility" (MI) and the Endoplasmic Reticulum (ER) Stress.

MI characterizes lean healthy subjects. It was first introduced by Kelly, from the University of Pittsburg, in 2000, who redefined the term four years later [172]. The main features of MI lie upon the idea that a healthy organism counts with a great adaptability to the fat from diet, so it is able to suitably metabolize this fat, while maintaining body weight. This process is mediated and/or conditioned by genetic and hormonal factors. On the contrary, metabolically inflexible subjects present decreased adaptability to fat ingestion, and when this occurs, a fat accumulation is promoted, and thus weight gain as food intake increases. Besides, neither the plasma levels of FFAs nor insulin oscillate depending on the postprandial state (absorptive/postabsorptive), both rather remain unchanged. In addition, consumption of local glucose at muscular tissue is increased and consumption of postprandial glucose is decreased. In this MI state, FFAs are stored in muscle and liver as triglycerides. Thus, although they do not directly interfere with carbohydrate metabolism, they can lead to IR by interfering with the insulin signaling cascade [173]. The Metabolic Flexibility is considered the ability to switch from fat to carbohydrate oxidation, what appears to be usually impaired in insulin-resistant subjects; however, this Metabolic Inflexibility is mostly the consequence of impaired cellular glucose uptake [174]. MI has been recently observed by Berk *et al.,* in postmenopausal Afro-American women [173], justifying the proneness of this population to suffer from MetS.

MI is closely related to IR, and both processes are intimately linked to a third one, which might be regarded as the metabolic cornerstone of Cardiometabolic Syndrome: Endoplasmic Reticulum Stress is the difficulty to discharge "old and useless" proteins that arises in the ER, probably as a consequence of MI and adiposopathy. This is likely to be due to the accumulation of dysfunctional fat, even though it really is a "protein catabolic dysfunction" [175]. ER is a critical cellular organelle, where protein, lipid, and glucose metabolism is integrated, and where lipoprotein secretion and calcium homeostasis takes place. Activation of chronic inflammation and impairment of ER and mitochondria function that may follow to adiposopathy can feed-forward and contribute to further deterioration of the already dysfunctional or unhealthy lipid profile, by reducing fatty acid oxidation, promoting lipolysis, and stimulating the lipogenesis process *de novo*.

Inflammatory mediators, as explained above, are increasingly secreted as fat accumulation grows, and can promote lipogenesis and impair mitochondrial respiratory chain function. On the other hand, altered lipid profile can also promote inflammation. Thus, they cross-interact and, in a synergic manner, enhance each other.

Finally, ER stress (Fig. **11**) activates inflammatory cascades such as JNK (c-jun N-terminal kinase) pathways, and increases the generation of ROS, leading to mitochondrial calcium overload, and activating lipogenesis. Mitochondrial dysfunction, oxidative stress, a low-grade systemic inflammation (metaflammation) and lipogenesis further exacerbate ER stress by impairing protein folding, protein overloading (acute phase proteins of inflammation) and lipid overloading (lipogenesis) [175].

Cytokines as TNF-α and IL-6, as well as fatty acids activate two main inflammatory pathways that lead to the disruption of insulin action: JNK/AP-1 (c-JUN NH2-terminal kinase-activator protein-1) and IKK-NF-κB (inhibitor κB kinase-nuclear factor κB). Both pathways are related to molecules involved in unfolded protein response (UPR) signaling. Moreover, ER is a major source of ROS, and oxidative stress emanating from the ER can also activate both JNK/AP-1 and IKK-NF-κB pathways, and thus potentially lead to IR [176]. ER stress is previous to IR, initiating the development of IR and inflammation of adipose tissue in obesity and T2DM [177].

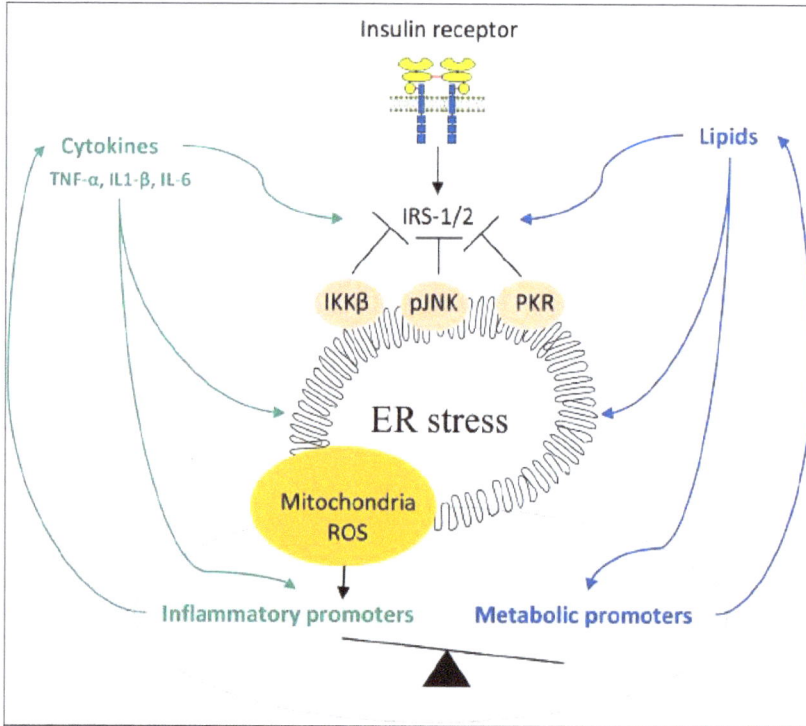

Figure 11: Metabolic Inflexibility: interactions among insulin resistance, metabolic promoters, inflammatory mediators and Endoplasmic Reticulum (ER) stress. Abbreviations: PKR-like endoplasmic reticulum localized kinase; JNK: c-jun N-terminal kinase; IKK: Inhibitor of IκB kinase. IRS-1/2: Insulin receptor substrates.

Hence, impaired lipid metabolism, systemic low grade inflammation, IR, MI and ER Stress that are present in obesity can trigger and develop a Cardiometabolic Disease, which encloses not only the dysfunctions that compose the MetS, but also cardiovascular disturbances with their own pathogenic mechanisms.

Endoplasmic Reticulum Stress in β-cell Dysfunction of T2DM and its relationship with GPR40 and Transcription Factors FOX01 and PDX-1

As previously discussed, proper folding, maturation, storage and transport of proteins take place in the endoplasmic reticulum (ER). Accumulation of unfolded proteins as well as extreme energy and nutrient fluctuations (glucolipotoxicity, hypoxia) may cause disturbances in the ER lumen and result in beta-cell stress. This activates the unfolded protein response (UPR), a complex signaling network, which tries to restore natural ER function through reduced translation and degradation of misfolded proteins, and increased transcription of ER chaperones in order to augment protein folding capacity. If UPR fails to recover normal ER function, it launches cellular apoptosis [178].

On the other hand, β-cell may become defective during IR only if there is a special susceptibility to develop diabetes mellitus, which occurs in about one third of obese patients. The earliest reaction to peripheral IR is to increase insulin production and release resulting in hyperinsulinemia, which promotes an increase in beta-cell mass as a result of increased beta-cell replication. However, animal and human models have shown that, after the onset of diabetes, there is a gradual deterioration in beta-cell function and mass.

In addition to ER stress, the Forkhead Transcription Factor (FOX01), oxidative stress and GPR40 receptor are also involved in β-cell dysfunction.

FOX Family (named Forkhead by a couple of ectopic structures in drosophila) is a set of proteins also called "winged helix" for his appearance in the crystallographic study. While they are genes in invertebrates, in mammals they are a family of transcription factors. Unlike other transcription factors, it does not contain homeodomains or zinc-fingers, but a distinct type of DNA-binding region including around 100 amino acids. The FOXO transcription factors in mammals are four: 1, 3, 4 and 6. FOX01 is involved in fundamental cellular processes such as apoptosis, responses to oxidative stress, cellular proliferation, cellular differentiation, and regulation of energy metabolism. On the other hand, oxidative stress and activation of the c-Jun N-terminal kinase (JNK) pathway induce the nucleocytoplasmic translocation of the pancreatic transcription factor PDX-1, which leads to pancreatic beta-cell dysfunction. The forkhead transcription factor FOXO1/FKHR plays a role as a mediator between the JNK pathway and PDX-1. Under oxidative stress conditions, FOXO1 changes its intracellular localization from the cytoplasm to the nucleus in the pancreatic beta-cell line HIT-T15. The overexpression of JNK also induces the nuclear localization of FOXO1, but in contrast, the suppression of JNK reduces the oxidative stress-induced nuclear localization of FOXO1, suggesting the involvement of the JNK pathway in FOXO1 translocation [179].

With regard to oxidative stress, high glucose concentrations promote oxidative stress through an increase in the production of ROS in a variety of cell types, including beta cells. When intracellular glucose concentrations exceed the glycolytic capacity of the β-cell, excess glucose is shunted to enolization pathways, resulting in superoxide (O^{2-}) production. In addition, beta cells express low levels of antioxidant enzymes, and therefore they are highly sensitive to oxidative stress [180].

Fatty acids may take part in β-cell dysfunction in two ways: a) a long term exposure to elevated levels of short and medium-chain FFAs impairs β-cell survival and insulin secretion, an alteration called "lipotoxicity". Intracellular FFA metabolism underlies the inhibitory effects of FFAs on beta-cell function. b) a short-term variety of physiological responses induced by the long-chain FFAs by means of the activation of GPR40 receptor. GPR40 (or free fatty acid 1 receptor [FFA1R]) is highly expressed in pancreatic β-cells. Deletion of GPR40 in transgenic mice results in impaired, but not suppressed, insulin release responses to intravenous glucose and lipids. This is further supported by the observation that loss-of-function mutations of the GPR40 gene in humans are associated with altered insulin secretion. Interestingly, GPR40 mediates FA-stimulated insulin secretion from the β-cell not only directly but also indirectly *via* regulation of incretin secretion (GLP1 and GIP). Nowadays, GPR40 agonists are under development as a therapy to treat T2DM [181].

The importance of cell-membrane receptors coupled to the G protein (GPCRs) is not limited to GPR40. Other GPCRs, expressed in beta cells and/or intestinal L cells, include the G protein-coupled receptors 119 (GPR119) and 120 (GPR120). Both receptors increase circulating insulin levels through a direct insulinotropic action on β-cells, and also mediating fatty acid stimulation of incretin secretion. Moreover, GPR19 could also act as a fat sensor [182].

Involvement of Muscle in Metabolic Dysregulation of Obese Patients

In a cardiometabolic context, muscular tissue may be considered as a large organ. Like most organs, except for endothelium and nerve tissue, striate muscle needs insulin to allow glucose getting into the cell. Until recently, skeletal muscle was strongly related to IR in T2DM [183], but not in obesity. Recent evidence has shown that a group of substances, named myokines or skeletal muscle-derived factors directly released by the muscle cells, play a major role in the IR related to overweight. Myokines can be divided into three groups according to their role in IR. Irisin helps to defend the muscle cell against the IR [184]. Musclin and IL-6 increase IR [185]. IL-6, with a dual origin (adipose and muscular tissue), plays a pivotal role in the pathophysiology of IR in the obese patient. Finally IL-15 and myostatin appear to be neutral. IL-15 is involved in immune response, but it has no proven action on metabolism. Meanwhile, myostatin, also known as "growth differentiating factor-8" or GDF-8, inhibits muscle growth in order to keep it within a certain limit [186], which might indirectly influence irisin levels.

Irisin

Physical exercise has been extensively related to a number of cardiovascular benefits independently of weight loss, including preservation of skeletal muscle, which plays an important role in fat metabolism. Irisin, a hormone secreted by the muscle has been considered an "exercise mimetic" [184], acting as a mediator of those benefits. In presence of obesity, irisin release is increased [187], attempting to counteract the associated IR. Irisin secretion is firstly expressed in muscle as the type I membrane protein precursor FNDC5, which is proteolytically cleaved and secreted into the circulation [188]. Irisin and FNDC5 secretion are increased in response to overexpression of PGC-1α (peroxisome proliferator-activated receptor gamma coactivator 1-alpha), as takes place after aerobic exercise-training [189]. After irisin exposition there is a brown-fat-like development in specific depots of white adipose tissue (WAT), which results in increased energy expenditure, leading to a modest but significant weight loss, and improved glucose tolerance [190]. So, lower circulating irisin levels have been associated with T2DM. In particular, obese subjects with T2DM present lower irisin levels than non-diabetics, which may contribute to increase IR in this subgroup [191]. One plausible explanation to this fact could be the lower abundance of PGC-1α in skeletal muscle, as patients with early-onset type 2 diabetes display abnormalities in the exercise-dependent pathway that regulates the expression of PGC-1α [192]. In the future, therapies targeting irisin could have a place as adjunct to training and weight loss therapies in obese patients. In addition, this myokine could exert positive actions in T2DM prevention.

Musclin

Musclin, released by type IIb muscle fibers, is markedly regulated by nutritional status and insulin levels [185, 193]. When circulating levels of insulin are increased, an obesity feature, the muscle secretes musclin as a regulatory mechanism, inducing a very special "protective" IR by activating Akt/protein kinase B [194]. This defensive mechanism against overaction of insulin is mediated by the FOXO1 (forkhead box O1) [195], a transcription factor usually associated with beneficial actions (*i.e.* antioxidant, anti-atherosclerosis and antiaging) [196]. The role of insulin in musclin secretion suggests a self-regulated phenomenon, so that musclin secretion would be also slowed by the IR itself. In the presence of malnutrition, musclin levels are reduced to facilitate the entrance of insulin into the cell.

The role of FOXO1 as a mediator of insulin in musclin secretion is not its only action with regard to the muscle tissue, as it is also involved in sterol regulatory element binding protein 1c (SREBP1c) and cathepsin-L expression. SREBP1c is a master regulator of lipogenic (triglycerides accumulation) liver gene expression in adipose tissue and skeletal muscle [197]. FOXO1 is inversely correlated to SREBP1c in muscle tissue. On the other hand, expression of cathepsin-L, a lysosomal cysteine protease associated to intracellular protein breakdown, is up-regulated in the skeletal muscle during starvation [198, 199], suggesting a role for the FOXO1/cathepsin L pathway in fasting-induced muscle atrophy [200].

Accordingly, an interesting question arises, why does FOXO1, usually working as a protector, increase the production of cathepsins and decrease the irisin levels? An attractive hypothesis could be a reduction in reticulum stress, being the atrophy action a side effect.

The Emerging Role of Endothelium in Adiposopathy

Once IR and Endothelial Dysfunction (ED) stata are settled, their pathological courses follow parallel ways, running towards type 2 diabetes mellitus and atherosclerosis respectively. Nevertheless, a remarkable author in the field of inflammation and obesity, John Yudkin (Washington Hospital, London) proposed an attractive theory in 1997, considering ED as a previous step to IR and atherosclerosis in a joint way. According to this theory, while ED plays a key role in the atherogenesis, in the case of capillaries and small veins, ED is actively engaged in the occurrence and onset of IR.

Nowadays there is strong evidence to support this theory. The blockage of the synthesis of Nitric Oxide (NO) by L-NMMA (an analogue of L-Arginine), has demonstrated not only to weaken the endothelium-dependent vasodilation (EDV), but also the glucose capture mediated by insulin [201]. These investigations are consistent with those obtained several years before in knock-out mice NOSe and NOSn (neuronal nitric oxide synthetase). Rodents lacking these enzymes developed IR in early states [202].

On the other hand, the production of Radical Oxygen Species (ROS) by the endothelium would attract macrophages. These release cytokines, which promotes IR, just as we have already seen regarding IL-6. The production of this pro-inflammatory mediators in diabetic subjects would result amplified as a consequence of an auto-oxidation process of the glucose. It would be induced by its free entrance through the GLUT-1 transporters, what does not require insulin. Thus, the production of ROS by the endothelium would add to that produced by the adipocyte itself [203]. On the other hand, as a consequence of the release of cytokines by the macrophages, a stimulation of the synthesis of NOSi can be induced and that overproduction could interfere with the action of insulin in the muscle cell.

THE "VASCULO-METABOLIC" THEORY (VMT)

This fascinating theory consists of two main pathogenic arms. On one hand, the Vascular Triad includes endothelial dysfunction, oxidative stress and vascular inflammation. On the other, the Metabolic Triad is composed by IR, MI and ER stress. The anatomical substrate remains the same as in the conventional paradigm, namely low-grade fat inflammation and activation of adipose tissue stroma, but according to this new theory, it is interpreted in a bidirectional way, what constitutes its added value (Fig. **12**)

The VMT understands vascular damage as occurring in a parallel way to metabolic damage, and not as a mere consequence of the first one. Moreover, this theory incorporates metabolic elements of paramount importance when compared with the conventional theory, which relies basically upon IR alone. The presence of MetS, which is much more prevalent in obese subjects, amplifies the pathogenic phenomena in both directions. In the case of T2DM, only present if there is a genetic susceptibility of β cells, it will enhance this even more due to the fact that this dysfunction incorporates a new key element, to configure an integrated "puzzle" of "health damage". This crucial element are the so called "Advanced Glycation End Products" (AGEs), whose interaction with AGEs from the endothelium increase oxidative stress, what explains the higher vulnerability of endothelium to hemodynamic phenomena and to the vascular damage exerted by oxidized LDL in diabetic patients.

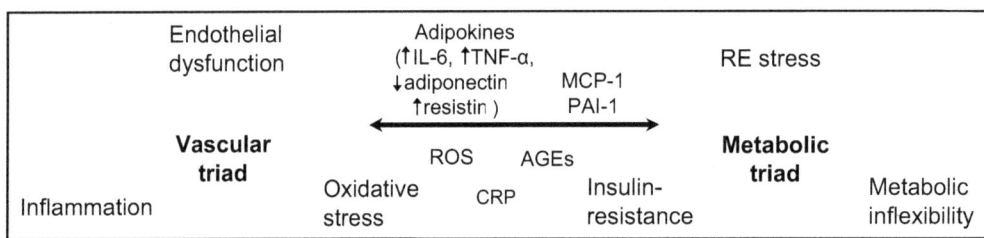

Figure 12: The VMT theory consists of two pathogenic arms: the Vascular Triad (endothelial dysfunction, oxidative stress, vascular inflammation) and the Metabolic Triad (metabolic inflexibility, reticule stress and insulin resistance). The "added value" of this newly coined theory is that although the anatomical substrate is the same as in the conventional one, hereby it is understood in a bidirectional way. Abbreviations: ROS: reactive oxygen species; AGEs: advanced glycation end products; CRP: C-Reactive Protein; RE: reticulum endoplasmic.

In both triads C-reactive protein (CRP) could take part in an active way. CRP, an acute-phase reactant predominantly synthesized in the liver, is an inflammatory marker that is also a classical and well-known biomarker of vascular disease. However, due to its anatomical proximity with fatty tissue, it could be reasonable to think that CRP is also involved in fat inflammation, amplifying alterations resulting from this inflammation such as the release of more adipokines. Baseline CRP levels are strongly associated with subsequent cardiovascular events independently of LDL-cholesterol and other known cardiovascular risk markers [204, 205]. Adipose tissue is a rich source of immune-related mediators, such as

IL-6 and TNF-α, that are involved in the inflammatory response. CRP is, in turn, under the control of these proinflammatory cytokines [120].

As a result, obesity is a major determinant of CRP in adults [206]. In 2000 Festa *et al.,* [207] studied the relationship between of CRP and the components of IR syndrome in the non-diabetic population of the Insulin Resistance Atherosclerosis Study (IRAS). CRP levels and a number of metabolic disorders were positively correlated. BMI, systolic blood pressure, and insulin sensitivity (IS) were also independently associated with CRP levels. On the other hand, population-based cohort studies of American children and adolescents have shown higher CRP concentrations in overweight subjects than in normal-weight subjects [208]. Several studies in obese children have also shown higher serum CRP levels in subjects with higher BMI and waist circumference [209, 210].

The response of cytokines to weight loss has shown mixed results, with most of studies showing at least trends towards improvement in adiponectin, leptin, TNF-α, IL-6, and CRP [211-215]. This reduction would certainly contribute to disable the two triads of vascular-metabolic theory. However, individual control of each risk factor seems also key to stop the process, especially the LDL-cholesterol, which plays a pivotal role in the vascular component of the endothelial dysfunction, on account of the high vulnerability of endothelium to even moderate levels of LDL-cholesterol, especially in obese diabetic patients [216].

Finally, within the VMT, the relevant role of circulating cathepsins in obesity-related cardiometabolic processes should be noted. As previously described, cathepsin is involved in skeletal muscle, but it also acts on the vascular wall. So, as extracellular proteases, contribute to extracellular matrix remodeling and interstitial matrix protein degradation, as well as to cell signaling and cell apoptosis in heart disease. Accordingly, both serum cathepsins S and L and cystatin C, an endogenous cathepsin inhibitor, have been proposed as promising biomarkers of coronary artery disease and aneurysm [217]. Even though the therapeutic use of cystatin C has not been assessed yet, other cathepsin inhibitors as proline-derived compounds have been already synthesized and successfully evaluated [218].

The Endothelial Dysfunction (ED) as a Cause of Insulin Resistance (IR)

Rodent models of endothelial dysfunction provide important insights into the relationship between ED and IR [219]. The pivotal role of endothelium in regulating metabolic actions of insulin is evident by the presence of IR and hypertension in eNOS knockout mice. These animals also present microvascular changes including rarefaction of capillary density and reduced insulin-mediated glucose disposal, increased triglyceride and FFA levels, decreased energy expenditure, defective beta-oxidation, and impaired mitochondrial function [220]. These findings suggest that endothelium-derived NO has additional and direct metabolic effects on mitochondrial function. Mice with partial eNOS deficiency (eNOS +/−) are insulin sensitive and normotensive, but when they are under a high-fat diet, also develop IR and hypertension [221]. Thus, partial defects in endothelial function characterized by reduced NO bioavailability are enough to cause cardio-metabolic abnormalities (insulin resistance and dyslipidemia) under pathogenic conditions (*e.g.,* caloric excess, physical inactivity, inflammation), as observed in humans. Several studies suggest that ED is an independent predictor for the incidence of diabetes [222-225]. In the Women's Health Initiative Observational Study higher levels of circulating E-selectin and intercellular adhesion molecule-1 (ICAM-1) were strongly related to increased risk of diabetes [224]. Similarly, in the Framingham Offspring Study, plasminogen activator inhibitor-1 (PAI-1) and von Willebrand factor (vWF), both circulating plasma markers of endothelial dysfunction, were independently associated with increased risk of diabetes [223].

The Insulin Resistance as a Cause of Endothelial Dysfunction (ED)

At the cellular level, the impairment in pathway-selective PI3K-dependent signaling pathways is a key feature of IR. Meanwhile other insulin signaling branches including Ras/MAPK-dependent pathways remain relatively unaffected. This fact has relevant pathophysiological implications because metabolic IR is typically accompanied by compensatory hyperinsulinemia to maintain normal values of plasma glucose. Hyperinsulinemia overdrives unaffected MAPK-dependent pathways, promoting an imbalance between PI3K- and MAPK-dependent functions of insulin. Lipotoxicity, glucotoxicity, and inflammation that contribute to IR states differentially affect PI3K and MAPK pathways through multiple independent and interdependent mechanisms in the endothelium. The imbalance between PI3K/Akt/eNOS/NO and MAPK/ET-1 vascular actions of insulin caused by hyperglycemia, dyslipidemia, and inflammatory cytokines may contribute to both altered metabolic and vascular actions of insulin [219]. So, compensatory hyperinsulinemia that typically accompanies pathway-selective insulin resistance (in PI3K pathways) activates unopposed MAPK pathways leading to ED and to increased pro-hypertensive pro-atherogenic actions of insulin [226].

Subjects with metabolic IR show simultaneous impairment in insulin ability to induce vasodilation. Diminished insulin-stimulated blood flow and glucose uptake is present in patients with various cardiovascular diseases such as essential hypertension, heart failure and microvascular angina. A diminished effect of insulin to induce vasodilation has been observed in subjects with obesity, T2DM and polycystic ovarian syndrome [227-230]. Thus, there may be similar genetic and acquired contributions to both IR and ED.

THERAPEUTIC IMPLICATIONS OF THE CARDIOMETABOLIC APPROACH TO OBESITY

Therapeutic strategy against obesity requires firstly a diagnosis of exclusion of secondary causes of obesity, such as Cushing's disease, hypothyroidism, binge eating disorder, Prader-Willi syndrome or hypothalamic tumour. Then it is time to design personalized targets as well as a stepped course of treatment from lifestyle changes to bariatric surgery when indicated, going through pharmacological therapy.

Bariatric surgery, such as Roux-en-Y bypass or gastric banding, is effective for weight loss as well as in the improvement of some of the obesity-related pathologies, since this techniques reduce adiposity and adiposopathy, recovering adipose tissue function [231]. However, due to all the concerns about perioperative mortality, surgical complications and frequent needing of reoperation, these methods are usually reserved for morbidly obese subjects.

Lifestyle Change Therapy

Lifestyle changes such as personalized diets and/or practicing physical exercise, frequently do not achieve good results as therapies for weight loss, mainly due to very low motivation and compliance, and most of the patients give them up [14]. When these methods are accompanied by psychological therapies, such as cognitive behavioural therapy, rate of success tends to be higher, but these treatments have intrinsic difficulties to be delivered on a mass scale and long-term results are frequently disappointing [232].

However, a challenge for the clinician and the patient is that public health initiatives promoting nutritional weight loss and physical activity, as well as commercial nutritional weight loss plans, have met with limited success in both individuals and populations [233]. Here, the following fact should be highlighted: searching and selecting personalized suitable treatments for obese subjects is medically justified, because even just a 5% weight loss in overweight patients may improve pathogenic adipose tissue responses, and subsequently a handful of metabolic dysfunctions and cardiovascular risk conditions [234, 235].

A number of studies in obese adults and children have shown that even moderate weight loss through dietary changes and physical exercise is effective in preventing and managing obesity-associated disorders [236]. However, only few studies have focused on the effect of hypocaloric diets on systemic inflammation [237-239]. Despite exceptions, most of them agree in the results: there is a decrease in leptin, TNF-α, IL-6, IL-8 and PAI-1 levels, as well in the complement C3, but adiponectin and MCP-1 do not show any changes. Also in overweigh/obese children and adolescents, significant reductions in IL-6, CRP or fibrinogen levels were found when hypocaloric diet and moderate physical activity were followed [239].

Beyond weight loss, a lifestyle change intervention should include improvements in diet and physical activity leading to achieve a reduction in cardiometabolic risk (hypertension, diabetes, metabolic syndrome and coronary risk) [56]. In this scenario, the biological impact of Mediterranean diet (MD) and regular physical exercise on cardiometabolic risk is outlined below.

The Mediterranean Diet as a Model of Healthy Eating

The Mediterranean diet (MD) has been widely considered as a model of healthy eating associated with a reduction in both total mortality and coronary heart disease (CHD) mortality [240, 241]. This is a current issue due to the PREDIMED Study

[242-244], even though it is focused just on certain components of the MD (olive oil and nuts) rather than in the MD as a global concept of diet. In this study the main target is not weight loss, but the behaviour of biomarkers and cardiovascular events, aiming to analyze for the first time in a large cohort study the biological impact of a type of diet in vascular health. Cardiometabolic benefits associated to the regular consumption of olive oil, rich in oleic acid (ω-9 monoinsaturated acid) and vitamin E, as well as nuts, high in vitamin E, omega-3 fatty acids (ω-3 fatty acids) and magnesium, were already known [245, 246].

However, the MD includes essentials aspects beyond those considered in the PREDIMED study:

a) The MD is low in saturated fat, which has metabolic and vascular implications. These fat acids induce insulin-resistance [247] and endothelial dysfunction [248]. On other hand, whereas most of western diets provide excessive amounts of omega-6 fatty acids respect to omega-3 fatty acids intake [249], the MD is rich in fatty fish with high content of ω-3. Eicosapentanoic acid, the most important ω-3 acid fat derived from fatty fish has demonstrated anti-inflammatory and antiplatelet actions [250], as well as an adiponectin-dependent anti-atherosclerotic effect that may be beneficial for the prevention of vascular complications in diabetic patients [251].

b) The MD is rich in fruits and vegetables, and thus high in antioxidants and flavonoids, which showed a clear cardiovascular preventive role in the INTERHEART study [252]. The MD is especially rich in lycopene, a carotene found in tomatoes, which has showed protective effects on coronary risk [253-255].

c) The MD is low in proteins, which was related in the DIOGENES Study to a lesser inflammatory status, as measured by high-sensitivity C-reactive protein [256].

d) Red wine is a usual component of MD, and its moderate consumption could play a role in preserving the endothelium [257].

Physical Activity Beyond Weight Loss

Traditionally a chapter dedicated to obesity addresses physical activity as a therapeutic tool to achieve weight reduction. This approach is as simple as wrong, since a number of studies, including the INTERHEART Study [252] have demonstrated that physical activity has cardiometabolic benefits beyond weight loss. So, maintaining or improving cardiorespiratory fitness has been related to a lower risk of all-cause and CVD mortality, as well as longevity regardless of changes in BMI [258]. Improved physical conditioning has been also associated with reduced arterial stiffness [259].

Regular aerobic exercise, and even modest physical activity, has shown to prevent the age-related decline in vascular endothelial function [260-262], suggesting an important mechanism by which regular aerobic exercise reduces the risk for cardiovascular disease. Physical activity has a beneficial impact on endothelial progenitor cells (EPC), which play an important role in repairing endothelial injury. Xia *et al.,* have demonstrated for the first time that physical exercise attenuates age-associated reduction in endothelium-reparative capacity of EPC by increasing CXCR4/JAK-2 signaling [263].

Anti-Obesity Drugs

General Considerations

In the last fifty years anti-obesity drugs (AOD) have emerged as a complementary approach to life-style changes, before resorting to surgery. Surgery should be always the last step in the therapeutic strategy, but an in-depth discussion on this subject exceeds the purpose of this chapter. ADO approach lies in the use of drugs which reduce the consumption of food or its absorption and/or increase energy expenditure [264]. Nevertheless, this way has also been quite disappointing, owing to the fact that many of these new drugs had at one point to be withdrawn from the market due to the occurrence of a great deal of unacceptable side-effects. In this scenario, advances in research on the neurological basis of appetite and energy homeostasis have resulted in the development of a handful of targets for potential AOD development [265].

Travelling back to the time when the anti-obesity drugs arrived to the market, we find that the first ones were the centrally-acting sympathomimetics, such as amphetamine derivatives like desosyephedrine, phentermine and diethylpropion [266], which were very popular in the 1950s and 1960s, but increasing concern about abuse potential and cardiovascular risk led to their decline in the 1970s [30]. In the 1980s their use was substituted by serotonin (5-HT)-releasing agents such as fenluramine and desfenfluramine [30]. From their start-point, this sort of drugs presented the potential to produce hyperpulmonary hypertension, but this side effect was "counteracted" by the benefit of the also important weight loss provided.

Phentermine: The Oldest Anti-Obesity Drug

Phentermine, approved only in US in 1959, is among the oldest AOD. Phentermine is an appetite suppressant agent, chemically related to amphetamine, but without its addictive potential. Phentermine has a medical use for short-term obesity treatment ($\leq$ 12 weeks) because it presents multiple adverse effects, although there is no large-scale studies on this issue. This sympathomimetic amine anorectic is indicated as a short-term adjunct in a regimen of weight loss based on lifestyle changes and caloric restriction in the management of obese patients with an initial BMI $\geq$ 30 kg/m^2 or $\geq$ 27 kg/m^2 in the presence of concomitant cardiovascular risk factors (*e.g.*, diabetes, hypertension, dyslipidemia) [267].

Phentermine is contraindicated in patients with unstable cardiovascular disease or cardiac dysrhythmias, uncontrolled high blood pressure and hyperthyroidism. In addition, phentermine is not recommended for patients with a history of drug and/or alcohol abuse or taking monoamine oxidase inhibitors, and it should be used with caution in patients under treatment with other agents acting on the CNS (*e.g.*, increasing adrenergic responses). Phentermine side effects include, palpitations, tachycardia and increased blood pressure, irritability, anxiety, diaphoresis, dizziness, insomnia, headache, euphoria, dysphoria, mouth dryness, diarrhoea and constipation [267].

In the early 1990s, the use of a combined treatment including phentermine plus fenfluramine started to be a general practice in the US [268]. But unfortunately, only a few years later, phentermine was reported to cause cardiac valvulopathy in combination with fenfluramine or dexfenfluramine. The role of phentermine in the etiology of valvulopathy has not been well established, as there were also cases of valvular heart disease in patients taking phentermine alone [269].

Studies on the possible effects of phentermine upon adiposopathy are very scarce, showing limited to effects upon adipogenesis, FFAs and adipose tissue endocrine and immune responses [270]. Short-term studies suggest that weight loss associated with phentermine may have some beneficial actions on lipid profile [88], with mixed effect on blood pressure [271].

Recently, in July of 2012, a combination of phentermine and topiramate has received the FDA approval to treat obesity under the trade name of Qsymia® [32]. This issue will be further discussed later in this chapter.

Amphetamines for Weight Loss: high efficacy but low tolerability

Amphetamines started to be used for weight loss purposes in 1938 [272]. Monoamine neurotransmitters reduce appetite by decreasing neuropeptide Y, and increasing pro-opiomelanocortin [273] and anorexigenic peptide, termed 'cocaine and amphetamine-regulated transcript' (CART), which is located in the hypothalamus, [274]. Amphetamine action mechanisms on central nervous system (CNS) include an increase in dopamine, norepinephrine and serotonin activity. Amphetamines are sympathomimetic agents which act upon obesity by increasing energy expenditure through diverse mechanisms, such as increasing thermogenesis [275], although this has been mainly studied in animals, while only a handful of clinical trials have shown that effects in humans [276-278]. Therefore, at least at doses prescribed for weight loss, the long-term effects of amphetamines on total energy balance still remain unclear. On the other hand, amphetamines have potential toxic effects for CNS and other adverse systemic effects, including increased blood pressure, tachycardia and euphoria, as well as a high potential for abuse and addiction [279].

The Main Anti-Obesity Drugs in the Last 12 Years

In Europe, three more agents were later approved for the long-term clinical management of obesity and related morbidities:

1. Sibutramine (Meridia[®] and Reductil[®]).

2. Rimonabant (Acomplia[®]).

3. Orlistart (Xenical[®] and Alli[®]).

Sibutramine

Sibutramine is a serotonin and norepinephrine reuptake inhibitor used for promoting weight loss in patients who have failed with lifestyle changes. In January 2010 it was suspended from the European market by the European Medicine Agency (EMEA), due to growing concerns about its potential negative effects on cardiovascular risk, according to the SCOUT study (Sibutramine Cardiovascular Outcome Trial) [280], a review of clinical trials including almost 10,000 overweight or obese patients at high risk of cardiovascular disease. The study randomly assigned patients to either treatment with sibutramine or placebo, and compared weight loss results assessing at the same time occurrence of cardiovascular events after a follow-up period of six years. As patients taking sibutramine presented significantly higher risk of cardiovascular events, the Committee for Medicinal Products for Human Use (CHMP) considered that it should not be prescribed in obese and overweight patients. In addition, subjects with previous cardiovascular conditions who were taking sibutramine had an increased risk of non-fatal myocardial infarction and non-fatal stroke, but not of cardiovascular death or death from any cause. In 2010, the FDA also withdrew sibutramine from the US market.

Sibutramine is a β-phenethylamine [281] that, when administered in doses ranging from 5 to 15 mg/day and combined with adequate lifestyle changes induces a significant body weight loss (around 5-10%). Sibutramine achieves weight loss by increasing satiety and reducing appetite. The selective inhibition of the reuptake of serotonine and noradrenaline within the hypothalamus [22] is the mechanism that underlies this effects. In addition, it has also demonstrated to lower plasma triglyceride levels, but unfortunately it has also been linked to increased blood pressure and heart rate [282]. Moreover, sibutramine has shown to reduce serum levels of proinflammatory mediators such as CRP, IL-6, and TNF-α when taken during 3 to 6 months [283].

Rimonabant

Human brain produces two different kinds of endocannabinoids: anandamide and 2-arachidonoylglycerol (2-AG) [284]. They are synthesized on demand and work in a reverse direction, from postsynaptic neurons where they are synthesized to presynaptic neurons where they bind to receptors. Two specific endocannabinoid receptors have been identified: CB_1 and CB_2 receptors. CB_1 receptor is thought to mediate the psychotropic actions of cannabis and be involved in the modulation of food intake and adipogenesis. It is expressed at high levels by brain cells and several peripheral tissues including heart and adipose tissue, gastrointestinal tract and adrenal gland. CB_1 knockout mice show a lean phenotype that appears to be resistant to diet-induced obesity and insulin resistance. On the contrary, CB_2 receptors are mainly located at immune tissues and blood cells. These receptors are usually located in the areas responsible for modulating energy balance, feeding behaviour, hepatic lipogenesis, and glucose homeostasis [285]. Endocannabinoid system stimulation promotes metabolic processes that lead to weight gain, lipogenesis, insulin resistance, dyslipidemia, and impaired glucose tolerance [286, 287].

Rimonabant, a CB-1endocannabinoid receptor inhibitor, showed not only to reduce excess body weight in obese subjects, but also a range of both central and metabolic peripheral effects [288], including decreased blood pressure in hypertensive patients, improved insulin sensitivity and dyslipidemia, also decreasing the prevalence of metabolic syndrome [289]. Rimonabant produced significant improvements in blood glucose control beyond what would be expected from its effects on weight loss [290]. So, metabolic and inflammatory benefits are not totally dependent on weight reduction and could be due to its direct action on abdominal fat or through neuroendocrine factors enabled or disabled by the drug [291]. The same argument has led to the use the topiramate not only as an anti-obesity drug, but also as an oral anti-diabetic drug, as discussed below.

Rimonabant, the first and only specific endocannabinoid inhibitor, was approved as an adjunct to diet and exercise for the treatment of obese or overweight patients by the EMEA in 2006. However the FDA never approved its use in the US due to concerns on serious adverse events. A meta-analysis reported that the 20 mg of rimonabant was associated with an increased risk of adverse events including psychiatric and nervous system adverse events [292]. As a result, in 2009 the EMEA withdrew the market authorisation for rimonabant in the European Union [293].

Orlistart

As explained above, the release of FFAs due to excessive fat accumulation at adipose tissue is one of the key inductors of pathogenesis in obese patients. One of the strategies of the anti-obesity pharmacology consists of the reduction in energy uptake by partially inhibiting the hydrolysis of dietary triglycerides into absorbable FFAs, thus decreasing lipid absorption in the gut by 30 percent [294]. In this category of drugs lies orlistart, a gastrointestinal lipase inhibitor that was firstly approved by the FDA for the treatment of obesity in 1999. The main advantage of these pharmacological agents is to avoid systemic-side effects, since they bind lipid molecules in the intestinal tract.

Orlistat is a synthetic drug derived from a natural lipase inhibitor. It does not directly act on appetite as sibutramine, but rather decreases fat absorption. This is achieved by binding to pancreatic lipase, the main enzyme that hydrolyses triglycerides [295]. The long-term efficacy of orlistat (120 mg three times daily) for weight loss has been demonstrated in several clinical trials with following periods from 2 to 4 years [296]. Additional evidence has been observed in several systematic reviews in adults [297] and a systematic review with 2 short-term studies in adolescents [298].

In average, the use of orlistart leads to around 5 to 10 % weight reduction in 50-60 % of patients after 12 months of treatment [17]. Moreover, in a trial assessing orlistat in the prevention of diabetes in obese subjects (the XENDOS Study), the risk of developing T2DM in obese subjects with impaired glucose tolerance was reduced [299]. Besides, this drug counts with an added value: several studies have evaluated the effects of orlistart on inflammatory markers in obese patients. Treatment with orlistart for up to 1 year showed a significant reduction of CRP levels [300]. For this reason, despite the modest weight loss achieved by orlistart, it is important to highlight that it confers some beneficial effects on cardiovascular risk, including plasma levels of LDL-cholesterol, blood pressure [301] and glycemia [299], as well as improving insulin resistance [299].

However, orlistart also produces relevant side effects, as the rest of anti-obesity drugs. Its main side effects include gastrointestinal disturbances such as abdominal pain, dyspepsia, flatulence, diarrhea and steatorrhea [295, 301]. Besides, it has been also related to severe liver injury [302]. After receiving 32 reports of serious liver injury in patients taking orlistat between 1999 and October 2008, including 6 cases of liver failure, the FDA carried out a safety review. In May 2010, these facts led to a label revision and the addition of a warning of severe liver injury.

Until 2012, when topiramate in combination with phentermine was approved by the FDA, orlistat was the only drug for weight loss that remained in the market.

Several new anti-obesity drugs are under research as monotherapy (Table **3**) or in combination (Table **4**). While these new drugs arrive to market, we are going to analyze the use of topiramate in the treatment of obesity as cardiometabolic disease.

Table 3: Novel obesity treatments in Phase II and III trials

Mode of Action	Drug Name	Company
5-HT2C agonist	Lorcaserin (ADP-356)	Arena
Amylin analogue	Pramlintide	Amylin Pharmaceuticals
CB1 receptor antagonist	CP 945598	Pfizer
CB1 receptor antagonist	Taranabant	Merck
CB1 receptor antagonist	AVE 1625 Surinabant	Sanofi-Aventis
Y2 receptor agonist	PYY3-36	Amylin, Nastech
Y4 receptor agonist	TM30339	7TM Pharma
Histamine Agonist	Betahistine	Obecure

Table 4: Novel combination obesity treatments in clinical trials

Mode of Action	Drug Name	Company
Bupropion + Naltrexone	Contrave	Orexigen
Bupropion + Zonisamide	Empatic (Excalia)	Orexigen
Pramlintide + Leptin		Amylin

Topiramate

Background

Topiramate (TPM) was serendipitously discovered in 1979 by Maryanoff and Gardocki when they were working on a new anti-diabetic agent [303]. TPM is a broad-spectrum anticonvulsant with useful neurological effects that derive from multiple central nervous system mechanisms of action. It is a "neurostabilizer" that attenuates the excitability of brain neuronal pathways. TPM is approved in many countries worldwide as monotherapy and adjunctive therapy for the treatment of epilepsy in adult and paediatric patients [304].

Besides its well-known antiepileptic properties, this drug is also used for prevention of migraine attacks [305, 306], and may have a potential role in the treatment of movement disorders [307]. Furthermore, TPM has been proposed to treat bipolar disorder [308], and due to its effects on stabilizing mood and reducing impulse control problems, as a treatment for obese patients with binge eating disorder [309-311]. So, it has been also associated with significant reductions in binge frequency, binge per day frequency, weight, body mass index and obsessive-compulsive scores. Moreover, it has also been used in patients with bulimia nervosa [312, 313], and even in patients with alcohol dependence and for tobacco abuse [314].

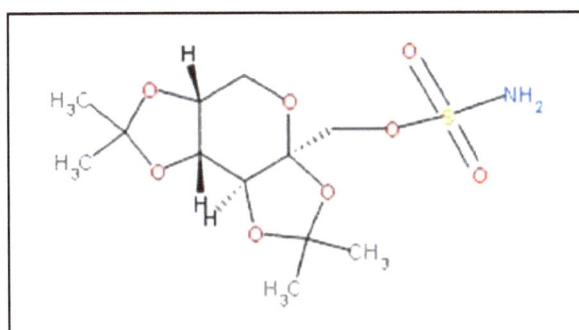

Figure 13: Topiramate chemical structure. Systematic (IUPAC) name: 2,3:4,5-Bis-O-(1-methylethylidene)-beta-D-fructopyranose sulfamate.

Pharmacology of Topiramate

Topiramate, a sulfamate-substituted monosaccharide derivative of the naturally occurring sugar monosaccharide D-fructose (Fig. **13**), is structurally different from other antiepileptic drugs (AEDs). It has a unique combination of actions at various receptor sites and ion channels. TPM enhances γ-aminobutyric acid (GABA)-mediated chloride flux at GABAA receptors [315], blocks the kainate/AMPA (α-amino-3-hydroxy-5-methylisoxazole-4-propionic acid) subtype of the glutamate receptor [316, 317], and there is also evidence that specific actions are taken on GluR5-kainate-receptors (Fig. **14**) [316].

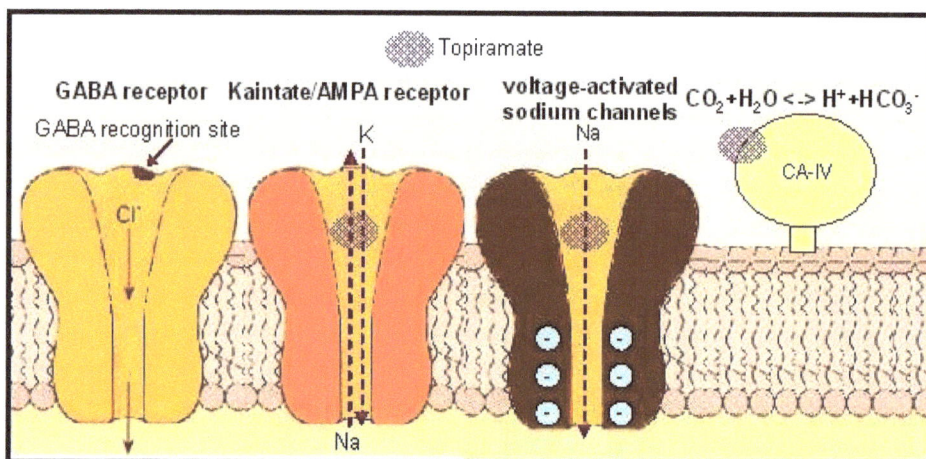

Figure 14: Topiramate activities at receptor sites (GABAA receptors and kainate/AMPA subtype of the glutamate receptor) and ion channels (voltage-activated sodium (Na) channels, high-voltage-activated calcium (Ca) currents, potassium (K) conductance). Inhibition of carbonic anhydrase (CA) isoenzymes (subtypes II and IV).

TPM is rapidly absorbed and its bioavailability after oral consumption is greater than 80%, reaching maximum plasma levels 1.3-1.7 hours after oral administration [315, 318]. TPM pharmacokinetics is dose proportional, reaching a steady state in 4-8 days in patients with normal renal function [319]. The extent of protein binding of TPM is around 15%. When administered as monotherapy, TPM is not extensively metabolized, with 50-80% of the drug being excreted unchanged in the urine [320], with an elimination half life of 19-23 hours.

TPM is not an inhibitor *in vitro* of the cytochrome P450 (CYP) isoenzymes CYP1A2, CYP2A6, CYP2B6, CYP2C9, CYP2D6, CYP2E1 and CYP3A4/5 [315, 321]. Therefore, no interactions involving changes in the pharmacokinetics of TPM are expected due to enzyme inhibition [322]. Moreover, predominantly renal elimination and low protein binding minimize the potential for clinically relevant interactions with other drugs. However, described TPM interaction with other drugs (*e.g.,* low-dose oral contraceptives, digoxin, hydrochlorothiazide, metformin, pioglytazone and risperidone) may require adjustments of TPM or the concomitant therapy or routine monitoring of clinical response. In patients taking oral contraceptives, it is important to consider that their efficacy may be reduced due to a decrease in circulating estrogens.

Topiramate: Mechanisms of Action and Metabolic Effects

Several potential mechanisms have been proposed to explain topiramate-induced weight loss, although the underlying mechanism remains still unclear. Studies in animal models suggest that the potential mechanisms of TPM-induced weight loss include decreased caloric intake and reduction in body fat gain [323]. During clinical trials in epilepsy, subjects taking TPM reported loss of appetite and hunger reduction [324-326] related to an increase in energy expenditure, even though the objective measurements of appetite may not be reduced during weight loss [327]. Regarding energy expenditure, TPM may decrease energy storage and usage efficiency, and thus increase energy consumption [328], theoretically by increasing thermogenesis [329].

With regard to adipocyte function, TPM may inhibit an adipocyte enzyme, the so called "mitochondrial carbonic anhydrase isoenzyme V" [330], and through this mechanism, inhibit the lipogenesis catalyzed by this enzyme [331]. TPM is also involved in the decrease of lipoprotein lipase (LPL) activity in white adipose tissue (WAT). This is a relevant fact regarding the potential pathogenicity of increased levels of free fatty acids (FFAs), what at the same time reduces lipogenesis [332]. On the contrary, TPM may increase lipoprotein lipase activity in brown adipose tissue [333], which may promote thermogenesis and lipoprotein lipase activity in skeletal muscle, supporting the potential for substrate oxidation [332, 334]. In addition, TPM may increase adiponectin levels [334], which favourably affects several peripheral physiologic processes related to metabolic disease. However, the effect of TPM on leptin in humans is controversial [332, 335].

The main potential mechanisms proposed to explain TPM-induced weight loss are summarized in the Fig. **15**.

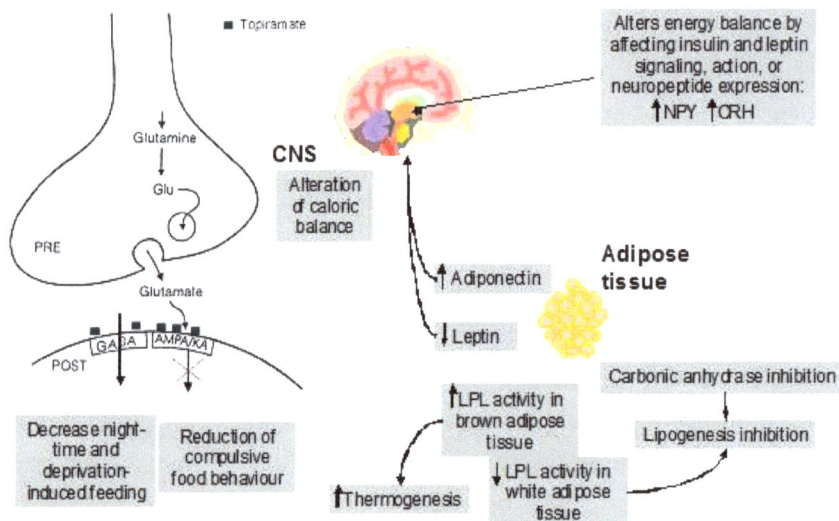

Figure 15: Anti-obesity topiramate proposed mechanisms of action. Topiramate enhances γ-aminobutyric acid (GABA)-mediated chloride flux at GABAA receptors, which may decrease night-time and deprivation-induced feeding and it blocks the kainate/AMPA subtype of the glutamate receptor, so it may reduce compulsive or addictive food behaviour. Topiramate may also increase levels of neuropeptide Y (NPY) in the hypothalamus and increase levels of hypothalamic corticotropic-releasing hormone (CRH), which may have catabolic activity. Thus it may have CNS effects which result in alteration of caloric balance. In the adipose tissue, topiramate inhibits lipogenesis, through the inhibition of mithocondrial carbonic anhydrase and also decreasing lipoprotein lipase (LPL) activity in white adipose tissue. TPM may decrease energy storage and usage efficiency, and thus increase energy expenditure, theoretically by increasing thermogenesis. Another effect of Topiramate is the increase of adiponectin levels and the decrease of leptin levels.

Efficacy and Tolerability of Topiramate as Anti-Obesity Drug

Early on, even at the time of its approval (in 1996 in the USA) as an antiepileptic drug, TPM was reported to promote dose-related weight loss [336]. Since then, clinical trial data have supported TPM as having weight loss effects [335, 337-345]. However, TPM does not have a regulatory for weight reduction [346], even though some clinicians have used it "off-label" for this purpose.

In a meta-analysis [347] of randomized controlled trials (3320 individuals), patients taking TPM lost around 5 kg of additional weight as compared with placebo. In addition, dosage and treatment duration were related to the efficacy of TPM to promote weight loss. Several factors have been studied as predictors of weight loss related to TPM intake. Among them, the baseline BMI and the duration of treatment appears to be the most closely related, whereas the role of gender and daily dosage is uncertain [327, 351-359]. With regard to the duration of TPM treatment, the weight loss occurred most frequently during the first months of treatment (4 to 6 months) and continued for at least 1 year [335, 348-350]. On the other hand, mixed results have been reported on the role of daily dosage. While some studies did not find a direct relationship between weight reduction and TPM dosage [351, 352], data from other studies support that the extent of the loss is directly related to final dose [325, 353]. As for gender, some results that suggested a greatest BMI decrease in females [351] have not been confirmed in other studies that did not find differences between adult males and females [354].

Several studies have been conducted to assess the safety of TPM for weight loss in obese subjects [337, 350]. The most frequent adverse events were related to the central and peripheral nervous system, including somnolence, paresthesia and memory loss, and were dose-related, occurring early in treatment, and they were usually resolved spontaneously. [350].

Efficacy and safety of TPM as an anti-obesity drug have been also tested in patients with T2DM [338, 355-357]. In a clinical trial, overweight/obese diabetic patients under diet and exercise alone or in combination with metformin were randomized to 175 mg/day of TPM or placebo [355]. Patients in the TPM group lost 6.0 kg *vs.* 2.5 in the placebo group, which respectively represented 5.8% and 2.3% of their baseline weight. Patients under TPM treatment showed a significant reduction in haemoglobin A1c from baseline (0.9% *vs.* 0.4% in the placebo group), along with reduced blood pressure and urinary albumin excretion. Adverse events were predominantly neuropsychiatric or related to the central and peripheral nervous system.

Topiramate in Combination Therapy for Weight Loss

Up to date, TPM alone does not have an indication for weight loss. However, a combination of TPM controlled-release with phentermine, known as Qsymia® (Vivus, Inc., CA, USA), has been recently approved (July 2012) in the US for the treatment of obesity [32].

Phentermine is among the oldest approved anti-obesity agents, indicated as an adjunct to appropriate nutrition and physical exercise for short-term (up to 12 weeks) treatment of obesity [358]. Due to its generic status, it is the most commonly prescribed appetite suppressant [358].

The combination of TPM and phentermine has shown synergistic potential for safe, effective and sustained weight loss [287, 302] (Fig. **16**). Lower doses of both agents also improve the intolerances and toxicities associated with higher doses of each one [359]. This fixed-dose combination is presented as a once-a-day single capsule of phentermine hydrochloride, which is readily absorbed to provide therapeutic effects early in the day, added to controlled release TPM, which provides persistent weight loss throughout the day.

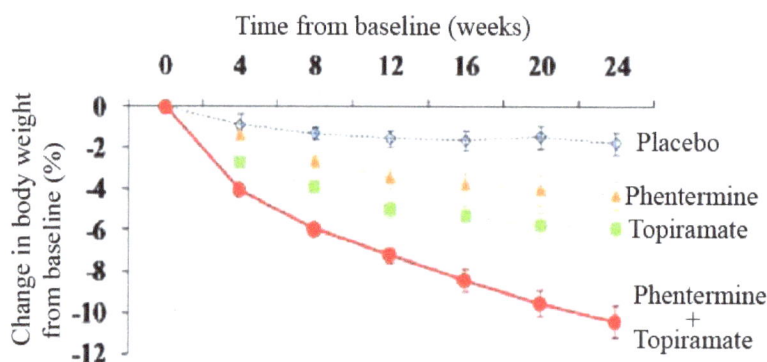

Figure 16: The combination (phentermine plus topiramate controlled-release) leads to greater changes in body weight from baseline than each agent alone or placebo. Source: A Study Comparing Multiple Doses of VI-0521 With Placebo and Their Single-agent Constituents for Treatment of Obesity in Adults. Vivis, Inc. ClinicalTrials.gov Identifier: NCT00563368.

Several clinical trials involving thousands of patients have demonstrated that the combination of phentermine and topiramate is effective in promoting weight loss and also in improving adiposopathy-associated metabolic diseases [358-363]. The weight loss achieved with combination therapy is greater than using either agent alone [364]. In a 1-year placebo-controlled clinical trial, phentermine plus topiramate combination in addition to lifestyle modification demonstrated clinically meaningful weight loss [362]. Moreover, when compared to placebo, combined treatment has been associated with favourable changes in cardiometabolic and anthropometric parameters (*e.g.,* HDL-cholesterol, blood pressure and waist circumference), also improving haemoglobin A1C levels in overweight and obese subjects with type 2 diabetes [365].

Cardiometabolic Implications of the Regular use of Topiramate

As discussed earlier in this chapter, the relentless rise in the prevalence of obesity predicts an exponential increase in the incidence of obesity-related cardiometabolic and non-cardiometabolic complications. A vigorous therapeutic strategy is needed to prevent and treat obesity-related comorbidities, thereby avoiding disability and premature death [366]. TPM actions on obesity should be evaluated not only by weight loss, but also according to the obesity-related comorbidities. If obesity is considered as a cardiometabolic disease, it should be mandatory to study not only the classical cardiovascular risk factors and cardiovascular events, but also the metabolic aspects related to insulin resistance, metabolic inflexibility and endoplasmic reticulum stress and adipokines, as well as inflammation, oxidative stress and endothelial biomarkers.

a) Classical Cardiovascular Risk Factors and Cardiovascular Events

TPM in combination with lifestyle measures, besides a demonstrated weight loss, may lead to a reduction in newly diagnosed type 2 diabetes mellitus as well an improvement in lipid profile and a reduction in blood pressure, and therefore a lower cardiovascular risk. However, data about these targets are sparse. In a study conducted in women with cryptogenic epilepsy receiving TPM, it was associated with lower HDL-cholesterol levels, which may increase vascular disease [367]. This important aspect of lipid metabolism should be clarified. Several studies have shown a beneficial decrease in total cholesterol and triglycerides, but also accompanied by a decrease in HDL-cholesterol [333, 335, 350, 368]. The influence of weight loss on LDL-cholesterol levels is poor, so limited reduction can be expected. In animal models, TPM has been reported to lower triglycerides and circulating free fatty acids [369, 370].

With regard to type 2 diabetes mellitus, a significant reduction in haemoglobin A1c from baseline has been reported in patients under TPM treatment [286], along with reduced blood pressure and urinary albumin excretion [338, 355-357].

Glucose tolerance, as measured during the oral glucose tolerance test, has been also observed to improve in obese subjects treated with TPM, but it may be secondary to weight loss [335]. However, although several studies in animal models have associated TPM with an increase in insulin sensitivity, enhancing insulin action in the adipose and muscle tissues [332, 368], this findings have not been confirmed in humans.

b) Metabolic Aspects Related to Insulin Resistance, Metabolic Inflexibility and Endoplasmic Reticulum Stress

Animal testing data show that TPM improves insulin resistance (IR) independently of weight loss [332, 368]. Recently, the potential hepatic molecular mechanistic cassette of the anti-insulin resistance effect of TPM has been reported [371]. The study demonstrated that IR acts at hepatic molecular level and that the TPM-mediated insulin sensitivity is ensued partly by the modulation of hepatic insulin receptor isoforms, activation of tyrosine kinase, induction of GLUT2 and elevation of adiponectin and adiponectin receptors, in addition to its known effects on improving lipid homeostasis and glucose tolerance [371].

In humans, IR, as measured by the HOMA index, was reduced after 20 weeks of treatment with an average dose of 100 mg TPM/day in patients with migraine [372]. Similarly, in premenopausal women with cryptogenic epilepsy taking TPM, a significant improvement in insulin resistance was found, although it was surprisingly accompanied by a HDL-cholesterol reduction when the expected effect should have been just the opposite [367]. With regard to MetS or IR syndrome -abdominal obesity, glucose intolerance, elevated triglycerides, low HDL-cholesterol and hypertension- in subjects under TPM treatment, most of the available data derive from studies carried out in epileptic patients [373]. There are no specific studies about insulin resistance, metabolic inflexibility and/or endoplasmic reticulum stress in obese subjects under TPM treatment.

c) Adipokines

In a study conducted in rats, TPM improved glucose homeostasis and lipid profile, as well as raised adiponectin levels in a dose-dependent manner [371].

In humans, TPM has shown to significantly reduce leptin levels from baseline in patients with migraine [372] and epilepsy [352]. In both types of patients, adiponectin as well as the leptin/adiponectin (L/A) ratio were also increased. The observed changes in leptin and adiponectin have also a positive cardiovascular profile, in addition to the metabolic improvements. However, other studies have not found a similar leptin reduction. So, in a prospective study carried out in patients with different types of refractory focal epilepsy who received TPM as adjunctive treatment, no significant reductions in serum leptin levels were observed [374]. Just like in the aforementioned study, no changes in leptin were found in premenopausal women with cryptogenic epilepsy [367].

d) Inflammatory Biomarkers

As previously described in this chapter, obesity is an established determinant of C-reactive protein (CRP) in adults [208, 375] and children [208-210, 376].

In a study evaluating the association between weight change and clinical markers of cardiovascular risk in subjects taking TPM or amitriptyline as migraine-preventive treatments, individuals from both treatment groups were divided into three groups: the 'major weight gain' group gained > 5% of their baseline body weight at the conclusion of the study; the 'major weight loss' group lost > 5% of their baseline body weight; and the third group had < 5% of weight change [377]. Those who gained weight presented significantly higher values of CRP, mean diastolic blood pressure, heart rate, haemoglobin A1c, total cholesterol, LDL-cholesterol and triglycerides than those with major weight loss. However, both groups experienced decreases in systolic blood pressure and HDL-cholesterol. Authors concluded that weight gain during migraine treatment is associated with deterioration of cardiovascular disease risk markers [377]. Nevertheless, no specific data are available on the effect in those just taking TPM.

Furthermore, although no particular studies linking CRP and TPM have been reported, a reduction in weight and body fat mass has been positively associated with lower plasma CRP levels [375]. In addition, the CRP response to lifestyle modifications, as well as drug treatment, may be genetically regulated. So, genetic variants on the CRP locus and other loci may be responsible for the interindividual variability of plasma CRP concentrations, which could have important implications for the development of more personalized preventive and therapeutic approaches to reduce cardiovascular disease in obese patients [378].

A study evaluating the effect on lipids and C-reactive protein of switching from enzyme-inducing antiepileptic drugs (carbamazepine or phenytoin) to TPM [379] showed that this therapy change resulted in a decrease in serum CRP around 50%, as well as a significant improvement of lipid profile. According to the authors, this finding provide evidence that CYP450 induction rises CRP levels and serum lipids, including LDL-cholesterol, and these effects are reversible upon deinduction [380]. Low-dose TPM appears not to induce the enzymes involved in cholesterol synthesis [379].

On the other hand, interleukin-6 (IL-6) and TNF-alpha (TNF-α), two adipokines with proinflammatory actions on both vascular and fat tissue, should be considered of paramount importance in obese subjects undergoing medical or surgical treatment, especially TNF-α because of its implication in insulin signaling impairment [381]. In animal models, a significant decrease in TNF-α have been observed in male rats when treated with TPM in a dose-dependent manner [371]. In humans, cytokines play an important role in obesity. IL-6 and/or TNF-α were unchanged in small samples of migraine patients receiving TPM therapy [372, 382].

e) Endothelial Biomarkers

Just one study assessing the relationship between TPM and endothelial biomarkers has been conducted in subjects suffering from migraine, obese and non-obese [372]. In this study, circulating vascular endothelial growth factor (VEGF) increased during the first 2-4 week followed by a continuous decrease. The role of increased VEGF concentrations prior to these metabolic changes is not clear and might, hypothetically, involve a centrally mediated effect of TPM on body weight regulation.

Our Preliminary Experience with TPM: Effects Upon Weight Loss and Inflammatory Markers (Adiponectin and IL-6)

Up to date, we have carried out two studies on the use of TPM as an anti-obesity agent. The results have not been published, but the work was presented at the

European Federation of Internal Medicine (EFIM) Congress (Madrid, October 2012).

In a first pilot trial, we aimed to assess the efficacy and tolerability of TPM when used as a weight loss agent in a sample of middle-aged overweight patients at moderate-high cardiovascular risk, who had been resistant to a lifestyle change for at least 6 months. Dosage was titrated upward by weekly increases of 25 mg/day over a 7-week period (according to Rosenstock [355]) and continued afterwards up to a target dose of 150-200 mg/day during the maintenance phase. Significant reductions in body weight (5.48 ± 4.12 kg; $p < 0.001$), BMI (2.0 ± 1.46 kg/m^2; $p < 0.001$) and body fat (2.7 ± 3.3 Kg, $p = 0.002$)) from baseline were observed in the sample population (n = 42). 9 out of 10 patients lost more than 5% of their initial body weight, and almost 2 out of 10 lost more than 10%. With regard to tolerance, 6 out of 10 patients suffered adverse events, being paresthesia the most frequent one (36% of the whole sample). Only 5 of the 42 patients abandoned the treatment, 4 of them due to moderate adverse events and only 1 due to inefficacy of treatment after a period of 6 months.

In a second phase, we aimed to assess the potential beneficial effects of TPM on metabolic factors and subsequently on cardiometabolic disease, usually associated to obesity. With this scope in mind, we also measured inflammatory markers such as IL-6 and adiponectin at baseline and after 9 months of treatment.

Subjects who were non-responders to lifestyle changes in usual clinical practice were treated with TPM in addition to lifestyle change measures (n = 15). In order to control the true potential TPM effects on haemodynamic, metabolic and biomarker parameters of TPM independently of the achieved weight reduction, these subjects were matched by sex and age with patients retrospectively selected who were responders to life-style changes with a clinically significant weight reduction (over 5%).

Main results of the study are summarized here. Subjects under TPM treatment showed significant weight loss, accompanied by a reduction in BMI and fat mass. In fact, 53.3% showed a weight reduction > 7%. These subjects also significantly reduced haemodynamic parameters, particularly systolic diastolic and mean blood pressure, whereas in the control group only relevant changes were observed in diastolic blood pressure. With regard to metabolic changes, haemoglobin A1c was significantly reduced in subjects treated with TPM but not so in the control group. Moreover, a downward trend was appreciated with regard to triglycerides in both groups, although it did not reach statistical significance. Regarding biomarkers, subjects under TPM treatment showed significant changes in IL-6 and adiponectin levels, unlike the life-style responder control group. Finally, drug tolerance was good overall and there were no patient withdrawals from the study. The most frequently reported side effects include paresthesia (35.7%) and insomnia (14.3%).

Our study confirms previous results [355] regarding the effectiveness of TPM as an anti-obesity drug in patients with moderate to high cardiovascular risk. In fact, it goes even further, obtaining an improvement in circulating cytokine levels (*i.e.* adiponectin and IL-6), which are related to vascular inflammation and pro-inflammatory activity of visceral fat and/or of the SVF (Stroma-Vascular Fraction - consisting of macrophages, endothelial cells, progenitor cells and leukocytes).

The effects of TPM on lowering blood pressure, IL-6 and adiponectin levels were not observed in subjects who achieved weight reduction based on recommended lifestyle changes given in usual clinical practice. This may suggest a favourable effect of the direct action of the drug, and not a weight-loss dependent effect. Patients under TPM treatment showed a more favourable cytokine profile, which underlines the probable anti-inflammatory effect of TPM. The effect of TPM on cytokine levels might be explained by its action at any of the following sites [315, 383]: GABA-activated chloride channels, inhibition of excitatory neurotransmission, kainate and AMPA receptors, or GluR5 kainate receptors. Thus, it is possible that some of these mechanisms may play a major role in the activity of macrophages and/or adipocytes. For example, TPM induced enhancement of GABA-activated chloride channels could interfere with autonomous nervous system functioning and, in turn, have major implications in the regulation of peripheral metabolism. So far, the only antiobesity drug that had demonstrated a peripheral metabolic effect was rimonabant, due to its action as a CB1 receptor blocker [384-386].

Despite of important limitations to our study, such as small sample size or the inclusion of a retrospectively selected control group, we believe these do not question the validity of our findings and observed tendencies, which should encourage the development of new prospective studies to clarify the mechanisms by which a drug, without granted peripheral action, could improve cytokine levels, and all the implications derived from this.

ACKNOWLEDGEMENTS

Declared none.

CONFLICT OF INTEREST

The authors confirm that this chapter contents have no conflict of interest.

REFERENCES

[1]   Grundy SM. Multifactorial causation of obesity: implications for prevention. Am J Clin Nutr, 1998; 67: 563S-72S.
[2]   Brownell KD, Frieden TR. Ounces of prevention--the public policy case for taxes on sugared beverages. N Engl J Med, 2009; 360: 1805-8.
[3]   Hammond RA, Levine R. The economic impact of obesity in the United States. Diabetes Metab Syndr Obes, 2010; 3: 285-95.
[4]   World Heath Organization [homepage on the Internet]. Obesity and overweight. Fact sheet N°311. [updated: March 2013; cited: 28/May/2013]. Available from: http://www.who.int/mediacentre/factsheets/fs311/en/
[5]   Ogden CL, Carroll MD, Kit BK, Flegal KM. Prevalence of obesity in the United States, 2009-2010. NCHS data brief, no 82. Hyattsville. [updated: 2012; cited: 28/May/2013]. Available from: http://www.cdc.gov/nchs/data/databriefs/db82.htm.
[6]   National Center for Health Statistics (US). Health, United States, 2010: With Special Feature on Death and Dying. Hyattsville. [updated: Feb/2011; cited: 28/May/2013]. Available from: http://www.ncbi.nlm.nih.gov/books/NBK54381/
[7]   World Health Organization Global Health Observatory (GHO). Overweight and obesity. [updated: 04/Apr/2011; cited: 28/May/2013]. Available from: http://www.who.int/gho/ncd/risk_factors/overweight/en/index.html.
[8]   Ju HW, Min JH, Chung MS, Kim CS. The atrzf1 mutation of the novel RING-type E3 ubiquitin ligase increases proline contents and enhances drought tolerance in Arabidopsis. Plant Sci, 2013; 203-204: 1-7.
[9]   Blackburn G. Effect of degree of weight loss on health benefits. Obes Res, 1995; 3 Suppl 2: 211s-216s.
[10]   Yanovski SZ, Bain RP, Williamson DF. Report of a National Institutes of Health--Centers for Disease Control and Prevention workshop on the feasibility of conducting a randomized clinical trial to estimate the long-term health effects of intentional weight loss in obese persons. Am J Clin Nutr, 1999; 69: 366-72.

[11] Kanders BS, Blackburn GL, Lavin P, Norton D. Weight loss outcome and health benefits associated with the Optifast program in the treatment of obesity. Int J Obes, 1989; 13 Suppl 2: 131-4.

[12] Follick MJ, Abrams DB, Smith TW, Henderson LO, Herbert PN. Contrasting short- and long-term effects of weight loss on lipoprotein levels. Arch Intern Med, 1984; 144: 1571-4.

[13] Wing RR. Long-term effects of a lifestyle intervention on weight and cardiovascular risk factors in individuals with type 2 diabetes mellitus: four-year results of the Look AHEAD trial. Arch Intern Med, 2010; 170: 1566-75.

[14] Tziomalos K, Dimitroula HV, Katsiki N, Savopoulos C, Hatzitolios AI. Effects of lifestyle measures, antiobesity agents, and bariatric surgery on serological markers of inflammation in obese patients. Mediators Inflamm, 2010; 2010: 364957.

[15] Snow V, Barry P, Fitterman N, Qaseem A, Weiss K. Pharmacologic and surgical management of obesity in primary care: a clinical practice guideline from the American College of Physicians. Ann Intern Med, 2005; 142: 525-31.

[16] Maggard MA, Shugarman LR, Suttorp M, Maglione M, Sugerman HJ, Livingston EH, *et al.,* Meta-analysis: surgical treatment of obesity. Ann Intern Med, 2005; 142: 547-59.

[17] Li Z, Maglione M, Tu W, Mojica W, Arterburn D, Shugarman LR, *et al.,* Meta-analysis: pharmacologic treatment of obesity. Ann Intern Med, 2005; 142: 532-46.

[18] Cummings DE. Metabolic surgery for type 2 diabetes. Nat Med, 2012; 18: 656-8.

[19] Henness S, Perry CM. Orlistat: a review of its use in the management of obesity. Drugs, 2006; 66: 1625-56.

[20] McClendon KS, Riche DM, Uwaifo GI. Orlistat: current status in clinical therapeutics. Expert Opin Drug Saf, 2009; 8: 727-44.

[21] Halford JC, Harrold JA, Boyland EJ, Lawton CL, Blundell JE. Serotonergic drugs : effects on appetite expression and use for the treatment of obesity. Drugs, 2007; 67: 27-55.

[22] Tziomalos K, Krassas GE, Tzotzas T. The use of sibutramine in the management of obesity and related disorders: an update. Vasc Health Risk Manag, 2009; 5: 441-52.

[23] Idelevich E, Kirch W, Schindler C. Current pharmacotherapeutic concepts for the treatment of obesity in adults. Ther Adv Cardiovasc Dis, 2009; 3: 75-90.

[24] Patel PN, Pathak R. Rimonabant: a novel selective cannabinoid-1 receptor antagonist for treatment of obesity. Am J Health Syst Pharm, 2007; 64: 481-9.

[25] Kintscher U. The cardiometabolic drug rimonabant: after 2 years of RIO-Europe and STRADIVARIUS. Eur Heart J, 2008; 29: 1709-10.

[26] Florentin M, Liberopoulos EN, Elisaf MS. Sibutramine-associated adverse effects: a practical guide for its safe use. Obes Rev, 2008; 9: 378-87.

[27] Christensen R, Kristensen PK, Bartels EM, Bliddal H, Astrup A. Efficacy and safety of the weight-loss drug rimonabant: a meta-analysis of randomised trials. Lancet, 2007; 370: 1706-13.

[28] Moreira FA, Grieb M, Lutz B. Central side-effects of therapies based on CB1 cannabinoid receptor agonists and antagonists: focus on anxiety and depression. Best Pract Res Clin Endocrinol Metab, 2009; 23: 133-44.

[29] Berridge KC, Ho CY, Richard JM, DiFeliceantonio AG. The tempted brain eats: pleasure and desire circuits in obesity and eating disorders. Brain Res, 2010; 1350: 43-64.

[30] Rodgers RJ, Tschop MH, Wilding JP. Anti-obesity drugs: past, present and future. Dis Model Mech, 2012; 5: 621-6.

[31]   Derosa G, Maffioli P. Anti-obesity drugs: a review about their effects and their safety. Expert Opin Drug Saf, 2012; 11: 459-71.

[32]   Cameron F, Whiteside G, McKeage K. Phentermine and topiramate extended release (qsymia): first global approval. Drugs, 2012; 72: 2033-42.

[33]   Loos RJ, Bouchard C. Obesity--is it a genetic disorder? J Intern Med, 2003; 254: 401-25.

[34]   Stunkard AJ, Foch TT, Hrubec Z. A twin study of human obesity. JAMA, 1986; 256: 51-4.

[35]   Bouchard C, Perusse L, Leblanc C, Tremblay A, Theriault G. Inheritance of the amount and distribution of human body fat. Int J Obes, 1988; 12: 205-15.

[36]   Frayling TM, Timpson NJ, Weedon MN, Zeggini E, Freathy RM, Lindgren CM, *et al.,* A common variant in the FTO gene is associated with body mass index and predisposes to childhood and adult obesity. Science, 2007; 316: 889-94.

[37]   Bray GA, Popkin BM. Dietary fat intake does affect obesity! Am J Clin Nutr, 1998; 68: 1157-73.

[38]   Ahima RS, Antwi DA. Brain regulation of appetite and satiety. Endocrinol Metab Clin North Am, 2008; 37: 811-23.

[39]   Harrold JA, Dovey TM, Blundell JE, Halford JC. CNS regulation of appetite. Neuropharmacology, 2012; 63: 3-17.

[40]   Suzuki K, Jayasena CN, Bloom SR. The gut hormones in appetite regulation. J Obes, 2011; 2011: 528401.

[41]   Lopez M, Tovar S, Vazquez MJ, Williams LM, Dieguez C. Peripheral tissue-brain interactions in the regulation of food intake. Proc Nutr Soc, 2007; 66: 131-55.

[42]   Muzik O, Mangner TJ, Granneman JG. Assessment of oxidative metabolism in brown fat using PET imaging. Front Endocrinol (Lausanne), 2012; 3: 15.

[43]   Fisher FM, Kleiner S, Douris N, Fox EC, Mepani RJ, Verdeguer F, *et al.,* FGF21 regulates PGC-1alpha and browning of white adipose tissues in adaptive thermogenesis. Genes Dev, 2012; 26: 271-81.

[44]   Beranger GE, Karbiener M, Barquissau V, Pisani DF, Scheideler M, Langin D, *et al., In vitro* brown and "brite"/"beige" adipogenesis: Human cellular models and molecular aspects. Biochim Biophys Acta, 2012.

[45]   Bays HE, Gonzalez-Campoy JM, Henry RR, Bergman DA, Kitabchi AE, Schorr AB, *et al.,* Is adiposopathy (sick fat) an endocrine disease? Int J Clin Pract, 2008; 62: 1474-83.

[46]   Chang SH, Beason, T.S., Hunleth, J.M., Colditz, G.A. A systematic review of body fat distribution and mortality in older people.. Maturitas., 2012; 72: 175-91.

[47]   Nedungadi TP, Clegg DJ. Sexual dimorphism in body fat distribution and risk for cardiovascular diseases. J Cardiovasc Transl Res, 2009; 2: 321-7.

[48]   Bays H. Adiposopathy: role of adipocyte factors in a new paradigm. Expert Rev Cardiovasc Ther, 2005; 3: 187-9.

[49]   Bays H, Dujovne, C.A. Adiposopathy is a more rational treatment target for metabolic disease than obesity alone. Curr Atheroscler Rep, 2006; 8: 144-56.

[50]   Howel D. Waist Circumference and Abdominal Obesity among Older Adults: Patterns, Prevalence and Trends. PLoS One, 2012; 7: e48528.

[51]   Prasad H, Ryan DA, Celzo MF, Stapleton D. Metabolic syndrome: definition and therapeutic implications. Postgrad Med, 2012; 124: 21-30.

[52]   Shah NR, Braverman ER. Measuring adiposity in patients: the utility of body mass index (BMI), percent body fat, and leptin. PLoS One, 2012; 7: e33308.

[53]   Goonasegaran AR, Nabila FN, Shuhada NS. Comparison of the effectiveness of body mass index and body fat percentage in defining body composition. Singapore Med J, 2012; 53: 403-8.

[54]   Coelho M, Oliveira T, Fernandes R. Biochemistry of adipose tissue: an endocrine organ. Arch Med Sci, 2013; 9: 191-200.

[55]   Ashwell M, Gunn P, Gibson S. Waist-to-height ratio is a better screening tool than waist circumference and BMI for adult cardiometabolic risk factors: systematic review and meta-analysis. Obes Rev, 2012; 13: 275-86.

[56]   Fung TT, Rexrode KM, Mantzoros CS, Manson JE, Willett WC, Hu FB. Mediterranean diet and incidence of and mortality from coronary heart disease and stroke in women. Circulation, 2009; 119: 1093-100.

[57]   Mitrou PN, Kipnis V, Thiebaut AC, Reedy J, Subar AF, Wirfalt E, *et al.,* Mediterranean dietary pattern and prediction of all-cause mortality in a US population: results from the NIH-AARP Diet and Health Study. Arch Intern Med, 2007; 167: 2461-8.

[58]   Iacobellis G, Ribaudo MC, Assael F, Vecci E, Tiberti C, Zappaterreno A, *et al.,* Echocardiographic epicardial adipose tissue is related to anthropometric and clinical parameters of metabolic syndrome: a new indicator of cardiovascular risk. J Clin Endocrinol Metab, 2003; 88: 5163-8.

[59]   Fluchter S, Haghi D, Dinter D, Heberlein W, Kuhl HP, Neff W, *et al.,* Volumetric assessment of epicardial adipose tissue with cardiovascular magnetic resonance imaging. Obesity (Silver Spring), 2007; 15: 870-8.

[60]   Willens HJ, Byers P, Chirinos JA, Labrador E, Hare JM, de Marchena E. Effects of weight loss after bariatric surgery on epicardial fat measured using echocardiography. Am J Cardiol, 2007; 99: 1242-5.

[61]   Jeong JW, Jeong MH, Yun KH, Oh SK, Park EM, Kim YK, *et al.,* Echocardiographic epicardial fat thickness and coronary artery disease. Circ J, 2007; 71: 536-9.

[62]   Rosito GA, Massaro JM, Hoffmann U, Ruberg FL, Mahabadi AA, Vasan RS, *et al.,* Pericardial fat, visceral abdominal fat, cardiovascular disease risk factors, and vascular calcification in a community-based sample: the Framingham Heart Study. Circulation, 2008; 117: 605-13.

[63]   Pettinelli P, Obregon AM, Videla LA. Molecular mechanisms of steatosis in nonalcoholic fatty liver disease. Nutr Hosp, 2011; 26: 441-50.

[64]   Araya J, Rodrigo R, Videla LA, Thielemann L, Orellana M, Pettinelli P, *et al.,* Increase in long-chain polyunsaturated fatty acid n - 6/n - 3 ratio in relation to hepatic steatosis in patients with non-alcoholic fatty liver disease. Clin Sci (Lond), 2004; 106: 635-43.

[65]   Delarue J, LeFoll C, Corporeau C, Lucas D. N-3 long chain polyunsaturated fatty acids: a nutritional tool to prevent insulin resistance associated to type 2 diabetes and obesity? Reprod Nutr Dev, 2004; 44: 289-99.

[66]   Robertson G, Leclercq I, Farrell GC. Nonalcoholic steatosis and steatohepatitis. II. Cytochrome P-450 enzymes and oxidative stress. Am J Physiol Gastrointest Liver Physiol, 2001; 281: G1135-9.

[67]   Licata A, Nebbia ME, Cabibbo G, Iacono GL, Barbaria F, Brucato V, *et al.,* Hyperferritinemia is a risk factor for steatosis in chronic liver disease. World J Gastroenterol, 2009; 15: 2132-8.

[68]   Beaton MD, Adams PC. Treatment of hyperferritinemia. Ann Hepatol, 2012; 11: 294-300.

[69]   Gautier A, Roussel R, Lange C, Piguel X, Cauchi S, Vol S, *et al.,* Effects of genetic susceptibility for type 2 diabetes on the evolution of glucose homeostasis traits before and after diabetes diagnosis: data from the D.E.S.I.R. Study. Diabetes, 2011; 60: 2654-63.

[70]   Kylin E. Studies of the hypertension-hyperglycemia-hyperuricemia syndrome. Zentralbl Inn Med 1923; 44: 105-127.

[71]   Sabán Ruiz J. Insulinresistencia e inflexibilidad metabólica. In: Sabán Ruiz J, Ed.Control Global del Riesgo Cardiometabólico. La disfunción endotelial como diana preferencial. 1st ed. Madrid. Editorial Díaz de Santos 2009; pp. 145-178.

[72]   Joseph T, Doyle, J.T., Dawber, T.R., Kannel, W.B., Heslin, M.S., Kahn, H.A.. Cigarette Smoking and Coronary Heart Disease — Combined Experience of the Albany and Framingham Studies. N Engl J Med 1962; 266: 796-801.

[73]   Himsworth HP. The syndrome of diabetes mellitus and its causes. Lancet, 1949; 1: 465-73.

[74]   Vague J. La differenciation sexuelle, facteur determinant des formes de l'obesity. Presse Med, 1947; 55: 339.

[75]   Vague J. The degree of masculine differentiation of obesities: a factor determining predisposition to diabetes, atherosclerosis, gout, and uric calculous disease. 1956. Nutrition, 1999; 15: 89-90; discussion 91.

[76]   Avogadro A, Crepaldi, G., Enzi, G., Tiengo, A.. Associazione di iperlipidemia, diabete mellito e obesità di medio grado.. Acta Diabetol Lat 1967; 4: 572-90.

[77]   DeFronzo RA, Tobin JD, Andres R. Glucose clamp technique: a method for quantifying insulin secretion and resistance. Am J Physiol, 1979; 237: E214-23.

[78]   Reaven GM, Chen YD. Role of insulin in regulation of lipoprotein metabolism in diabetes. Diabetes Metab Rev, 1988; 4: 639-52.

[79]   Kaplan NM. The deadly quartet. Upper-body obesity, glucose intolerance, hypertriglyceridemia, and hypertension. Arch Intern Med, 1989; 149: 1514-20.

[80]   Hanefeld M, Leonhardt, W. Das metabolische syndrom. Dt Gesundh Wesen 1981; 36: 545-51.

[81]   DeFronzo RA. Insulin resistance: a multifaceted syndrome responsible for NIDDM, obesity, hypertension, dyslipidaemia and atherosclerosis. Neth J Med, 1997; 50: 191-7.

[82]   Del Prato S, Matsuda M, Simonson DC, Groop LC, Sheehan P, Leonetti F, *et al.,* Studies on the mass action effect of glucose in NIDDM and IDDM: evidence for glucose resistance. Diabetologia, 1997; 40: 687-97.

[83]   Yuan M, Konstantopoulos N, Lee J, Hansen L, Li ZW, Karin M, *et al.,* Reversal of obesity- and diet-induced insulin resistance with salicylates or targeted disruption of Ikkbeta. Science, 2001; 293: 1673-7.

[84]   Lonardo A, Lombardini S, Ricchi M, Scaglioni F, Loria P. Review article: hepatic steatosis and insulin resistance. Aliment Pharmacol Ther, 2005; 22 Suppl 2: 64-70.

[85]   McLaughlin T, Abbasi F, Cheal K, Chu J, Lamendola C, Reaven G. Use of metabolic markers to identify overweight individuals who are insulin resistant. Ann Intern Med, 2003; 139: 802-9.

[86]   Ferrannini E, Natali A, Capaldo B, Lehtovirta M, Jacob S, Yki-Jarvinen H. Insulin resistance, hyperinsulinemia, and blood pressure: role of age and obesity. European Group for the Study of Insulin Resistance (EGIR). Hypertension, 1997; 30: 1144-9.

[87]   Abouchacra S, Baines AD, Zinman B, Skorecki KL, Logan AG. Insulin blunts the natriuretic action of atrial natriuretic peptide in hypertension. Hypertension, 1994; 23: 1054-8.

[88]   Han TS, Williams K, Sattar N, Hunt KJ, Lean ME, Haffner SM. Analysis of obesity and hyperinsulinemia in the development of metabolic syndrome: San Antonio Heart Study. Obes Res, 2002; 10: 923-31.

[89]   Erzen B, Sabovic M. In young post-myocardial infarction male patients elevated plasminogen activator inhibitor-1 correlates with insulin resistance and endothelial dysfunction. Heart Vessels, 2012.

[90]   Meigs JB, D'Agostino RB, Sr., Wilson PW, Cupples LA, Nathan DM, Singer DE. Risk variable clustering in the insulin resistance syndrome. The Framingham Offspring Study. Diabetes, 1997; 46: 1594-600.

[91]   Purkayastha S, Zhang G, Cai D. Uncoupling the mechanisms of obesity and hypertension by targeting hypothalamic IKK-beta and NF-kappaB. Nat Med, 2011; 17: 883-7.

[92]   Reaven G. All obese individuals are not created equal: insulin resistance is the major determinant of cardiovascular disease in overweight/obese individuals. Diab Vasc Dis Res, 2005; 2: 105-12.

[93]   de las Fuentes L, de Simone G, Arnett DK, Davila-Roman VG. Molecular determinants of the cardiometabolic phenotype. Endocr Metab Immune Disord Drug Targets, 2010; 10: 109-23.

[94]   Henneman P, Aulchenko YS, Frants RR, van Dijk KW, Oostra BA, van Duijn CM. Prevalence and heritability of the metabolic syndrome and its individual components in a Dutch isolate: the Erasmus Rucphen Family study. J Med Genet, 2008; 45: 572-7.

[95]   Bellia A, Giardina E, Lauro D, Tesauro M, Di Fede G, Cusumano G, *et al.,* "The Linosa Study": epidemiological and heritability data of the metabolic syndrome in a Caucasian genetic isolate. Nutr Metab Cardiovasc Dis, 2009; 19: 455-61.

[96]   Zhang S, Liu X, Yu Y, Hong X, Christoffel KK, Wang B, *et al.,* Genetic and environmental contributions to phenotypic components of metabolic syndrome: a population-based twin study. Obesity (Silver Spring), 2009; 17: 1581-7.

[97]   Unger RH, Orci L. Lipoapoptosis: its mechanism and its diseases. Biochim Biophys Acta, 2002; 1585: 202-12.

[98]   LeRoith D. Beta-cell dysfunction and insulin resistance in type 2 diabetes: role of metabolic and genetic abnormalities. Am J Med, 2002; 113 Suppl 6A: 3S-11S.

[99]   Klein S. The case of visceral fat: argument for the defense. J Clin Invest, 2004; 113: 1530-2.

[100]   Jensen MD. Is visceral fat involved in the pathogenesis of the metabolic syndrome? Human model. Obesity (Silver Spring), 2006; 14 Suppl 1: 20S-24S.

[101]   Johnson JA, Fried SK, Pi-Sunyer FX, Albu JB. Impaired insulin action in subcutaneous adipocytes from women with visceral obesity. Am J Physiol Endocrinol Metab, 2001; 280: E40-9.

[102]   Bays HE, Fox KM, Grandy S. Anthropometric measurements and diabetes mellitus: clues to the "pathogenic" and "protective" potential of adipose tissue. Metab Syndr Relat Disord, 2010; 8: 307-15.

[103]   Storlien L, Oakes ND, Kelley DE. Metabolic flexibility. Proc Nutr Soc, 2004; 63: 363-8.

[104]   Bays HE. "Sick fat," metabolic disease, and atherosclerosis. Am J Med, 2009; 122: S26-37.

[105]   Chavez JA, Holland WL, Bar J, Sandhoff K, Summers SA. Acid ceramidase overexpression prevents the inhibitory effects of saturated fatty acids on insulin signaling. J Biol Chem, 2005; 280: 20148-53.

[106] Bergman M. Pathophysiology of prediabetes and treatment implications for the prevention of type 2 diabetes mellitus. Endocrine, 2012.

[107] Lee Y, Hirose H, Ohneda M, Johnson JH, McGarry JD, Unger RH. Beta-cell lipotoxicity in the pathogenesis of non-insulin-dependent diabetes mellitus of obese rats: impairment in adipocyte-beta-cell relationships. Proc Natl Acad Sci U S A, 1994; 91: 10878-82.

[108] Tanaka H, Dinenno FA, Monahan KD, Clevenger CM, DeSouza CA, Seals DR. Aging, habitual exercise, and dynamic arterial compliance. Circulation, 2000; 102: 1270-5.

[109] Xia WH, Li J, Su C, Yang Z, Chen L, Wu F, *et al.*, Physical exercise attenuates age-associated reduction in endothelium-reparative capacity of endothelial progenitor cells by increasing CXCR4/JAK-2 signaling in healthy men. Aging Cell, 2012; 11: 111-9.

[110] Payne GA, Kohr MC, Tune JD. Epicardial perivascular adipose tissue as a therapeutic target in obesity-related coronary artery disease. Br J Pharmacol, 2012; 165: 659-69.

[111] Martinez de Morentin PB, Varela L, Ferno J, Nogueiras R, Dieguez C, Lopez M. Hypothalamic lipotoxicity and the metabolic syndrome. Biochim Biophys Acta, 2010; 1801: 350-61.

[112] Son NH, Yu S, Tuinei J, Arai K, Hamai H, Homma S, *et al.*, PPARgamma-induced cardiolipotoxicity in mice is ameliorated by PPARalpha deficiency despite increases in fatty acid oxidation. J Clin Invest, 2010; 120: 3443-54.

[113] Payne GA, Borbouse L, Kumar S, Neeb Z, Alloosh M, Sturek M, *et al.*, Epicardial perivascular adipose-derived leptin exacerbates coronary endothelial dysfunction in metabolic syndrome *via* a protein kinase C-beta pathway. Arterioscler Thromb Vasc Biol, 2010; 30: 1711-7.

[114] Choi SY, Kim D, Oh BH, Kim M, Park HE, Lee CH, *et al.*, General and abdominal obesity and abdominal visceral fat accumulation associated with coronary artery calcification in Korean men. Atherosclerosis, 2010; 213: 273-8.

[115] Corr PB, Yamada KA. Selected metabolic alterations in the ischemic heart and their contributions to arrhythmogenesis. Herz, 1995; 20: 156-68.

[116] Bluher M. Clinical relevance of adipokines. Diabetes Metab J, 2012; 36: 317-27.

[117] Kershaw EE, Flier JS. Adipose tissue as an endocrine organ. J Clin Endocrinol Metab, 2004; 89: 2548-56.

[118] Greenwood JP, Malik I, Jennings P, Stevenson RN. Haemodynamic and electrocardiographic consequences of severe nicorandil toxicity. Emerg Med J, 2003; 20: 98-100.

[119] Boyce SH, Stevenson J, Jamieson IS, Campbell S. Impact of a newly opened prison on an accident and emergency department. Emerg Med J, 2003; 20: 48-51.

[120] Trayhurn P, Wood IS. Adipokines: inflammation and the pleiotropic role of white adipose tissue. Br J Nutr, 2004; 92: 347-55.

[121] Bastard JP, Maachi M, Lagathu C, Kim MJ, Caron M, Vidal H, *et al.*, Recent advances in the relationship between obesity, inflammation, and insulin resistance. Eur Cytokine Netw, 2006; 17: 4-12.

[122] Bays H, Rodbard HW, Schorr AB, Gonzalez-Campoy JM. Adiposopathy: treating pathogenic adipose tissue to reduce cardiovascular disease risk. Curr Treat Options Cardiovasc Med, 2007; 9: 259-71.

[123] Primeau V, Coderre L, Karelis AD, Brochu M, Lavoie ME, Messier V, *et al.*, Characterizing the profile of obese patients who are metabolically healthy. Int J Obes (Lond), 2011; 35: 971-81.

[124] Ortega FB, Lee DC, Katzmarzyk PT, Ruiz JR, Sui X, Church TS, *et al.*, The intriguing metabolically healthy but obese phenotype: cardiovascular prognosis and role of fitness. Eur Heart J, 2012.

[125] Arita Y, Kihara S, Ouchi N, Takahashi M, Maeda K, Miyagawa J, *et al.*, Paradoxical decrease of an adipose-specific protein, adiponectin, in obesity. Biochem Biophys Res Commun, 1999; 257: 79-83.

[126] Corgosinho FC, de Piano A, Sanches PL, Campos RM, Silva PL, Carnier J, *et al.*, The role of PAI-1 and adiponectin on the inflammatory state and energy balance in obese adolescents with metabolic syndrome. Inflammation, 2012; 35: 944-51.

[127] Ouchi N, Kihara S, Arita Y, Okamoto Y, Maeda K, Kuriyama H, *et al.*, Adiponectin, an adipocyte-derived plasma protein, inhibits endothelial NF-kappaB signaling through a cAMP-dependent pathway. Circulation, 2000; 102: 1296-301.

[128] Iwashima Y, Katsuya T, Ishikawa K, Ouchi N, Ohishi M, Sugimoto K, *et al.*, Hypoadiponectinemia is an independent risk factor for hypertension. Hypertension, 2004; 43: 1318-23.

[129] Stevenson WG, Epstein LM. Predicting sudden death risk for heart failure patients in the implantable cardioverter-defibrillator age. Circulation, 2003; 107: 514-6.

[130] Coleman HM, de Lima B, Morton V, Stevenson PG. Murine gammaherpesvirus 68 lacking thymidine kinase shows severe attenuation of lytic cycle replication *in vivo* but still establishes latency. J Virol, 2003; 77: 2410-7.

[131] Belz GT, Liu H, Andreansky S, Doherty PC, Stevenson PG. Absence of a functional defect in CD8+ T cells during primary murine gammaherpesvirus-68 infection of I-A(b-/-) mice. J Gen Virol, 2003; 84: 337-41.

[132] Stevenson M. Tat's seductive side. Nat Med, 2003; 9: 163-4.

[133] Stevenson MR, Rimajova M, Edgecombe D, Vickery K. Childhood drowning: barriers surrounding private swimming pools. Pediatrics, 2003; 111: E115-9.

[134] Stevenson K, Ion V, Merry M, Sinfield P. Primary care. More than words. Health Serv J, 2003; 113: 26-8.

[135] Verma S, Li SH, Wang CH, Fedak PW, Li RK, Weisel RD, *et al.*, Resistin promotes endothelial cell activation: further evidence of adipokine-endothelial interaction. Circulation, 2003; 108: 736-40.

[136] Stevenson RJ, Case TI. Preexposure to the stimulus elements, but not training to detect them, retards human odour-taste learning. Behav Processes, 2003; 61: 13-25.

[137] Anand D, Stevenson CJ, West CR, Pharoah PO. Lung function and respiratory health in adolescents of very low birth weight. Arch Dis Child, 2003; 88: 135-8.

[138] Stevenson CW, Sullivan RM, Gratton A. Effects of basolateral amygdala dopamine depletion on the nucleus accumbens and medial prefrontal cortical dopamine responses to stress. Neuroscience, 2003; 116: 285-93.

[139] Inadera H. The usefulness of circulating adipokine levels for the assessment of obesity-related health problems. Int J Med Sci, 2008; 5: 248-62.

[140] Kim SO, Yun SJ, Jung B, Lee EH, Hahm DH, Shim I, *et al.*, Hypolipidemic effects of crude extract of adlay seed (Coix lachrymajobi var. mayuen) in obesity rat fed high fat diet: relations of TNF-alpha and leptin mRNA expressions and serum lipid levels. Life Sci, 2004; 75: 1391-404.

[141] Camerino C. Low sympathetic tone and obese phenotype in oxytocin-deficient mice. Obesity (Silver Spring), 2009; 17: 980-4.

[142] Rahmouni K, Haynes WG. Endothelial effects of leptin: implications in health and diseases. Curr Diab Rep, 2005; 5: 260-6.

[143] Younus S, Rodgers G. Biomarkers associated with cardiometabolic risk in obesity. Am Heart Hosp J, 2011; 9: E28-32.

[144] Pescatello LS, VanHeest JL. Physical activity mediates a healthier body weight in the presence of obesity. Br J Sports Med, 2000; 34: 86-93.

[145] Egger G, Dixon J. Obesity and chronic disease: always offender or often just accomplice? Br J Nutr, 2009; 102: 1238-42.

[146] Rutkowski JM, Davis KE, Scherer PE. Mechanisms of obesity and related pathologies: the macro- and microcirculation of adipose tissue. FEBS J, 2009; 276: 5738-46.

[147] Weisberg SP, McCann D, Desai M, Rosenbaum M, Leibel RL, Ferrante AW, Jr. Obesity is associated with macrophage accumulation in adipose tissue. J Clin Invest, 2003; 112: 1796-808.

[148] Xu H, Barnes GT, Yang Q, Tan G, Yang D, Chou CJ, *et al.,* Chronic inflammation in fat plays a crucial role in the development of obesity-related insulin resistance. J Clin Invest, 2003; 112: 1821-30.

[149] Harwood HJ, Jr. The adipocyte as an endocrine organ in the regulation of metabolic homeostasis. Neuropharmacology, 2012; 63: 57-75.

[150] Johnson AR, Milner JJ, Makowski L. The inflammation highway: metabolism accelerates inflammatory traffic in obesity. Immunol Rev, 2012; 249: 218-38.

[151] Berges-Gimeno MP, Simon RA, Stevenson DD. Long-term treatment with aspirin desensitization in asthmatic patients with aspirin-exacerbated respiratory disease. J Allergy Clin Immunol, 2003; 111: 180-6.

[152] Stevenson A, Macdonald J, Roberts M. Cloning and characterisation of type 4 fimbrial genes from Actinobacillus pleuropneumoniae. Vet Microbiol, 2003; 92: 121-34.

[153] Gormley GJ, Corrigan M, Steele WK, Stevenson M, Taggart AJ. Joint and soft tissue injections in the community: questionnaire survey of general practitioners' experiences and attitudes. Ann Rheum Dis, 2003; 62: 61-4.

[154] Deboer MD. Obesity, systemic inflammation, and increased risk for cardiovascular disease and diabetes among adolescents: A need for screening tools to target interventions. Nutrition, 2012.

[155] Dandona P, Aljada A, Bandyopadhyay A. Inflammation: the link between insulin resistance, obesity and diabetes. Trends Immunol, 2004; 25: 4-7.

[156] Hube F, Hauner H. The role of TNF-alpha in human adipose tissue: prevention of weight gain at the expense of insulin resistance? Horm Metab Res, 1999; 31: 626-31.

[157] Eckel RH. Insulin resistance: an adaptation for weight maintenance. Lancet, 1992; 340: 1452-3.

[158] Hotamisligil GS. Mechanisms of TNF-alpha-induced insulin resistance. Exp Clin Endocrinol Diabetes, 1999; 107: 119-25.

[159] Yudkin JS. Inflammation, obesity, and the metabolic syndrome. Horm Metab Res, 2007; 39: 707-9.

[160] Fried SK, Bunkin DA, Greenberg AS. Omental and subcutaneous adipose tissues of obese subjects release interleukin-6: depot difference and regulation by glucocorticoid. J Clin Endocrinol Metab, 1998; 83: 847-50.

[161] Bastard JP, Maachi M, Van Nhieu JT, Jardel C, Bruckert E, Grimaldi A, *et al.,* Adipose tissue IL-6 content correlates with resistance to insulin activation of glucose uptake both *in vivo* and *in vitro*. J Clin Endocrinol Metab, 2002; 87: 2084-9.

[162]   Bastard JP, Jardel C, Bruckert E, Blondy P, Capeau J, Laville M, *et al.,* Elevated levels of interleukin 6 are reduced in serum and subcutaneous adipose tissue of obese women after weight loss. J Clin Endocrinol Metab, 2000; 85: 3338-42.

[163]   Kroder G, Bossenmaier B, Kellerer M, Capp E, Stoyanov B, Muhlhofer A, *et al.,* Tumor necrosis factor-alpha- and hyperglycemia-induced insulin resistance. Evidence for different mechanisms and different effects on insulin signaling. J Clin Invest, 1996; 97: 1471-7.

[164]   Jung DY, Ko HJ, Lichtman EI, Lee E, Lawton E, Ong H, *et al.,* Short-Term Weight Loss Attenuates Local Tissue Inflammation and Improves Insulin Sensitivity without Affecting Adipose Inflammation in Obese Mice. Am J Physiol Endocrinol Metab, 2013.

[165]   Shah R, Lu Y, Hinkle CC, McGillicuddy FC, Kim R, Hannenhalli S, *et al.,* Gene profiling of human adipose tissue during evoked inflammation *in vivo*. Diabetes, 2009; 58: 2211-9.

[166]   Bouloumie A, Curat CA, Sengenes C, Lolmede K, Miranville A, Busse R. Role of macrophage tissue infiltration in metabolic diseases. Curr Opin Clin Nutr Metab Care, 2005; 8: 347-54.

[167]   Frayn KN, Summers LK, Fielding BA. Regulation of the plasma non-esterified fatty acid concentration in the postprandial state. Proc Nutr Soc, 1997; 56: 713-21.

[168]   Bays H, Mandarino L, DeFronzo RA. Role of the adipocyte, free fatty acids, and ectopic fat in pathogenesis of type 2 diabetes mellitus: peroxisomal proliferator-activated receptor agonists provide a rational therapeutic approach. J Clin Endocrinol Metab, 2004; 89: 463-78.

[169]   Kelley DE, Goodpaster BH. Skeletal muscle triglyceride. An aspect of regional adiposity and insulin resistance. Diabetes Care, 2001; 24: 933-41.

[170]   Grill V, Persson G, Carlsson S, Norman A, Alvarsson M, Ostensson CG, *et al.,* Family history of diabetes in middle-aged Swedish men is a gender unrelated factor which associates with insulinopenia in newly diagnosed diabetic subjects. Diabetologia, 1999; 42: 15-23.

[171]   Bays HE. Current and investigational antiobesity agents and obesity therapeutic treatment targets. Obes Res, 2004; 12: 1197-211.

[172]   Kelly AS, Wetzsteon RJ, Kaiser DR, Steinberger J, Bank AJ, Dengel DR. Inflammation, insulin, and endothelial function in overweight children and adolescents: the role of exercise. J Pediatr, 2004; 145: 731-6.

[173]   Berk ES, Kovera AJ, Boozer CN, Pi-Sunyer FX, Albu JB. Metabolic inflexibility in substrate use is present in African-American but not Caucasian healthy, premenopausal, nondiabetic women. J Clin Endocrinol Metab, 2006; 91: 4099-106.

[174]   Astrup A. The relevance of increased fat oxidation for body-weight management: metabolic inflexibility in the predisposition to weight gain. Obes Rev, 2011; 12: 859-65.

[175]   Adolph TE, Niederreiter L, Blumberg RS, Kaser A. Endoplasmic reticulum stress and inflammation. Dig Dis, 2012; 30: 341-6.

[176]   Varma V, Yao-Borengasser A, Rasouli N, Nolen GT, Phanavanh B, Starks T, *et al.,* Muscle inflammatory response and insulin resistance: synergistic interaction between macrophages and fatty acids leads to impaired insulin action. Am J Physiol Endocrinol Metab, 2009; 296: E1300-10.

[177]   Hummasti S, Hotamisligil GS. Endoplasmic reticulum stress and inflammation in obesity and diabetes. Circ Res, 2010; 107: 579-91.

[178]   Oyadomari S, Araki E, Mori M. Endoplasmic reticulum stress-mediated apoptosis in pancreatic beta-cells. Apoptosis, 2002; 7: 335-45.

[179] Kawamori D, Kaneto H, Nakatani Y, Matsuoka TA, Matsuhisa M, Hori M, *et al.,* The forkhead transcription factor Foxo1 bridges the JNK pathway and the transcription factor PDX-1 through its intracellular translocation. J Biol Chem, 2006; 281: 1091-8.

[180] Lenzen S. Oxidative stress: the vulnerable beta-cell. Biochem Soc Trans, 2008; 36: 343-7.

[181] Feng XT, Leng J, Xie Z, Li SL, Zhao W, Tang QL. GPR40: A therapeutic target for mediating insulin secretion (Review). Int J Mol Med, 2012; 30: 1261-6.

[182] Hansen HS, Rosenkilde MM, Holst JJ, Schwartz TW. GPR119 as a fat sensor. Trends Pharmacol Sci, 2012; 33: 374-81.

[183] Garaulet M, Corbalan-Tutau MD, Madrid JA, Baraza JC, Parnell LD, Lee YC, *et al.,* PERIOD2 variants are associated with abdominal obesity, psycho-behavioral factors, and attrition in the dietary treatment of obesity. J Am Diet Assoc, 2010; 110: 917-21.

[184] Kim KS, Moon HJ, Choi CH, Baek EK, Lee SY, Cha BK, *et al.,* The Frequency and Risk Factors of Colorectal Adenoma in Health-Check-up Subjects in South Korea: Relationship to Abdominal Obesity and Age. Gut Liver, 2010; 4: 36-42.

[185] Gristina AG, Shibata Y, Giridhar G, Kreger A, Myrvik QN. The glycocalyx, biofilm, microbes, and resistant infection. Semin Arthroplasty, 1994; 5: 160-70.

[186] Girinsky TA, Pallardy M, Comoy E, Benassi T, Roger R, Ganem G, *et al.,* Peripheral blood corticotropin-releasing factor, adrenocorticotropic hormone and cytokine (interleukin beta, interleukin 6, tumor necrosis factor alpha) levels after high- and low-dose total-body irradiation in humans. Radiat Res, 1994; 139: 360-3.

[187] Shan T, Liu W, Kuang S. Fatty acid binding protein 4 expression marks a population of adipocyte progenitors in white and brown adipose tissues. FASEB J, 2013; 27: 277-87.

[188] Mwimanzi P, Markle TJ, Ogata Y, Martin E, Tokunaga M, Mahiti M, *et al.,* Dynamic range of Nef functions in chronic HIV-1 infection. Virology, 2013; 439: 74-80.

[189] Liao Y, Huang X, Wu Q, Yang C, Kuang W, Du M, *et al.,* Is depression a disconnection syndrome? Meta-analysis of diffusion tensor imaging studies in patients with MDD. J Psychiatry Neurosci, 2013; 38: 49-56.

[190] Perlis N, Turker P, Bostrom PJ, Kuk C, Mirtti T, Kulkarni G, *et al.,* Upper urinary tract and urethral recurrences following radical cystectomy: review of risk factors and outcomes between centres with different follow-up protocols. World J Urol, 2013; 31: 161-7.

[191] Zhang LL, Wang HE, Li J, Kuang YW, Wen DZ. Physiological responses and accumulation of pollutants in woody species under *in situ* polluted condition in Southern China. J Plant Res, 2013; 126: 95-103.

[192] Wallin L, Bostrom AM, Gustavsson JP. Capability beliefs regarding evidence-based practice are associated with application of EBP and research use: validation of a new measure. Worldviews Evid Based Nurs, 2012; 9: 139-48.

[193] van Rhijn BW, Liu L, Vis AN, Bostrom PJ, Zuiverloon TC, Fleshner NE, *et al.,* Prognostic value of molecular markers, sub-stage and European Organisation for the Research and Treatment of Cancer risk scores in primary T1 bladder cancer. BJU Int, 2012; 110: 1169-76.

[194] Takata Y, Hamada D, Miyatake K, Nakano S, Shinomiya F, Scafe CR, *et al.,* Genetic association between the PRKCH gene encoding protein kinase Ceta isozyme and rheumatoid arthritis in the Japanese population. Arthritis Rheum, 2007; 56: 30-42.

[195] Ishikawa N, Takano A, Yasui W, Inai K, Nishimura H, Ito H, *et al.,* Cancer-testis antigen lymphocyte antigen 6 complex locus K is a serologic biomarker and a therapeutic target for lung and esophageal carcinomas. Cancer Res, 2007; 67: 11601-11.

[196]　Burnham RS, Yasui Y. An alternate method of radiofrequency neurotomy of the sacroiliac joint: a pilot study of the effect on pain, function, and satisfaction. Reg Anesth Pain Med, 2007; 32: 12-9.

[197]　Ikeda M, Sekimoto M, Takiguchi S, Yasui M, Danno K, Fujie Y, *et al.,* Total splenic vein thrombosis after laparoscopic splenectomy: a possible candidate for treatment. Am J Surg, 2007; 193: 21-5.

[198]　Akiyama H, Gotoh A, Shin RW, Koga T, Ohashi T, Sakamoto W, *et al.,* A novel role for hGas7b in microtubular maintenance: possible implication in tau-associated pathology in Alzheimer disease. J Biol Chem, 2009; 284: 32695-9.

[199]　Mercer JF, Barnes N, Stevenson J, Strausak D, Llanos RM. Copper-induced trafficking of the cU-ATPases: a key mechanism for copper homeostasis. Biometals, 2003; 16: 175-84.

[200]　Hata T, Ikeda M, Ikenaga M, Yasui M, Shingai T, Yamamoto H, *et al.,* Castleman's disease of the rectum: report of a case. Dis Colon Rectum, 2007; 50: 389-94.

[201]　Baron AD, Zhu JS, Marshall S, Irsula O, Brechtel G, Keech C. Insulin resistance after hypertension induced by the nitric oxide synthesis inhibitor L-NMMA in rats. Am J Physiol, 1995; 269: E709-15.

[202]　Shankar RR, Wu Y, Shen HQ, Zhu JS, Baron AD. Mice with gene disruption of both endothelial and neuronal nitric oxide synthase exhibit insulin resistance. Diabetes, 2000; 49: 684-7.

[203]　Lin Y, Luo E, Chen X, Liu L, Qiao J, Yan Z, *et al.,* Molecular and cellular characterization during chondrogenic differentiation of adipose tissue-derived stromal cells *in vitro* and cartilage formation *in vivo.* J Cell Mol Med, 2005; 9: 929-39.

[204]　Ridker PM, Cushman M, Stampfer MJ, Tracy RP, Hennekens CH. Inflammation, aspirin, and the risk of cardiovascular disease in apparently healthy men. N Engl J Med, 1997; 336: 973-9.

[205]　Ridker PM, Hennekens CH, Buring JE, Rifai N. C-reactive protein and other markers of inflammation in the prediction of cardiovascular disease in women. N Engl J Med, 2000; 342: 836-43.

[206]　Santos AC, Lopes C, Guimaraes JT, Barros H. Central obesity as a major determinant of increased high-sensitivity C-reactive protein in metabolic syndrome. Int J Obes (Lond), 2005; 29: 1452-6.

[207]　Festa A, D'Agostino R, Jr., Howard G, Mykkanen L, Tracy RP, Haffner SM. Chronic subclinical inflammation as part of the insulin resistance syndrome: the Insulin Resistance Atherosclerosis Study (IRAS). Circulation, 2000; 102: 42-7.

[208]　Visser M, Bouter LM, McQuillan GM, Wener MH, Harris TB. Low-grade systemic inflammation in overweight children. Pediatrics, 2001; 107: E13.

[209]　Wu DM, Chu NF, Shen MH, Chang JB. Plasma C-reactive protein levels and their relationship to anthropometric and lipid characteristics among children. J Clin Epidemiol, 2003; 56: 94-100.

[210]　Lopez-Jaramillo P, Herrera E, Garcia RG, Camacho PA, Castillo VR. Inter-relationships between body mass index, C-reactive protein and blood pressure in a Hispanic pediatric population. Am J Hypertens, 2008; 21: 527-32.

[211]　Kern PA, Saghizadeh M, Ong JM, Bosch RJ, Deem R, Simsolo RB. The expression of tumor necrosis factor in human adipose tissue. Regulation by obesity, weight loss, and relationship to lipoprotein lipase. J Clin Invest, 1995; 95: 2111-9.

[212] Laimer M, Ebenbichler CF, Kaser S, Sandhofer A, Weiss H, Nehoda H, *et al.,* Markers of chronic inflammation and obesity: a prospective study on the reversibility of this association in middle-aged women undergoing weight loss by surgical intervention. Int J Obes Relat Metab Disord, 2002; 26: 659-62.

[213] Monzillo LU, Hamdy O, Horton ES, Ledbury S, Mullooly C, Jarema C, *et al.,* Effect of lifestyle modification on adipokine levels in obese subjects with insulin resistance. Obes Res, 2003; 11: 1048-54.

[214] Kopp HP, Krzyzanowska K, Mohlig M, Spranger J, Pfeiffer AF, Schernthaner G. Effects of marked weight loss on plasma levels of adiponectin, markers of chronic subclinical inflammation and insulin resistance in morbidly obese women. Int J Obes (Lond), 2005; 29: 766-71.

[215] Manigrasso MR, Ferroni P, Santilli F, Taraborelli T, Guagnano MT, Michetti N, *et al.,* Association between circulating adiponectin and interleukin-10 levels in android obesity: effects of weight loss. J Clin Endocrinol Metab, 2005; 90: 5876-9.

[216] Grundy SM, Cleeman JI, Merz CN, Brewer HB, Jr., Clark LT, Hunninghake DB, *et al.,* Implications of recent clinical trials for the National Cholesterol Education Program Adult Treatment Panel III Guidelines. J Am Coll Cardiol, 2004; 44: 720-32.

[217] Lee HW, Kim MJ, Park MY, Han KH, Kim J. The Conserved Proline Residue in the LOB Domain of LBD18 Is Critical for DNA-Binding and Biological Function. Mol Plant, 2013.

[218] Kim GB, Nam YW. A novel Delta(1)-pyrroline-5-carboxylate synthetase gene of Medicago truncatula plays a predominant role in stress-induced proline accumulation during symbiotic nitrogen fixation. J Plant Physiol, 2013; 170: 291-302.

[219] Muniyappa R, Iantorno M, Quon MJ. An integrated view of insulin resistance and endothelial dysfunction. Endocrinol Metab Clin North Am, 2008; 37: 685-711, ix-x.

[220] Le Gouill E, Jimenez M, Binnert C, Jayet PY, Thalmann S, Nicod P, *et al.,* Endothelial nitric oxide synthase (eNOS) knockout mice have defective mitochondrial beta-oxidation. Diabetes, 2007; 56: 2690-6.

[221] Cook S, Hugli O, Egli M, Menard B, Thalmann S, Sartori C, *et al.,* Partial gene deletion of endothelial nitric oxide synthase predisposes to exaggerated high-fat diet-induced insulin resistance and arterial hypertension. Diabetes, 2004; 53: 2067-72.

[222] Meigs JB, Hu FB, Rifai N, Manson JE. Biomarkers of endothelial dysfunction and risk of type 2 diabetes mellitus. JAMA, 2004; 291: 1978-86.

[223] Meigs JB, O'Donnell C J, Tofler GH, Benjamin EJ, Fox CS, Lipinska I, *et al.,* Hemostatic markers of endothelial dysfunction and risk of incident type 2 diabetes: the Framingham Offspring Study. Diabetes, 2006; 55: 530-7.

[224] Song Y, Manson JE, Tinker L, Rifai N, Cook NR, Hu FB, *et al.,* Circulating levels of endothelial adhesion molecules and risk of diabetes in an ethnically diverse cohort of women. Diabetes, 2007; 56: 1898-904.

[225] Donahue RP, Rejman K, Rafalson LB, Dmochowski J, Stranges S, Trevisan M. Sex differences in endothelial function markers before conversion to pre-diabetes: does the clock start ticking earlier among women? The Western New York Study. Diabetes Care, 2007; 30: 354-9.

[226] Kim JA, Montagnani M, Koh KK, Quon MJ. Reciprocal relationships between insulin resistance and endothelial dysfunction: molecular and pathophysiological mechanisms. Circulation, 2006; 113: 1888-904.

[227] Paradisi G, Steinberg HO, Hempfling A, Cronin J, Hook G, Shepard MK, *et al.,* Polycystic ovary syndrome is associated with endothelial dysfunction. Circulation, 2001; 103: 1410-5.

[228] Clerk LH, Vincent MA, Jahn LA, Liu Z, Lindner JR, Barrett EJ. Obesity blunts insulin-mediated microvascular recruitment in human forearm muscle. Diabetes, 2006; 55: 1436-42.

[229] Hermann TS, Li W, Dominguez H, Ihlemann N, Rask-Madsen C, Major-Pedersen A, *et al.,* Quinapril treatment increases insulin-stimulated endothelial function and adiponectin gene expression in patients with type 2 diabetes. J Clin Endocrinol Metab, 2006; 91: 1001-8.

[230] Goldfine AB, Beckman JA, Betensky RA, Devlin H, Hurley S, Varo N, *et al.,* Family history of diabetes is a major determinant of endothelial function. J Am Coll Cardiol, 2006; 47: 2456-61.

[231] Eilat-Adar S, Eldar M, Goldbourt U. Association of intentional changes in body weight with coronary heart disease event rates in overweight subjects who have an additional coronary risk factor. Am J Epidemiol, 2005; 161: 352-8.

[232] Wing AM. More grip, less force. Occup Health Saf, 2006; 75: 64, 66, 68-72.

[233] Keogh JB, Brinkworth GD, Noakes M, Belobrajdic DP, Buckley JD, Clifton PM. Effects of weight loss from a very-low-carbohydrate diet on endothelial function and markers of cardiovascular disease risk in subjects with abdominal obesity. Am J Clin Nutr, 2008; 87: 567-76.

[234] Seshadri P, Iqbal N, Stern L, Williams M, Chicano KL, Daily DA, *et al.,* A randomized study comparing the effects of a low-carbohydrate diet and a conventional diet on lipoprotein subfractions and C-reactive protein levels in patients with severe obesity. Am J Med, 2004; 117: 398-405.

[235] Mazzali G, Di Francesco V, Zoico E, Fantin F, Zamboni G, Benati C, *et al.,* Interrelations between fat distribution, muscle lipid content, adipocytokines, and insulin resistance: effect of moderate weight loss in older women. Am J Clin Nutr, 2006; 84: 1193-9.

[236] Tuomilehto J, Lindstrom J, Eriksson JG, Valle TT, Hamalainen H, Ilanne-Parikka P, *et al.,* Prevention of type 2 diabetes mellitus by changes in lifestyle among subjects with impaired glucose tolerance. N Engl J Med, 2001; 344: 1343-50.

[237] Arvidsson E, Viguerie N, Andersson I, Verdich C, Langin D, Arner P. Effects of different hypocaloric diets on protein secretion from adipose tissue of obese women. Diabetes, 2004; 53: 1966-71.

[238] Heggen E, Klemsdal TO, Haugen F, Holme I, Tonstad S. Effect of a Low-Fat *Versus* a Low-Gycemic-Load Diet on Inflammatory Biomarker and Adipokine Concentrations. Metab Syndr Relat Disord, 2012.

[239] Garanty-Bogacka B, Syrenicz M, Goral J, Krupa B, Syrenicz J, Walczak M, *et al.,* Changes in inflammatory biomarkers after successful lifestyle intervention in obese children. Endokrynol Pol, 2011; 62: 499-505.

[240] Kim DH, Sandoval D, Reed JA, Matter EK, Tolod EG, Woods SC, *et al.,* The role of GM-CSF in adipose tissue inflammation. Am J Physiol Endocrinol Metab, 2008; 295: E1038-46.

[241] Poirier H, Shapiro JS, Kim RJ, Lazar MA. Nutritional supplementation with trans-10, cis-12-conjugated linoleic acid induces inflammation of white adipose tissue. Diabetes, 2006; 55: 1634-41.

[242] Reed JA, Clegg DJ, Smith KB, Tolod-Richer EG, Matter EK, Picard LS, *et al.,* GM-CSF action in the CNS decreases food intake and body weight. J Clin Invest, 2005; 115: 3035-44.

[243] Takahashi Y, Takahashi M, Carpino N, Jou ST, Chao JR, Tanaka S, *et al.,* Leukemia inhibitory factor regulates trophoblast giant cell differentiation *via* Janus kinase 1-signal transducer and activator of transcription 3-suppressor of cytokine signaling 3 pathway. Mol Endocrinol, 2008; 22: 1673-81.

[244] Moriggl R, Marine JC, Topham DJ, Teglund S, Sexl V, McKay C, *et al.,* Differential roles of cytokine signaling during T-cell development. Cold Spring Harb Symp Quant Biol, 1999; 64: 389-95.

[245] Prieto RM, Fiol M, Perello J, Estruch R, Ros E, Sanchis P, *et al.,* Effects of Mediterranean diets with low and high proportions of phytate-rich foods on the urinary phytate excretion. Eur J Nutr, 2010; 49: 321-6.

[246] Salas-Salvado J, Fernandez-Ballart J, Ros E, Martinez-Gonzalez MA, Fito M, Estruch R, *et al.,* Effect of a Mediterranean diet supplemented with nuts on metabolic syndrome status: one-year results of the PREDIMED randomized trial. Arch Intern Med, 2008; 168: 2449-58.

[247] Zhao L, Jin Y, Ma C, Song H, Li H, Wang Z, *et al.,* Physico-chemical characteristics and free fatty acid composition of dry fermented mutton sausages as affected by the use of various combinations of starter cultures and spices. Meat Sci, 2011; 88: 761-6.

[248] DeGrado TR, Kitapci MT, Wang S, Ying J, Lopaschuk GD. Validation of 18F-fluoro-4-thia-palmitate as a PET probe for myocardial fatty acid oxidation: effects of hypoxia and composition of exogenous fatty acids. J Nucl Med, 2006; 47: 173-81.

[249] Wang H, Cronan JE. Haemophilus influenzae Rd lacks a stringently conserved fatty acid biosynthetic enzyme and thermal control of membrane lipid composition. J Bacteriol, 2003; 185: 4930-7.

[250] Wang JC, Park JK, Whang LM. Comparison of fatty acid composition and kinetics of phosphorus-accumulating organisms and glycogen-accumulating organisms. Water Environ Res, 2001; 73: 704-10.

[251] Loizou CL, Ozanne SE, Martensz ND, Petry CJ, Wang CL, Hales CN. Early growth restriction, membrane phospholipid fatty acid composition, and insulin sensitivity. Metabolism, 2001; 50: 1070-7.

[252] Gerstein HC, Islam S, Anand S, Almahmeed W, Damasceno A, Dans A, *et al.,* Dysglycaemia and the risk of acute myocardial infarction in multiple ethnic groups: an analysis of 15,780 patients from the INTERHEART study. Diabetologia, 2010; 53: 2509-17.

[253] Rosengren A, Subramanian SV, Islam S, Chow CK, Avezum A, Kazmi K, *et al.,* Education and risk for acute myocardial infarction in 52 high, middle and low-income countries: INTERHEART case-control study. Heart, 2009; 95: 2014-22.

[254] Karthikeyan G, Teo KK, Islam S, McQueen MJ, Pais P, Wang X, *et al.,* Lipid profile, plasma apolipoproteins, and risk of a first myocardial infarction among Asians: an analysis from the INTERHEART Study. J Am Coll Cardiol, 2009; 53: 244-53.

[255] Anand SS, Islam S, Rosengren A, Franzosi MG, Steyn K, Yusufali AH, *et al.,* Risk factors for myocardial infarction in women and men: insights from the INTERHEART study. Eur Heart J, 2008; 29: 932-40.

[256] Karppi J, Nurmi T, Kurl S, Rissanen TH, Nyyssonen K. Lycopene, lutein and beta-carotene as determinants of LDL conjugated dienes in serum. Atherosclerosis, 2010; 209: 565-72.

[257] Rissanen TH, Voutilainen S, Nyyssonen K, Salonen R, Kaplan GA, Salonen JT. Serum lycopene concentrations and carotid atherosclerosis: the Kuopio Ischaemic Heart Disease Risk Factor Study. Am J Clin Nutr, 2003; 77: 133-8.

[258] Hoek JB, Cahill A, Pastorino JG. Alcohol and mitochondria: a dysfunctional relationship. Gastroenterology, 2002; 122: 2049-63.

[259] Volicer BJ, Cahill MH, Neuburger E, Arntz G. Randomized response estimates of problem use of alcohol among employed females. Alcohol Clin Exp Res, 1983; 7: 321-6.

[260] Cahill MH, Volicer BJ. Male and female differences in severity of problems with alcohol at the workplace. Drug Alcohol Depend, 1981; 8: 143-56.

[261] Gates PE, Tanaka H, Graves J, Seals DR. Left ventricular structure and diastolic function with human ageing. Relation to habitual exercise and arterial stiffness. Eur Heart J, 2003; 24: 2213-20.

[262] Huffman MD, Lloyd-Jones DM, Ning H, Labarthe DR, Guzman Castillo M, O'Flaherty M, *et al.,* Quantifying Options for Reducing Coronary Heart Disease Mortality By 2020. Circulation, 2013.

[263] Tsuru M, Soejima T, Shiba N, Kimura K, Sato K, Toyama Y, *et al.,* Proline/Arginine-Rich End Leucine-Rich Repeat Protein Converts Stem Cells to Ligament Tissue and Zn(II) Influences Its Nuclear Expression. Stem Cells Dev, 2013.

[264] Sargent BJ, Moore NA. New central targets for the treatment of obesity. Br J Clin Pharmacol, 2009; 68: 852-60.

[265] Halford JC, Boyland EJ, Blundell JE, Kirkham TC, Harrold JA. Pharmacological management of appetite expression in obesity. Nat Rev Endocrinol, 2010; 6: 255-69.

[266] Wilding JP. Treatment strategies for obesity. Obes Rev, 2007; 8 Suppl 1: 137-44.

[267] Tsuchida A, Yamauchi T, Kadowaki T. Nuclear receptors as targets for drug development: molecular mechanisms for regulation of obesity and insulin resistance by peroxisome proliferator-activated receptor gamma, CREB-binding protein, and adiponectin. J Pharmacol Sci, 2005; 97: 164-70.

[268] Weintraub M. Long-term weight control study: conclusions. Clin Pharmacol Ther, 1992; 51: 642-6.

[269] Connolly HM, Crary JL, McGoon MD, Hensrud DD, Edwards BS, Edwards WD, *et al.,* Valvular heart disease associated with fenfluramine-phentermine. N Engl J Med, 1997; 337: 581-8.

[270] Dixit VD. Adipose-immune interactions during obesity and caloric restriction: reciprocal mechanisms regulating immunity and health span. J Leukoc Biol, 2008; 84: 882-92.

[271] Aronne LJ, Halseth AE, Burns CM, Miller S, Shen LZ. Enhanced weight loss following coadministration of pramlintide with sibutramine or phentermine in a multicenter trial. Obesity (Silver Spring); 18: 1739-46.

[272] Lesses MF, Myerson A. Human autonomic pharmacology. XVI. Benzedrine sulfate as an aid in the treatment of obesity. 1938. Obes Res, 1994; 2: 286-92.

[273] Jaworska L, Budziszewska B, Lason W. The effect of repeated amphetamine administration on the proopiomelanocortin mRNA level in the rat pituitary: an *in situ* hybridization study. Drug Alcohol Depend, 1994; 36: 123-7.

[274] Menyhert J, Wittmann G, Lechan RM, Keller E, Liposits Z, Fekete C. Cocaine- and amphetamine-regulated transcript (CART) is colocalized with the orexigenic neuropeptide Y and agouti-related protein and absent from the anorexigenic alpha-melanocyte-stimulating hormone neurons in the infundibular nucleus of the human hypothalamus. Endocrinology, 2007; 148: 4276-81.

[275] Lang SS, Danforth E, Jr., Lien EL. Anorectic drugs which stimulate thermogenesis. Life Sci, 1983; 33: 1269-75.

[276] Pasquali R, Casimirri F, Melchionda N, Grossi G, Bortoluzzi L, Morselli Labate AM, *et al.,* Effects of chronic administration of ephedrine during very-low-calorie diets on energy expenditure, protein metabolism and hormone levels in obese subjects. Clin Sci (Lond), 1992; 82: 85-92.

[277] Lorello C, Goldfield GS, Doucet E. Methylphenidate hydrochloride increases energy expenditure in healthy adults. Obesity (Silver Spring), 2008; 16: 470-2.

[278] Jones JR, Caul WF, Hill JO. The effects of amphetamine on body weight and energy expenditure. Physiol Behav, 1992; 51: 607-11.

[279] Bray GA, Greenway FL. Current and potential drugs for treatment of obesity. Endocr Rev, 1999; 20: 805-75.

[280] James WP, Caterson ID, Coutinho W, Finer N, Van Gaal LF, Maggioni AP, *et al.,* Effect of sibutramine on cardiovascular outcomes in overweight and obese subjects. N Engl J Med, 2010; 363: 905-17.

[281] Lavie CJ, Milani RV, Ventura HO. Obesity and cardiovascular disease: risk factor, paradox, and impact of weight loss. J Am Coll Cardiol, 2009; 53: 1925-32.

[282] Rucker D, Padwal R, Li SK, Curioni C, Lau DC. Long term pharmacotherapy for obesity and overweight: updated meta-analysis. Bmj, 2007; 335: 1194-9.

[283] Jung SH, Park HS, Kim KS, Choi WH, Ahn CW, Kim BT, *et al.,* Effect of weight loss on some serum cytokines in human obesity: increase in IL-10 after weight loss. J Nutr Biochem, 2008; 19: 371-5.

[284] Devane WA, Breuer A, Sheskin T, Jarbe TU, Eisen MS, Mechoulam R. A novel probe for the cannabinoid receptor. J Med Chem, 1992; 35: 2065-9.

[285] Di Marzo V, Matias I. Endocannabinoid control of food intake and energy balance. Nat Neurosci, 2005; 8: 585-9.

[286] Chen Y, Barry T, Giasson J. Rapid weight loss and decrease in hemoglobin A1c after treatment with topiramate in a patient with status epilepticus. Endocr Pract, 2011; 17: 658-9.

[287] Cosentino G, Conrad AO, Uwaifo GI. Phentermine and topiramate for the management of obesity: a review. Drug Des Devel Ther, 2013; 7: 267-78.

[288] Ioannides-Demos LL, Piccenna L, McNeil JJ. Pharmacotherapies for obesity: past, current, and future therapies. J Obes, 2011; 2011: 179674.

[289] Pi-Sunyer FX, Aronne LJ, Heshmati HM, Devin J, Rosenstock J. Effect of rimonabant, a cannabinoid-1 receptor blocker, on weight and cardiometabolic risk factors in overweight or obese patients: RIO-North America: a randomized controlled trial. JAMA, 2006; 295: 761-75.

[290] Rosenstock J, Hollander P, Chevalier S, Iranmanesh A. SERENADE: the Study Evaluating Rimonabant Efficacy in Drug-naive Diabetic Patients: effects of monotherapy with rimonabant, the first selective CB1 receptor antagonist, on glycemic control, body weight, and lipid profile in drug-naive type 2 diabetes. Diabetes Care, 2008; 31: 2169-76.

[291] Van Gaal LF, Scheen AJ, Rissanen AM, Rossner S, Hanotin C, Ziegler O. Long-term effect of CB1 blockade with rimonabant on cardiometabolic risk factors: two year results from the RIO-Europe Study. Eur Heart J, 2008; 29: 1761-71.

[292] Chavez-Tapia NC, Tellez-Avila FI, Bedogni G, Croce LS, Masutti F, Tiribelli C. Systematic review and meta-analysis on the adverse events of rimonabant treatment: considerations for its potential use in hepatology. BMC Gastroenterol, 2009; 9: 75.

[293] Sam AH, Salem V, Ghatei MA. Rimonabant: From RIO to Ban. J Obes, 2011; 2011: 432607.

[294] Borgstrom B. Mode of action of tetrahydrolipstatin: a derivative of the naturally occurring lipase inhibitor lipstatin. Biochim Biophys Acta, 1988; 962: 308-16.

[295] Padwal RS, Majumdar SR. Drug treatments for obesity: orlistat, sibutramine, and rimonabant. Lancet, 2007; 369: 71-7.

[296] Hutton B, Fergusson D. Changes in body weight and serum lipid profile in obese patients treated with orlistat in addition to a hypocaloric diet: a systematic review of randomized clinical trials. Am J Clin Nutr, 2004; 80: 1461-8.

[297] Franz MJ, VanWormer JJ, Crain AL, Boucher JL, Histon T, Caplan W, *et al.*, Weight-loss outcomes: a systematic review and meta-analysis of weight-loss clinical trials with a minimum 1-year follow-up. J Am Diet Assoc, 2007; 107: 1755-67.

[298] Czernichow S, Lee CM, Barzi F, Greenfield JR, Baur LA, Chalmers J, *et al.*, Efficacy of weight loss drugs on obesity and cardiovascular risk factors in obese adolescents: a meta-analysis of randomized controlled trials. Obes Rev; 11: 150-8.

[299] Torgerson JS, Hauptman J, Boldrin MN, Sjostrom L. XENical in the prevention of diabetes in obese subjects (XENDOS) study: a randomized study of orlistat as an adjunct to lifestyle changes for the prevention of type 2 diabetes in obese patients. Diabetes Care, 2004; 27: 155-61.

[300] Derosa G, Cicero AF, D'Angelo A, Fogari E, Maffioli P. Effects of 1-year orlistat treatment compared to placebo on insulin resistance parameters in patients with type 2 diabetes. J Clin Pharm Ther, 2012; 37: 187-95.

[301] Li M, Cheung BM. Pharmacotherapy for obesity. Br J Clin Pharmacol, 2009; 68: 804-10.

[302] Halpern B, Faria AM, Halpern A. Fixed-dose combination of phentermine-topiramate for the treatment of obesity. Expert Rev Clin Pharmacol, 2013; 6: 235-41.

[303] Maryanoff BE. Sugar sulfamates for seizure control: discovery and development of topiramate, a structurally unique antiepileptic drug. Curr Top Med Chem, 2009; 9: 1049-62.

[304] Beydoun A. Monotherapy trials of new antiepileptic drugs. Epilepsia, 1997; 38 Suppl 9: S21-31.

[305] Adelman J, Freitag FG, Lainez M, Shi Y, Ascher S, Mao L, *et al.*, Analysis of safety and tolerability data obtained from over 1,500 patients receiving topiramate for migraine prevention in controlled trials. Pain Med, 2008; 9: 175-85.

[306] Silberstein SD, Neto W, Schmitt J, Jacobs D. Topiramate in migraine prevention: results of a large controlled trial. Arch Neurol, 2004; 61: 490-5.

[307] Ondo WG, Jankovic J, Connor GS, Pahwa R, Elble R, Stacy MA, *et al.*, Topiramate in essential tremor: a double-blind, placebo-controlled trial. Neurology, 2006; 66: 672-7.

[308] Suppes T. Review of the use of topiramate for treatment of bipolar disorders. J Clin Psychopharmacol, 2002; 22: 599-609.

[309] Tata AL, Kockler DR. Topiramate for binge-eating disorder associated with obesity. Ann Pharmacother, 2006; 40: 1993-7.

[310] McElroy SL, Arnold LM, Shapira NA, Keck PE, Jr., Rosenthal NR, Karim MR, *et al.*, Topiramate in the treatment of binge eating disorder associated with obesity: a randomized, placebo-controlled trial. Am J Psychiatry, 2003; 160: 255-61.

[311] Rosenfeld WE, Sachdeo RC, Faught RE, Privitera M. Long-term experience with topiramate as adjunctive therapy and as monotherapy in patients with partial onset seizures: retrospective survey of open-label treatment. Epilepsia, 1997; 38 Suppl 1: S34-6.

[312] Nickel C, Tritt K, Muehlbacher M, Pedrosa Gil F, Mitterlehner FO, Kaplan P, *et al.,* Topiramate treatment in bulimia nervosa patients: a randomized, double-blind, placebo-controlled trial. Int J Eat Disord, 2005; 38: 295-300.

[313] Hoopes SP, Reimherr FW, Hedges DW, Rosenthal NR, Kamin M, Karim R, *et al.,* Treatment of bulimia nervosa with topiramate in a randomized, double-blind, placebo-controlled trial, part 1: improvement in binge and purge measures. J Clin Psychiatry, 2003; 64: 1335-41.

[314] Baltieri DA, Daro FR, Ribeiro PL, Andrade AG. Effects of topiramate or naltrexone on tobacco use among male alcohol-dependent outpatients. Drug Alcohol Depend, 2009; 105: 33-41.

[315] Sachdeo RC, Sachdeo SK, Levy RH, Streeter AJ, Bishop FE, Kunze KL, *et al.,* Topiramate and phenytoin pharmacokinetics during repetitive monotherapy and combination therapy to epileptic patients. Epilepsia, 2002; 43: 691-6.

[316] Braga MF, Aroniadou-Anderjaska V, Li H, Rogawski MA. Topiramate reduces excitability in the basolateral amygdala by selectively inhibiting GluK1 (GluR5) kainate receptors on interneurons and positively modulating GABAA receptors on principal neurons. J Pharmacol Exp Ther, 2009; 330: 558-66.

[317] De Simone G, Scozzafava A, Supuran CT. Which carbonic anhydrases are targeted by the antiepileptic sulfonamides and sulfamates? Chem Biol Drug Des, 2009; 74: 317-21.

[318] Sachdeo RC, Sachdeo SK, Walker SA, Kramer LD, Nayak RK, Doose DR. Steady-state pharmacokinetics of topiramate and carbamazepine in patients with epilepsy during monotherapy and concomitant therapy. Epilepsia, 1996; 37: 774-80.

[319] Bialer M, Doose DR, Murthy B, Curtin C, Wang SS, Twyman RE, *et al.,* Pharmacokinetic interactions of topiramate. Clin Pharmacokinet, 2004; 43: 763-80.

[320] D'Amico D, Grazzi L, Bussone G. Topiramate in the prevention of migraine: a review of its efficacy, tolerability, and acceptability. Neuropsychiatr Dis Treat, 2006; 2: 261-7.

[321] Lyseng-Williamson KA, Yang LP. Topiramate: a review of its use in the treatment of epilepsy. Drugs, 2007; 67: 2231-56.

[322] Verrotti A, Scaparrotta A, Agostinelli S, Di Pillo S, Chiarelli F, Grosso S. Topiramate-induced weight loss: a review. Epilepsy Res, 2011; 95: 189-99.

[323] Liang Y, She P, Wang X, Demarest K. The messenger RNA profiles in liver, hypothalamus, white adipose tissue, and skeletal muscle of female Zucker diabetic fatty rats after topiramate treatment. Metabolism, 2006; 55: 1411-9.

[324] Klein KM, Theisen F, Knake S, Oertel WH, Hebebrand J, Rosenow F, *et al.,* Topiramate, nutrition and weight change: a prospective study. J Neurol Neurosurg Psychiatry, 2008; 79: 590-3.

[325] Biton V. Effect of antiepileptic drugs on bodyweight: overview and clinical implications for the treatment of epilepsy. CNS Drugs, 2003; 17: 781-91.

[326] Biton V, Montouris GD, Ritter F, Riviello JJ, Reife R, Lim P, *et al.,* A randomized, placebo-controlled study of topiramate in primary generalized tonic-clonic seizures. Topiramate YTC Study Group. Neurology, 1999; 52: 1330-7.

[327] Tremblay A, Chaput JP, Berube-Parent S, Prud'homme D, Leblanc C, Almeras N, *et al.,* The effect of topiramate on energy balance in obese men: a 6-month double-blind randomized placebo-controlled study with a 6-month open-label extension. Eur J Clin Pharmacol, 2007; 63: 123-34.

[328] Picard F, Deshaies Y, Lalonde J, Samson P, Richard D. Topiramate reduces energy and fat gains in lean (Fa/?) and obese (fa/fa) Zucker rats. Obes Res, 2000; 8: 656-63.

[329] Richard D, Picard F, Lemieux C, Lalonde J, Samson P, Deshaies Y. The effects of topiramate and sex hormones on energy balance of male and female rats. Int J Obes Relat Metab Disord, 2002; 26: 344-53.

[330] Winum JY, Scozzafava A, Montero JL, Supuran CT. Sulfamates and their therapeutic potential. Med Res Rev, 2005; 25: 186-228.

[331] Poulsen SA, Wilkinson BL, Innocenti A, Vullo D, Supuran CT. Inhibition of human mitochondrial carbonic anhydrases VA and VB with para-(4-phenyltriazole-1-yl)-benzenesulfonamide derivatives. Bioorg Med Chem Lett, 2008; 18: 4624-7.

[332] Richard D, Ferland J, Lalonde J, Samson P, Deshaies Y. Influence of topiramate in the regulation of energy balance. Nutrition, 2000; 16: 961-6.

[333] Astrup A, Caterson I, Zelissen P, Guy-Grand B, Carruba M, Levy B, *et al.,* Topiramate: long-term maintenance of weight loss induced by a low-calorie diet in obese subjects. Obes Res, 2004; 12: 1658-69.

[334] Kadowaki T, Yamauchi T, Kubota N, Hara K, Ueki K, Tobe K. Adiponectin and adiponectin receptors in insulin resistance, diabetes, and the metabolic syndrome. J Clin Invest, 2006; 116: 1784-92.

[335] Ben-Menachem E, Axelsen M, Johanson EH, Stagge A, Smith U. Predictors of weight loss in adults with topiramate-treated epilepsy. Obes Res, 2003; 11: 556-62.

[336] Ramsay E, Faught E, Krumholz A, Naritoku D, Privitera M, Schwarzman L, *et al.,* Efficacy, tolerability, and safety of rapid initiation of topiramate *versus* phenytoin in patients with new-onset epilepsy: a randomized double-blind clinical trial. Epilepsia, 2010; 51: 1970-7.

[337] Wilding J, Van Gaal L, Rissanen A, Vercruysse F, Fitchet M. A randomized double-blind placebo-controlled study of the long-term efficacy and safety of topiramate in the treatment of obese subjects. Int J Obes Relat Metab Disord, 2004; 28: 1399-410.

[338] Stenlof K, Rossner S, Vercruysse F, Kumar A, Fitchet M, Sjostrom L. Topiramate in the treatment of obese subjects with drug-naive type 2 diabetes. Diabetes Obes Metab, 2007; 9: 360-8.

[339] Kanner AM, Wuu J, Faught E, Tatum WOt, Fix A, French JA. A past psychiatric history may be a risk factor for topiramate-related psychiatric and cognitive adverse events. Epilepsy Behav, 2003; 4: 548-52.

[340] Faught E. Clinical studies of topiramate. Drugs Today (Barc), 1999; 35: 49-57.

[341] Tatum WOt, French JA, Faught E, Morris GL, 3rd, Liporace J, Kanner A, *et al.,* Postmarketing experience with topiramate and cognition. Epilepsia, 2001; 42: 1134-40.

[342] Khan A, Faught E, Gilliam F, Kuzniecky R. Acute psychotic symptoms induced by topiramate. Seizure, 1999; 8: 235-7.

[343] Martin R, Kuzniecky R, Ho S, Hetherington H, Pan J, Sinclair K, *et al.,* Cognitive effects of topiramate, gabapentin, and lamotrigine in healthy young adults. Neurology, 1999; 52: 321-7.

[344] Kuzniecky R, Hetherington H, Ho S, Pan J, Martin R, Gilliam F, *et al.,* Topiramate increases cerebral GABA in healthy humans. Neurology, 1998; 51: 627-9.

[345] Rosenfeld WE. Topiramate: a review of preclinical, pharmacokinetic, and clinical data. Clin Ther, 1997; 19: 1294-308.

[346] Leombruni P, Lavagnino L, Fassino S. Treatment of obese patients with binge eating disorder using topiramate: a review. Neuropsychiatr Dis Treat, 2009; 5: 385-92.

[347] Kramer CK, Leitao CB, Pinto LC, Canani LH, Azevedo MJ, Gross JL. Efficacy and safety of topiramate on weight loss: a meta-analysis of randomized controlled trials. Obes Rev, 2011; 12: e338-47.

[348] Arroyo S, Dodson WE, Privitera MD, Glauser TA, Naritoku DK, Dlugos DJ, *et al.,* Randomized dose-controlled study of topiramate as first-line therapy in epilepsy. Acta Neurol Scand, 2005; 112: 214-22.

[349] Guerrini R, Carpay J, Groselj J, van Oene J, Schreiner A, Lahaye M, *et al.,* Topiramate monotherapy as broad-spectrum antiepileptic drug in a naturalistic clinical setting. Seizure, 2005; 14: 371-80.

[350] Bray GA, Hollander P, Klein S, Kushner R, Levy B, Fitchet M, *et al.,* A 6-month randomized, placebo-controlled, dose-ranging trial of topiramate for weight loss in obesity. Obes Res, 2003; 11: 722-33.

[351] Reiter E, Feucht M, Hauser E, Freilinger M, Seidl R. Changes in body mass index during long-term topiramate therapy in paediatric epilepsy patients--a retrospective analysis. Seizure, 2004; 13: 491-3.

[352] Li HF, Zou Y, Xia ZZ, Gao F, Feng JH, Yang CW. Effects of topiramate on weight and metabolism in children with epilepsy. Acta Paediatr, 2009; 98: 1521-5.

[353] Schreiner A, Stollhoff K, Ossig W, Unkelbach S, Luer W, Bogdanow M, *et al.,* Conversion from valproic acid onto topiramate in adolescents and adults with epilepsy. Acta Neurol Scand, 2009; 119: 304-12.

[354] Alberici A, Borroni B, Manelli F, Griffini S, Zavarise P, Padovani A, *et al.,* Topiramate weight loss in migraine patients. J Neurol Sci, 2009; 278: 64-5.

[355] Rosenstock J, Hollander P, Gadde KM, Sun X, Strauss R, Leung A. A randomized, double-blind, placebo-controlled, multicenter study to assess the efficacy and safety of topiramate controlled release in the treatment of obese type 2 diabetic patients. Diabetes Care, 2007; 30: 1480-6.

[356] Toplak H, Hamann A, Moore R, Masson E, Gorska M, Vercruysse F, *et al.,* Efficacy and safety of topiramate in combination with metformin in the treatment of obese subjects with type 2 diabetes: a randomized, double-blind, placebo-controlled study. Int J Obes (Lond), 2007; 31: 138-46.

[357] Eliasson B, Gudbjornsdottir S, Cederholm J, Liang Y, Vercruysse F, Smith U. Weight loss and metabolic effects of topiramate in overweight and obese type 2 diabetic patients: randomized double-blind placebo-controlled trial. Int J Obes (Lond), 2007; 31: 1140-7.

[358] Bays H. Phentermine, topiramate and their combination for the treatment of adiposopathy ('sick fat') and metabolic disease. Expert Rev Cardiovasc Ther, 2010; 8: 1777-801.

[359] Bays HE, Gadde KM. Phentermine/topiramate for weight reduction and treatment of adverse metabolic consequences in obesity. Drugs Today (Barc), 2011; 47: 903-14.

[360] Garvey WT, Ryan DH, Look M, Gadde KM, Allison DB, Peterson CA, *et al.,* Two-year sustained weight loss and metabolic benefits with controlled-release phentermine/topiramate in obese and overweight adults (SEQUEL): a randomized, placebo-controlled, phase 3 extension study. Am J Clin Nutr, 2012; 95: 297-308.

[361] Powell AG, Apovian CM, Aronne LJ. The combination of phentermine and topiramate is an effective adjunct to diet and lifestyle modification for weight loss and measures of

comorbidity in overweight or obese adults with additional metabolic risk factors. Evid Based Med, 2012; 17: 14-5.

[362] Gadde KM, Allison DB, Ryan DH, Peterson CA, Troupin B, Schwiers ML, *et al.,* Effects of low-dose, controlled-release, phentermine plus topiramate combination on weight and associated comorbidities in overweight and obese adults (CONQUER): a randomised, placebo-controlled, phase 3 trial. Lancet, 2011; 377: 1341-52.

[363] Allison DB, Gadde KM, Garvey WT, Peterson CA, Schwiers ML, Najarian T, *et al.,* Controlled-release phentermine/topiramate in severely obese adults: a randomized controlled trial (EQUIP). Obesity (Silver Spring), 2012; 20: 330-42.

[364] Shin JH, Gadde KM. Clinical utility of phentermine/topiramate (Qsymia) combination for the treatment of obesity. Diabetes Metab Syndr Obes, 2013; 6: 131-9.

[365] Colman E, Golden J, Roberts M, Egan A, Weaver J, Rosebraugh C. The FDA's assessment of two drugs for chronic weight management. N Engl J Med, 2012; 367: 1577-9.

[366] Aylwin S, Al-Zaman Y. Emerging concepts in the medical and surgical treatment of obesity. Front Horm Res, 2008; 36: 229-59.

[367] Genc BO, Dogan EA, Dogan U, Genc E. Anthropometric indexes, insulin resistance, and serum leptin and lipid levels in women with cryptogenic epilepsy receiving topiramate treatment. J Clin Neurosci, 2010; 17: 1256-9.

[368] Narula PK, Rehan HS, Unni KE, Gupta N. Topiramate for prevention of olanzapine associated weight gain and metabolic dysfunction in schizophrenia: a double-blind, placebo-controlled trial. Schizophr Res, 2010; 118: 218-23.

[369] Wilkes JJ, Nelson E, Osborne M, Demarest KT, Olefsky JM. Topiramate is an insulin-sensitizing compound *in vivo* with direct effects on adipocytes in female ZDF rats. Am J Physiol Endocrinol Metab, 2005; 288: E617-24.

[370] Wilkes JJ, Nguyen MT, Bandyopadhyay GK, Nelson E, Olefsky JM. Topiramate treatment causes skeletal muscle insulin sensitization and increased Acrp30 secretion in high-fat-fed male Wistar rats. Am J Physiol Endocrinol Metab, 2005; 289: E1015-22.

[371] El-Abhar HS, Schaalan MF. Topiramate-induced modulation of hepatic molecular mechanisms: an aspect for its anti-insulin resistant effect. PLoS One, 2012; 7: e37757.

[372] Schutt M, Brinkhoff J, Drenckhan M, Lehnert H, Sommer C. Weight reducing and metabolic effects of topiramate in patients with migraine--an observational study. Exp Clin Endocrinol Diabetes, 2010; 118: 449-52.

[373] Kim JY, Lee HW. Metabolic and hormonal disturbances in women with epilepsy on antiepileptic drug monotherapy. Epilepsia, 2007; 48: 1366-70.

[374] Theisen FM, Beyenburg S, Gebhardt S, Kluge M, Blum WF, Remschmidt H, *et al.,* A prospective study of body weight and serum leptin levels in patients treated with topiramate. Clin Neuropharmacol, 2008; 31: 226-30.

[375] Tchernof A, Nolan A, Sites CK, Ades PA, Poehlman ET. Weight loss reduces C-reactive protein levels in obese postmenopausal women. Circulation, 2002; 105: 564-9.

[376] Ford ES, Galuska DA, Gillespie C, Will JC, Giles WH, Dietz WH. C-reactive protein and body mass index in children: findings from the Third National Health and Nutrition Examination Survey, 1988-1994. J Pediatr, 2001; 138: 486-92.

[377] Bigal ME, Lipton RB, Biondi DM, Xiang J, Hulihan J. Weight change and clinical markers of cardiovascular disease risk during preventive treatment of migraine. Cephalalgia, 2009; 29: 1188-96.

[378]   Shen J, Ordovas JM. Impact of genetic and environmental factors on hsCRP concentrations and response to therapeutic agents. Clin Chem, 2009; 55: 256-64.

[379]   Mintzer S, Skidmore CT, Rankin SJ, Chervoneva I, Pequinot E, Capuzzi DM, *et al.,* Conversion from enzyme-inducing antiepileptic drugs to topiramate: effects on lipids and C-reactive protein. Epilepsy Res, 2012; 98: 88-93.

[380]   Mintzer S, Skidmore CT, Abidin CJ, Morales MC, Chervoneva I, Capuzzi DM, *et al.,* Effects of antiepileptic drugs on lipids, homocysteine, and C-reactive protein. Ann Neurol, 2009; 65: 448-56.

[381]   Tsuchida A, Yamauchi T, Takekawa S, Hada Y, Ito Y, Maki T, *et al.,* Peroxisome proliferator-activated receptor (PPAR)alpha activation increases adiponectin receptors and reduces obesity-related inflammation in adipose tissue: comparison of activation of PPARalpha, PPARgamma, and their combination. Diabetes, 2005; 54: 3358-70.

[382]   Kocer A, Memisogullari R, Domac FM, Ilhan A, Kocer E, Okuyucu S, *et al.,* IL-6 levels in migraine patients receiving topiramate. Pain Pract, 2009; 9: 375-9.

[383]   Kugler SL, Sachdeo RC. Topiramate efficacy in infancy. Pediatr Neurol, 1998; 19: 320-2.

[384]   Shi RF, Wang KL, Li QH, Zheng HC, Yang HF, Tang HX, *et al.,* [Changes of body weight and galanin in epileptic children treated with topiramate]. Zhonghua Er Ke Za Zhi, 2007; 45: 199-202.

[385]   Yang W, Li M. [Changes of the event related potential P300 following topiramate treatment in children with epilepsy]. Zhongguo Dang Dai Er Ke Za Zhi, 2008; 10: 583-5.

[386]   Chen J, Quan QY, Yang F, Wang Y, Wang JC, Zhao G, *et al.,* Effects of lamotrigine and topiramate on hippocampal neurogenesis in experimental temporal-lobe epilepsy. Brain Res, 2010; 1313: 270-82.

CHAPTER 2

Estrogen is Protective Against Obesity and Obesity Related Co-Morbidities; Cardiovascular Diseases and Malignancies

Zsuzsanna Suba[*]

National Institute of Oncology, Department of Surgical and Molecular Pathology, Budapest, Hungary

Abstract: Obesity is a heterogeneous disorder predisposing patients to a variety of diseases such as; metabolic syndrome, type 2 diabetes, cardiovascular lesions and malignancies. Adipose tissue is principally deposited subcutaneously and centrally. The predominance of central, viscerally deposited fat may alter the immunological, metabolic and endocrine milieu. Visceral adipose tissue mass secretes a number of proinflammatory cytokines, adipokines and growth factors leading to low grade inflammatory process and insulin resistance.

In the first phase of insulin resistance a compensatory hyperinsulinemia develops. Insulin is not only the mediator of glucose uptake and metabolic processes but also a growth factor. Excessive insulin production enhances the secretion and mitotic activity of insulin-like growth factors as well. Moreover, insulin is a potent effector of sexual steroid hormone production and obesity associated hyperinsulinemia stimulates ovarian and adrenal androgen production at the expense of reduced estrogen synthesis.

Metabolic syndrome is a partially compensated phase of insulin resistance. This is a quartet of elevated fasting glucose, high serum triglyceride, low HDL-cholesterol and hypertension being characteristic of viscerally obese patients. Each of these symptoms is strong risk for obesity associated morbidity. Type-2 diabetes is the final uncompensated phase of insulin resistance with a disruption of metabolic processes causing serious damages in all biological structures even at a molecular level.

Estrogens and estrogen receptor signals have diverse anti-obesity impacts. Estrogen has positive regulatory effects on the serum lipid profile, insulin sensitivity and energy homeostasis and on advantageous body fat distribution. Estrogen ensures the healthy balance of adipocytokine secretion in the adipose tissue and increases insulin sensitivity. Moreover, it preserves the functional activity of pancreatic beta cell mass improving the biosynthesis and secretion of insulin.

Premenopausal obesity is frequently associated with defective estrogen synthesis, androgen excess, anovulation and infertility. Hyperandrogenism of obese young women

---

*Address correspondence to Zsuzsanna Suba: National Institute of Oncology, Department of Surgical and Molecular Pathology, Address: H-1122 Ráth György str. 7-9, Budapest, Hungary; Tel: 00 36 1 224 86 00; Fax: 0036 1 224 86 20; E-mail: subazdr@gmail.com is common risk for both premature cardiovascular diseases and malignancies in the female organ triad; breast, endometrium and ovarium. After menopause, increasing prevalence of obesity and insulin resistance is well known in women. Hormone replacement in obese postmenopausal women improves insulin resistance and decreases the accumulation of visceral fatty tissue.

Antiobesity treatment may be completed by estrogen administration in order to restore the metabolic and sexual hormone equilibrium and to protect patients from obesity related co-morbidities.

Keywords: Cancer, cardiovascular disease, estrogen loss, hyperandrogenism, hyperinsulinism, insulin resistance, menopause, metabolic syndrome, obesity, type 2 diabetes.

INTRODUCTION

Obesity is an excessive deposition of adipose tissue caused by a complex interaction between genetic, metabolic, hormonal, behavioral and environmental factors. The deleterious effects of obesity are diverse, ranging from an increased risk of life threatening diseases, such as; type-2 diabetes, cardiovascular lesions and malignancies to several non-fatal diseases with an adverse impact on life quality [1, 2].

Obesity has become a crucial public health problem in many parts of the world. In the past decades disadvantageous changes in lifestyle caused a steady increase in average body weight, especially in the economically developed countries [3]. Obesity and overweight may also be associated with malnutrition attributed to the excessive fat and carbohydrate intake in the developing countries and those under going economic and political transitions.

Since the early 1980s fairly increased prevalence of obesity has been observed in the United States [1]. By the year 2000 nearly two-thirds of adults in the United States were overweight or obese [4]. The incidence of type-2 diabetes during the same time period similarly increased, mirroring a presumed co-morbidity of the obesity epidemic [5]. Incidence of obesity is also enhanced in other parts of the world including the Caribbean region, South America and Southeast Asia [6, 7].

Trends in obesity from 1999 to 2008 and the prevalence of obesity and overweight for the years 2007-2008 were examined in the United States [8]. Over the 10-year period, prevalence of obesity showed no significant trend among women, whereas for men, there was a significant linearly increasing trend. In 2007-2008, the prevalence of obesity was shockingly high; 32.2% among adult men and 35.5% among adult women.

Obesity is a multifaceted disorder and emerging research delineates the specific role of excessive visceral adiposity as opposed to predominantly subcutaneous fat deposition in morbidity and mortality of obese people [9]. Adipose tissue, particularly visceral fat is a metabolically active endocrine organ inducing insulin resistance with associated dysmetabolism and hormonal imbalance. The self-generating insulin resistance mediates the obesity-associated serious illnesses, such as metabolic syndrome, type-2 diabetes, cardiovascular disease and malignancy [10].

High prevalence of obesity plays pivotal role in both cardiovascular disease and cancer related mortality. Researchers speculate that cancer may share a similar disease and risk factor interaction mechanism with that of cardiovascular disease [11]. Correlations among body mass index, diabetes, hypertension and short term mortality were examined in a population based observational study in 2000-2006, in a representative, contemporary United States sample [12]. Severe obesity (but not overweight) was associated with increased premature mortality, an association accounted for by coexisting diabetes and hypertension.

In the United States, overweight and obesity were associated with 90 000 deaths from cancer per year and 280,000-325,000 deaths from all causes per year before 2000. [13, 14]. In the European Union, annual deaths from all causes attributed to overweight and obesity have been estimated at 279,000-304,000 [15]. Some studies estimate that the impact of overweight and obesity in terms of both mortality and health-care costs equals or exceeds that associated with tobacco use [16].

Estrogens and their signaling pathways have well identified roles in the promotion, maintenance and control of the ideal body fat distribution [17]. In premenopausal women, the protective impact of female sexual steroids against cardiovascular diseases is well known, even in the vast majority of obese cases.

By contrast, after menopause, the abrupt loss of beneficial estrogen effect equalizes the gender-related differences in cardiovascular disease morbidity [18]. Nevertheless, concepts on the links between the circulating estrogen level and obesity associated malignancies are highly controversial [19]. In obese postmenopausal women, the mistakenly presumed excessive endogenous estrogen production is regarded as strong cancer risk for the highly hormone dependent breast, endometrium and ovary. On the other hand, the defective estrogen synthesis in obese premenopausal cases is erroneously supposed to be a cancer protective agent [20].

Obesity and overweight are deleterious alterations in both male and female patients. In women, obesity associated dysmetabolism and sexual hormone imbalance with androgen excess seem to be pathogenic in both pre- and postmenopausal cases [20]. These findings disqualify the myth of diseases caused by excessive estrogen level. Results of studies on gender and age related differences in obesity associated co-morbidities justify the health advantage of hormonal equilibrium over defective estrogen synthesis [21].

There are many efforts globally to reduce the rapidly increasing prevalence of obesity. Nevertheless, the prerequisite of successful anti-obesity fight would be the revelation of exact mechanisms by which obesity develops and induces the high morbidity and mortality of life threatening diseases.

PATHOGENETIC MECHANISMS AS LINKS BETWEEN OBESITY AND THE ADIPOSITY RELATED CO-MORBIDITIES

Clinical and experimental evidences prove that obesity, particularly visceral fatty tissue deposition leads to insulin resistance, associated with diverse immunologic, metabolic and hormonal alterations mediating life threatening diseases (Fig. **1**). The main stream of obesity related alterations is a self-generating, progressive insulin resistance in thorough interplay with the dysmetabolism and inflammation of adipose tissue mass and with an imbalance of sexual steroid production in the endocrine organs.

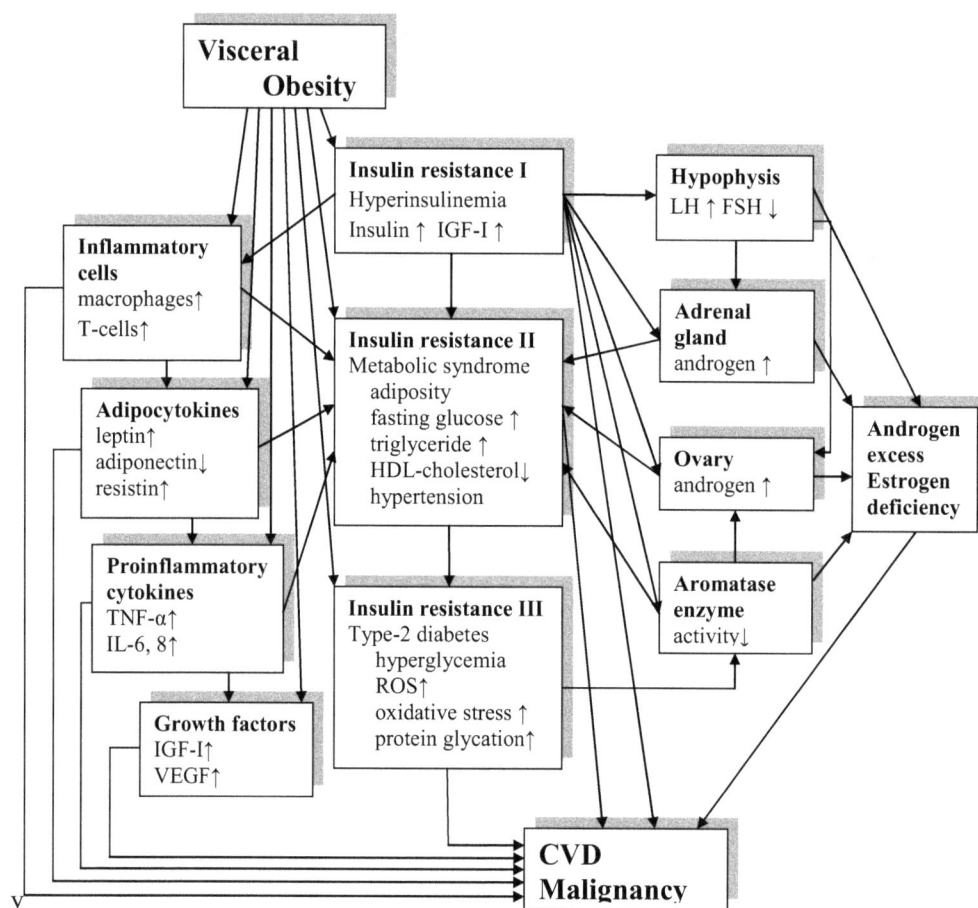

Figure 1: Pathogenetic mechanisms of obesity-related co-morbidities; cardiovascular diseases (CVDs) and malignancies. (Adapted from: Suba Z. Circulatory estrogen level protects against breast cancer in obese women. Recent Pat Anticancer Drug Discov 2013; 8(2): 154-67. Review).

Obesity Related Insulin Resistant States

Insulin resistance (IR) is a defect of insulin-mediated cellular glucose uptake, which may elicit many disorders in the gene regulation of cellular metabolism, growth, differentiation and mitotic activity. The progression of this disorder predisposes patients to a variety of diseases, such as metabolic syndrome, type-2 diabetes, cardiovascular lesions and malignancies at different sites [22].

Reactive hyperinsulinemia in the first, compensated phase of insulin resistance maintains serum glucose level within the normal range by means of an increased secretory capacity of insular β-cells [23]. Insulin has diverse metabolic effects and at the same time functions as a growth factor with strong mitogenic capacity. High insulin level in itself may be regarded as cancer risk by the excessive stimulation of multiple cellular signaling cascades [24]. Hyperinsulinemia increases the hepatic synthesis and mitogenic activity of other, insulin-like growth factors, such as IGF-I. High levels of insulin and IGF-I have important role in the alterations of cell proliferation and in tumor induction, particularly in breast, prostate and colon [25, 26]. Evidences suggest, that certain lifestyle factors, such as diet with high energy intake, may also increase circulating IGF-I levels and increases the risk for cancer [25]. A recent patent introduced somatostatin analogues and IGF-I inhibition for the prevention and treatment of preneoplastic lesions and cancers of the breast [27].

Metabolic syndrome (prediabetes) develops in the second, partially uncompensated phase of insulin resistance when the enhanced insulin synthesis of pancreatic islet cells is not enough to maintain euglycemia. This is a quartet of elevated fasting glucose, high serum triglyceride, low HDL cholesterol level and hypertension, being characteristic of viscerally obese patients [28]. Each of these symptoms alone is risk factor for both cardiovascular diseases and cancers, and together they mean a multiple risk [28-30].

Hyperglycemia is advantageous for the unrestrained DNA synthesis of tumor cells. It provokes deliberation of free radicals causing derangements in both DNA and enzymes having important role in repair mechanisms [31, 32]. High serum glucose level leads to a non-enzymatic glycation of protein structures, and the glycated products enhance the deliberation of free radicals, cytokines and growth factors [33]. These signaling molecules play pivotal role in the inflammatory vascular damage and the atherogenic processes [34]. A prospective study on the role of glucose metabolism in breast cancer incidence justified that hyperglycemia among insulin resistant women exhibits direct correlation with mammary cancer risk [35].

Dyslipidemia is a complex disturbance of the lipid metabolism associated with insulin resistance and hyperinsulinemia [36]. Serum level of triglycerides shows close parallelism with insulin resistance, serum insulin level and BMI, whereas being inversely correlated with the high density lipoprotein (HDL) level.

Dyslipidemia in patients with metabolic syndrome have a great role in the development of cardiovascular diseases [37]. Correlation of dyslipidemia and malignant tumors was thoroughly studied in colorectal and breast cancer cases [38, 39]. Results of clinical examinations justified the close association between hypertriglyceridemia and breast cancer [40].

Hypertension usually shows close positive correlation with obesity, insulin resistance and hyperinsulinemia [41, 42]. Elevated insulin level is closely associated with increased activity of the sympathetic nervous system resulting in adrenergic vasoconstriction and hypertension [23, 43]. There are further crossroads between obesity and hypertension by means of hormonal regulation. Activation of the renin-angiotensin-aldosterone system and subsequent elevations in angiotensin II and aldosterone levels are frequently seen in metabolic syndrome [44]. In postmenopausal hypertension, changes in androgen/estrogen ratios favoring for androgens have been implicated to play an important causal role. After menopause, hypertension proved to be a strong risk factor for hormone dependent tumors as well, separately from obesity [45].

Metabolic syndrome is associated with increased risk for CVD and cancer risk and means increased mortality risk in postmenopausal cases [46-48]. Time-dependent covariate analyses indicated a positive association between the metabolic syndrome and breast cancer, due primarily to positive associations with serum glucose, serum triglycerides, and diastolic blood pressure [49].

Type-2 diabetes is the uncompensated phase of insulin resistance when the secretory capacity of insular β-cells becomes exhausted and the decreased serum insulin level results in hyperglycemia. The disrupted glucose homeostasis, the excessive formation of free radicals and the protein glycation depress the activities of the antioxidant scavengers and enzymes. These noxious processes cause serious damages in all biological structures even at a molecular level and promote the development of cardiovascular lesions [31, 50, 51]. The role of free radicals and oxidative stress in the process of carcinogenesis is a well-known fact [52, 53]. Type-2 diabetes seems to be an independent risk for cancer development [54-56].

Obesity Related Alterations in the Sexual Steroid Production

Obesity related insulin resistance and excessive insulin synthesis in women may contribute to ***hyperandrogenism*** and anovulatory infertility through several pathways as insulin is a potent regulator of sexual steroid production in the endocrine organs [57]. Hyperinsulinemia and excessive IGF-I supply stimulates *ovarian androgen production* at the expense of reduced estrogen synthesis [58]. High insulin level was found to increase the testosterone biosynthesis of human ovarian thecal cells deriving from insulin resistant, infertile women with polycystic ovarian syndrome (PCOS) [59]. Therapeutic improvement of insulin sensitivity and effective reduction of insulin secretion decreased ovarian cytochrome P450c17 alpha activity and normalized serum free testosterone level [60, 61]. A recent patent introduced a new metformin derivative as a therapeutic agent for treating metabolic syndrome, type-2 diabetes, PCOS and cancers depleted of gene P53 [62].

Hyperinsulinemia promotes *adrenal androgen synthesis* as well by means of increased adrenal sensitivity to adrenocorticotropin. At the same time, high insulin level may favor the *luteinizing hormone(LH) secretion of pituitary*. Increased LH level also stimulates androgen biosynthesis by the activation of adrenal gland and ovarian theca cells [63, 64]. Loss of the protective effects of estrogen in women with androgen excess may mediate premature cardiovascular lesions [18]. According to earlier hypotheses, breast cancer risk is increased not only in hyperandrogenic postmenopausal women, but also in premenopausal cases with mild hyperandrogenism and apparently normal (ovulatory) menstrual cycles [65]. In centrally obese, either premenopausal or postmenopausal women, excessive ovarian production of testosterone seems to be a genetically determined risk for breast cancer [66, 67].

Insulin resistance, hyperinsulinemia and excessive IGF-I activity mediate **defective estrogen synthesis** by counteraction to aromatase enzyme gene expression at cellular level. The aromatase enzyme complex catalyzes the conversion of androgens to estrogens in a wide variety of tissues. In premenopausal women, the ovaries are the principle sources of estradiol; by contrast, in postmenopausal women when the ovaries cease to produce estrogen, it is synthesized in a number of extragonadal sites [68]. These sites include the adipose tissue, breast, endometrium, bone, endothelium, aortic smooth muscle cells, and numerous locations in the brain. All these tissues, particularly breast and endometrium, have high estrogen demand and a local hormone synthesis helps to preserve their structural integrity and functional activity in spite of low circulatory estrogen levels [69].

In premenopausal insulin resistant women with type-2 diabetes, the ovaries exhibit decreased capacity to convert androgen to estrogen, probably due to a reduction of ovarian aromatase activity [70]. Conversely, in patients with either estrogen deficiency (aromatase deficiency) or estrogen resistance (estrogen receptor mutation) glucose intolerance, hyperinsulinemia and lipid abnormalities are concomittant alterations associated with excessive gonadotropin and androgen levels [71].

Estrogens decrease low grade inflammatory reactions and may in parallel reduce the glucocorticoid responses. Low estrogen levels after menopause allow the predominance of glucocorticoids and the manifestation of the metabolic syndrome. These observations suggest that the disturbed equilibrium between sex hormones and glucocorticoids may be a critical element in the manifestation of metabolic syndrome-related pathologies [72].

Inflammatory and Metabolic Dysfunctions of Adipose Tissue in Visceral Obesity

Visceral adipose tissue has important functions in energy homeostasis, metabolic equilibrium, immune responses and in the regulation of cell proliferation. Secretion of signaling molecules; adipokines regulates the cellular microenvironment both locally and systemically [9, 73, 74].

The chronic low grade inflammation associated with obesity is an important player in the development of vascular lesions [75]. Increased IGF-I level may mediate the inflammation of adipose tissue *via* its effects on immunologically active cells including macrophages and T cells. [76]. IGF-I may provoke macrophage migration and invasion and increased production of proinflammatory cytokines having great role in tumor development and progression.

Adipokines include unique products of fatty tissue known as *adipocytokines*; such as leptin, adiponectin resist in, *etc.* [77]. Healthy equilibrium of adipocytokines means protective effect against cardiovascular diseases [78]. Leptin biosynthesis is in close direct correlation with insulin level and this may explain the increased leptin levels observed in obesity [79]. High leptin concentrations may constitute a possible link relating obesity and breast cancer promoting the invasion and migration of tumor cells [80]. Conversely, obesity may downregulate the secretion of adiponectin, an adipokine with anti-inflammatory, insulin sensitizing and anti-tumor properties [81]. The balances of lept in as well as the adiponect in concentrations are critical factors in obesity related cancer genesis [82].

Proinflammatory cytokines (TNF-α, IL-6, IL-8) formed in excessive adipose tissue mass increase the production of nitric oxide (NO) and other members of reactive oxygen species (ROS). Accumulation of cytokines and ROS further contributes to insulin resistance resulting in elevated circulating glucose and free fatty acid levels, which may contribute to atherosclerotic vascular lesions [83]. All signaling molecules of fatty tissue including cytokines, hormones and growth factors are involved in the regulation of the proliferation, invasion and metastatic spread of tumor cells [84]. Proinflammatory cytokines within the tumor microenvironment correlate with growth, increased invasiveness and poor prognosis in many types of cancer [85].

PROTECTIVE EFFECTS OF ESTROGEN AGAINST OBESITY AND OBESITY ASSOCIATED ALTERATIONS

Out of several hormones affecting body mass and adipose tissue deposition, estrogens promote, maintain and control the ideal distribution of body fat [82]. These steroids are known to regulate differentiation and metabolism of adipocytes as well. Estrogen deficiency and defective estrogen signaling results in obesity with increasing adipose tissue mass, preferentially in visceral location [21, 86].

Anti-Obesity Effects of Estrogen

Estrogen regulates the metabolism, differentiation, growth and cell kinetic mechanisms of adipocytes. In healthy premenopausal women central adipocytes show higher insulin sensitivity and exhibit a higher turnover rate despite similar fat content as compared with male cases [87]. Conversely, after menopause, decreased ovarian estrogen synthesis results in increasing insulin resistance in central adipocytes and higher fasting insulin levels conferring increased risk for metabolic and cardiovascular diseases [88, 89]. In experiments, estradiol is able to inhibit the glucocorticoid production in rodent adipocytes of mesenteric origin, providing novel insight into the anti-obesity mechanism of estrogen effect [90].

Obesity and overweight are important concomitants of insulin resistance and they are strongly associated with disturbed equilibrium of male to female sexual hormone concentrations in women [91]. Healthy estrogen predominance in women induces subcutaneous gluteofemoral adipose tissue deposition [88]. Conversely, androgen excess and deficient estrogen synthesis exhibits close correlation with visceral obesity both in pre- and postmenopausal women [92]. In young women with PCOS, there are several advantages of treatment with oral contraceptives, including protection from the development of endometrial carcinoma, regularization of menses, amelioration of hirsutism, acne and obesity [93]. Similarly, in obese postmenopausal women with or without type-2 diabetes, HRT reduces abdominal adiposity and insulin resistance [94] and decreases the risk for obesity associated breast cancer [95].

Anti-Atherogenic and Anti-Hypertensive Effects of Estrogen

Healthy premenopausal women are typically protected from cardiovascular diseases and hypertension as compared with men and this has been hypothesized to be because of the protective effects of estrogens. Conversely, obese, diabetic young women, and postmenopausal cases may lose this protected state as their bioavailable estradiol levels are strongly reduced [18].

Estrogen may have crucial role in the maintenance of normal serum lipid levels. Postmenopausal women have higher total cholesterol, LDL cholesterol and triglyceride levels, whereas lower HDL cholesterol levels as compared with premenopausal cases. These changes may be regarded as a shift toward a more atherogenic lipid profile in estrogen deficient milieu [96]. Postmenopausal estrogen therapy may reduce the risk of cardiovascular disease and this beneficial effect may be mediated in part by favorable changes in plasma lipid levels [97].

Estrogens have important regulatory role in the hepatic lipid metabolism as well. In aged rats, estradiol administration lowered the level of lipid peroxidation and improved the dysfunction parameters of the liver [98].

Estradiol has cardiovascular protective impact by its anti-hypertensive activity as well. Estrogens can downregulate components of the renin-angiotensin system (RAS) and reduce the expression and activity of angiotensin I-converting enzyme [99, 100]. Estradiol inhibits the excessive synthesis of vasoconstrictor endothelin and improves endothelial dysfunction in ovariectomized female spontaneously hypertensive rats [96, 101]. In the pathogenesis of postmenopausal hypertension increased androgen to estrogen ratio may be associated with the activation of renin-angiotensin and endothelin systems [102].

Clinical and experimental studies support that estradiol has also antioxidant activities [103, 104] that may be effective against inflammatory lesions, atherosclerotic vessel injuries and malignancies.

Antidiabetogenic Impacts of Estrogen

Estrogens have beneficial effects on the energy metabolism and glucose homeostasis by means of several pathways [105]. Estrogens advantageously regulate the insulin production capacity of the *pancreatic islet cells* [89]. Estrogen receptor alpha (ER-α) activation promotes β-cell mass survival and insulin biosynthesis in diabetic and obese cases, whereas ERβ activation improves glucose stimulated insulin secretion [106]. Estrogen administration seems to be a therapeutic avenue to preserve functional β-cell mass in patients with diabetes mellitus.

In the liver, estrogen regulates insulin sensitivity by the balanced activation of glycogen synthase and glycolytic enzymes to maintain the equilibrium of glycogen synthesis and glycogenolysis. In ER-α knockout mice, hepatic insulin resistance was associated with decreased glucose uptake in skeletal muscles [107].

In the peripheral tissues ERs advantageously modulate the insulin stimulated glucose uptake through regulation of the phosphorylation of insulin receptor protein. In hyperinsulinemia, high concentrations of estradiol can inhibit the excessive insulin signaling in adipocytes [108], which may be a safety impact both against pathological glucose uptake and dangerous mitogenic activity.

ERs have crucial roles in cellular glucose uptake by regulation of intracellular glucose transporters (GLUTs) and enhancing both GLUT4 expression and translocation [109]. In human adipocytes GLUT4 abundance is highly correlated with insulin responsiveness. In women with PCOS, decrease in insulin stimulated glucose uptake was associated with reduced amount of GLUT4 on adipocyte membrane [110].

Estrogens and ER signals have pivotal role in the regulation of growth hormone (GH) activity by means of modulation of its secretion and cellular GH receptor function. Estrogens play a major and positive role in the regulation of GH-IGF-I axis in both genders [111], which may be in close correlation with their antidiabetogenic and anticancer capacities.

Postmenopausal hormone replacement therapy (HRT) reduced abdominal obesity, insulin resistance, new-onset diabetes, hyperlipidemia, blood pressure, adhesion molecules and procoagulant factors in women without diabetes and reduced insulin resistance and fasting glucose in women with diabetes [94].

Regulation of Adipokine Secretion, Inflammatory Reactions and Growth Factor Activity by Estrogen

Low grade systemic inflammation may be associated with estrogen deficient states, namely menopause and ovariectomy. At early stages of estrogen deficiency estrogen administration decreased the inflammation associated risk of developing cardiovascular disease [112]. Nevertheless, estradiol may contribute even to the vascular healing process and to the prevention of lumen restenosis in atherogenic arteries. It improves reendothelialization through ER-α activation and decreases smooth muscle cell migration and proliferation through ER-β stimulation [113].

Phytoestrogens may advantageously influence the level of adipokines in insulin resistant women. In postmenopausal cases, diet, physical exercise and daily oral intake of soy isoflavones had a beneficial lowering effect on serum leptin, and TNF-α levels and showed a significant increase in mean serum levels of adiponectin [114]. Epidemiologic studies support that phytoestrogen rich foods may be beneficial consumed before or during adolescence for the prevention of breast cancer [115].

Estrogen advantageously regulates serum levels of available growth factors. In clinical studies estradiol lowered, whereas testosteron increased total IGF-I level and estradiol specifically suppressed unbound, free IGF-I level [116]. Crosstalk between estrogen receptors and growth factor (IGF-I, EGF, VEGF) receptor signaling pathways is well-known both in healthy tissues and malignancies [117, 118]. Nevertheless, estradiol may induce both growth stimulation and growth inhibition depending on the ratio and activity of ERs and GFRs [119].

The presumed synergistic contribution of ERs and GFRs to cancer development and progression would be a permanent danger without contraregulatory impact. Inhibition of growth factor signaling in apparently ER-negative breast cancer cells successfully restored ER expression suggesting a dynamic, inverse relationship between the two receptor systems [120]. Moreover, excessive EGF predominance suppressed both ER-α protein concentration and gene transcription activity in the human breast cancer cell line MCF-7 [121]. These results suggest rather an alternative role of estrogen and growth factor actions in tumor cell proliferation.

CORRELATIONS BETWEEN GRADE AND DISTRIBUTION OF ADIPOSITY AND OBESITY RELATED MORBIDITY

Fat deposition is thoroughly affected by male to female sexual steroid level [88]. Circulating estrogen level may be the key regulator in mediating differences in adipose tissue distribution between pre- and postmenopausal women [122]. In *obese premenopausal women*, peripheral, subcutaneous adiposity is typical and there is a lower incidence of obesity associated dysmetabolism. By contrast, in *obese postmenopausal cases*, circulating levels of estrogen are dramatically decreased and adipose tissue distribution becomes more male-like. Predominance of visceral adiposity and the associated metabolic and hormonal disorders mean high risk for obesity related diseases, included cancers [9].

The most important data characterizing the grade of obesity are body mass index (BMI) and weight in kilogram [123-125] reflecting general adiposity. Knowing the hormonal and metabolic background of the diverse distribution of adipose tissue, BMI or body weight in kilogram may not correctly reflect the correlations among obesity, hormonal disturbances and cancer risk in young women [126]. Body circumference measurements; such as hip (HC), waist (WC) and waist to hip ratio (WHR) inform about the regional distribution of fatty tissue deposition [127-129] so as to quantify the mass of visceral abdominal fat and the metabolic risk of patients.

Magnetic resonance imaging (MRI) was used to quantify separately the mass of visceral and subcutaneous abdominal fat depositions in obese adolescent girls [130]. Mass of visceral fat was highly correlated with insulin secretion and insulin resistance. Conversely, abdominal subcutaneous fat mass measured by MRI did not show close correlation with the quantified indicators of insulin resistance.

In conclusion, neither BMI nor circumference measurement may exactly separate the metabolically indifferent, subcutaneous fat and the dangerous visceral fat, which may partially explain the controversial correlations between obesity grade and cancer risk.

LIFELONG CHANGES IN THE HORMONAL STATUS OF OBESE WOMEN AND THEIR RELATION TO OBESITY ASSOCIATED MORBIDITIES

Circulating female sexual steroid levels and fertility continuously decrease during the life of women. The ability to conceive is at its peak in young women under 30 years of age with a continuous decline from the fourth decade, which suggests decreasing fertility even in the premenopausal phase [131]. Menopause at 50-51 years of age means a sudden break in ovarian estrogen synthesis and confers further decline in the circulating hormone level.

In premenopausal women, the good equilibrium of sex steroid synthesis defines somatic health and reproductive capacity, whereas good, symptom-free adaptation to the estrogen deficient environment is a prerequisite of postmenopausal health. Changes in the hormonal equilibrium during women's lives strongly influence the obesity associated risk for CVD and malignancies (Table **1**).

Table 1: Lifelong changes in the hormonal status of obese women and their risk for CVD and malignancies (Adapted from: Suba Z. Circulatory estrogen level protects against breast cancer in obese women. Recent Pat Anticancer Drug Discov 2013; 8(2): 154-67. Review)

Life Periods of Obese Women	Estrogen Level	Insulin Resistance	Risk for CVD and Malignancies
Children	↓	↑	↑
Adolescent Girls	↓↓	↑↑	↑↑
Premenopausal Women			
type-2 diabetes	↓	↑	↑
anovulation	↓	↑	↑
nulliparity	↓	↑	↑
contraceptive use	↑	↓	↓
multiparity	↑	↓	↓
in vitro fertililization	↑	↓	↓
Postmenopausal Women			
HRT user	↑	↓	↓
non HRT user	↓	↑	↑
type-2 diabetes	↓↓	↑↑	↑↑
hysterectomy	↓↓	↑↑	↑↑

Obesity Associated Hormonal Alterations in Childhood and Adolescence and their Prediction for Obesity Related Diseases

Obesity is a detrimental disorder and may not be protective against malignancies even in children. *Childhood obesity* is associated with insulin resistance and hyperinsulinemia mediating risks for chronic diseases and cancer in the adult life [132]. Many factors of metabolic syndrome, such as elevated glucose level, hypertension, high triglyceride and low HDL-cholesterol level even type-2 diabetes might occur in these young prepubertal obese cases [133].

Before menopause, breast cancer incidence is relatively low and adiposity in childhood is erroneously regarded as a protective factor against this tumor conferred by the obesity associated defective estrogen-synthesis [20]. Some studies suppose a definite key age; for example 10 years when breast cancer "protective" obesity turns to harmful between the ages of 10 and 20 years as a prediction of elevated breast cancer risk in the premenopausal life [134]. Nevertheless, finding a key age at which obesity in young girls turns from a cancer protective to a cancer promoting agent seemed to be unsuccessful.

Obesity in puberty with extreme somatic growth and explosion-like sexual development means a great challenge for the entire metabolic and hormonal systems. In obese children, puberty becomes a more serious danger for insulin resistant states as compared with normal weight cases [135, 136]. In obese adolescent patients, increased insulin resistance does not return to prepubertal values at the end of puberty and represents high risk for adult metabolic syndrome, type-2 diabetes and for their complications [133, 137].

In adolescent girls, obesity associated metabolic storms are related to abnormal ovarian sexual steroidgenesis as well, resulting in excessive androgen and defective estrogen production and greater frequency of irregular, anovulatory cycles [138-140]. High serum androgen concentrations developing in puberty are preserved into adulthood and are reflected by defective fertility patterns at least until 30 years of age [139, 140]. This observation may be in concordance with an increased premenopausal breast cancer risk of delayed first childbearing [141, 142].

Equilibrium of sexual hormone production and the development of regular cycles are prerequisites not only for reproduction but also for somatic health in women [21, 143-145]. Pathological alterations in the critical period of puberty, such as obesity endangering both the fertility and survival of women might not be protective against cancer initiation in either pre- or postmenopausal cases. In conclusion, obesity related endocrine alterations in children, adolescents and at young age might really be defining factors for later diseases, being not protective, but rather highly dangerous [20].

Correlations Between Obesity and Estrogen Deficient States in Premenopausal Women

Premenopausal obesity is frequently associated with decreased estrogen level, anovulation and infertility. In premenopausal women there are many pathologic states predisposing to mild or moderate estrogen deficiency. Clinical signs of ovarian insufficiency are the long or irregular menstrual cycles [19].

In obese premenopausal women with type-2 diabetes, cycle anomalies or amenorrhoea are typical findings as the insulin resistance associated defective ovarian aromatase activity results in decreased circulating estrogen levels [70].

Nulliparity may be associated with ovulatory disorders in the majority of cases and means an increased breast cancer risk [146, 147]. Coexistence of nulliparity and overweight or obesity may amplify each other's effect on increasing breast cancer risk having strong synergism [146]. By contrast, multiparity in women means a protective effect against cancers of the highly estrogen dependent breast, endometrium and ovaries [148, 149]. This may be attributed to the healthy equilibrium of female sexual steroid production associated with good fertility. Recent results suggest health protective effects of fertility medication as well. Before *in vitro* fertilization (IVF) overall cancer risk was found to be markedly increased among infertile women in a great study in Sweden [150]. Conversely, after IVF assisted childbirth, cancer risk was significantly decreased mainly due to a lower than expected risk for breast and cervical cancers.

Obesity and overweight are characteristic concomitants of polycystic ovarian syndrome (PCOS), more than 50% of such cases are obese. PCOS is a complex disorder that is presumably caused by a large number of different genetic abnormalities and it is the most common endocrinopathy of women in the reproductive age [23]. It seems to be a pathological model of hormonal and metabolic alterations of postmenopausal status in premenopausal women. PCOS may usually be manifested by menstrual disorders, anovulation, infertility, and obesity or overweight. Nevertheless, polycystic ovaries are common findings in symptom-free women with normal menses as well, only the laboratory findings of hyperinsulinemia and hyperandrogenism reveal the early phase of metabolic and hormonal alterations [151, 152].

Dysmetabolism and hyperandrogenism of obese PCOS cases mean high risk for premature hypertension, cardiovascular disease and malignancies in the highly estrogen dependent female organ triad; the endometrium, breast and ovaries [20, 144]. In young, obese, infertile, nulliparous women the high prevalence of endometrial cancer is frequently associated with synchronous primary cancers of the ovary or breast [153, 154].

Earlier, some authors presumed that elevated estrogen levels unopposed by progestin continuously stimulate estrogen receptors in women with PCOS. It seemed to be an explanation for the high risk of endometrial and breast cancers observed in these cases based on the concept of the carcinogenic capacity of estrogen [155]. Recently, insulin resistance and hyperinsulinemia in PCOS patients are regarded as concomitants of high ovarian and adrenal androgen synthesis at the expense of estrogen deficiency [156].

How can we explain the preferential cancer risk of breast, endometrium and ovaries in obese women with fertility disorders? In premenopausal cases, slight or moderate decrease in circulating female sexual steroid levels may be enough to block the delicate mechanism of ovulation. At the same time, a slightly estrogen deficient milieu confers preferential cancer risk for the female organ triad having high estrogen demand [20, 21, 144].

In PCOS cases, hormone treatment by oral contraceptives reduces the volume of cystic ovaries, decreases testosterone secretion and there are favorable effects on carbohydrate and lipid metabolism as well [157]. Epidemiologic studies have confirmed that combined oral contraceptives provide substantial protection against endometrial and ovarian cancers in the endangered anovulatory women [158]. A recent patent disclosed a method for treating hyperandrogenism and associated conditions, including PCOS by a fatty acid ester of estrogen or an estrogen derivative compound [159]. This therapy seems to be more advantageous against the dangerous dysmetabolism of PCOS cases than oral contraceptive administration.

Hyperprolactinemia is also associated with obesity, cycle disorders, reproductive dysfunction and hyperandrogenism in women, however, it should be delineated from PCOS and other disorders related to androgen excess. Weight gain and obesity is characteristic in hyperprolactinemia, suggesting that prolactin or the associated hormonal disturbances might also be modulators of body composition and body weight [160]. In a population based cohort study the allover cancer risk was elevated in patients with hyperprolactinemia [161]. Central obesity and fatty liver is common in women with Turner syndrome suffering of premature ovarian failure and estrogen deficiency when compared with age matched normal controls [162].

Summarizing the pathologies in estrogen deficient premenopausal women, a high prevalence of weight gain and obesity are the characteristic, common concomitants of sexual hormonal imbalance in spite of the diverse etiologies.

Correlations Between Obesity and Estrogen Loss at Menopause

For women aged 55-65 years, weight gain is one of their major health risks [2]. Many studies have focused on the question of whether midlife weight gain is simply an age related alteration or may be attributed to the hormonal changes that occur in relation to menopause [163, 164]. Effects of the loss of ovarian hormone production on body weight and body composition are thoroughly studied in both animal models and human populations.

In experimental mice, loss of ovarian function promoted a diet-independent increase in adipose tissue mass and associated dysmetabolic pathologies. Oophorectomized mice exhibit decreased energy expenditure without concomitant change in energy intake, resulting in hypertrophy and inflammation of adipose tissue as well as development of fatty liver [165]. By contrast, estradiol supplementation in oophorectomized mice supplied protection from hepatic steatosis, insulin resistance and adipose tissue hypertrophy [166].

Preferential accumulation of central fat is a special consequence of estrogen deficiency that was supported by studies on aromatase gene knock-out (ArKO) mice, being incapable of synthesizing endogenous estrogens [167]. Estradiol replacement in female ArKO mice reduced the volume of adipocytes without changes in their fatty acid synthesis. This observation suggests that the lower lipid uptake from the circulation may be the main mechanism by which estradiol regulates fat accumulation.

The prevalence of abdominal obesity is almost double that of general obesity and shows an increasing trend as women age. In the US, 65.5% of women aged 40-59 years and 73.8% of women over the age of 60 exhibited central adiposity in 2008 [8]. Studies on the correlation between menopause and changes in body composition in Chinese women suggest that menopause has an independent effect on the increase in both fat mass and abdominal adiposity [168].

Results of studies on both experimental animals and postmenopausal women justified that loss of ovarian function promotes a diet-independent increase in adipose tissue deposition particularly in the metabolically dangerous abdominal location [2]. Increasing body weight during the menopausal transition aggravates the menopausal symptoms as well. Obesity proved to be an independent risk factor for severe menopausal symptoms [169] suggesting that excessive fat mass disturbs the hormonal and metabolic adaptation to the menopausal transition.

Good hormonal equilibrium in premenopausal cases may be associated with later age at natural menopause. A later menopause has been associated with non-smoking, regular alcohol consumption and strenuous exercise, which all are advantageous for estrogen synthesis. By contrast, as smoking and type-2 diabetes have a decreasing effect on estrogen production they may predict an earlier menopause [170].

Bilateral oophorectomy is applied as a supposed risk reduction strategy in BRCA mutation carrier women, although data on its long term effects are not available. The joint effect of obesity and early oophorectomy on mortality was significantly greater than expected. Obese women who had an oophorectomy at less than 40 years were more than twice more likely to die than their age matched non obese controls, attributed particularly to CVD [171]. Obesity associated defective estrogen synthesis and a further sudden estrogen loss caused by early artificial menopause may explain this increased mortality.

The results of studies on women using HRT show a marked reduction in central adiposity [172, 173]. Studies mostly indicate a decrease in overall fat mass with both estrogen and estrogen-progestin therapy, improved insulin sensitivity and a lower rate of development of type-2 diabetes [174, 175].

CHANGING CONCEPTS CONCERNING THE ASSOCIATIONS OF HORMONE REPLACEMENT THERAPY AND WOMEN'S HEALTH

From the early 80s clinical and epidemiological studies increasingly pointed to elevated breast, endometrial and ovarian cancer risk of hormone replacement therapy (HRT) for postmenopausal women [144]. Principal results from the Women's Health Initiative (WHI) randomized controlled trial in 2002 established that overall health risks, particularly that of breast cancer exceeded benefits from use of combined estrogen plus progestin therapy among postmenopausal US women [176]. This publication led to a sharp decline in postmenopausal HRT use and many women unnecessarily refused hormone treatment.

A breakthrough in breast cancer research came in 2010 when in San Antonio Canadian scientists reported on the re-evaluation of the earlier results of original WHI Hormone Replacement Therapy Trial. After a proper selection of same patients and controls according to their risk factors, HRT use proved to be not only safe but strongly protective against breast cancer as well as for many other aspects of women's health [177]. Recently, great HRT studies on homogenously selected hysterectomised cases and controls yielded a strikingly unexpected breast cancer protective effect of one-armed estrogen treatment [178, 179]. As the health risk of women after hysterectomy may be near uniformly high because of their abrupt, shocking hormone deprivation, these methodologically strong studies resulted in correct conclusions [Ciculatory, Interplay].

The Global Consensus Statement on Menopausal Hormone Therapy means a milestone in core recommendations regarding HRT [180]. Representatives of major regional menopause societies cautiously but progressively established that in women with premature ovarian insufficiency, systemic HRT is recommended at least until the average age of natural menopause. Moreover, standard-dose estrogen-alone HRT use was regarded as advantageous measure to decrease coronary heart disease and all-cause mortality in postmenopausal women.

CORRELATIONS BETWEEN ESTROGEN SIGNALING AND LIFESTYLE FACTORS AFFECTING BODY WEIGHT

The dramatic increase in the occurrence of overweight and obesity over the past several decades is attributed in part to changes in dietary and lifestyle habits, such as rapidly changing diets, increased availability of high-energy foods, and reduced physical activity of people in both developed and developing countries [181, 182].

As estrogens have beneficial effects on energy metabolism and glucose homeostasis, sufficient estrogen exposure and intact signal transduction of estrogen receptors (ERs) have great role in defensive processes against obesity and insulin resistance [183]. Body mass and insulin sensitivity are highly defined by food intake and physical activity and both of them are in close correlation with estrogenic regulation. These associations explain the impact of defective estrogen signaling on the increased risk of obesity, type 2 diabetes, cardiovascular disease and malignancy in both infertile young and postmenopausal women [21].

In the central nervous system hypothalamic nuclei are the key regulators of food intake and energy expenditure by means of their estrogen receptors [184]. In animal experiments ERα activation results in a decrease in food intake [185], whereas silencing of ERα and predominance of ERβ leads to hyperphagia, obesity, decreased glucose tolerance and reduced energy expenditure [186]. Central effects of ERs seem to have a balanced interplay regarding the maintenance of ideal body mass with continuous adaptation to the changing intra- and extracellular stimuli [183]. Emerging evidences suggest that diets rich in phytoestrogens (isoflavones and lignans), namely soy protein and flaxseed, may have beneficial effects on many aspects of diabetes and obesity [187, 188]. These findings suggest that long-term substitution of animal protein by vegetable protein in a low-energy diet may provide additional benefit for weight reduction in obese subjects. Several nutritional intervention studies in animals and humans indicate that consumption of soy protein reduces body weight and fat mass in addition to lowering plasma cholesterol and triglyceride levels [189].

In animal models of obesity, soy protein ingestion limits or reduces body fat accumulation and improves insulin resistance. In ovariectomized monkeys, both dietary soy protein and estrogen replacement therapy improved cardiovascular risk factors and decreased aortic cholesterol ester content [190].

In obese people, dietary soy protein also reduces body weight and body fat mass in addition to reducing plasma lipid levels and improving insulin sensitivity [189]. Phytoestrogens, such as isoflavones and lignans may also exert beneficial effects on tissue lipid content through their antioxidant actions [188].

Soy in diet seems to be beneficial and preventive against breast cancer if consumed in early life before puberty or during adolescence based on the results of immigrant and epidemiological studies [115]. Prepubertal estradiol and genistein exposures may reduce later breast cancer risk even in BRCA gene mutation carrier cases by inducing a persistent, effective upregulation of the tumor suppressor gene [191]. Phytoestrogen containing diet is highly protective as regards breast cancer in adult women as well, based on epidemiological observations [192]. Soybean extract with phytoestrogen component also proved to be useful as therapeutic agent for solid cancers, such as mammary malignancies [193].

Skeletal muscle mass is responsible for 75% of the insulin-mediated glucose uptake in the body and consequently, physical activity is in direct correlation with insulin sensitivity [194]. The majority of literary data support the fact that strong physical exercise has beneficial effect on insulin sensitivity in normal as well as insulin resistant populations [195, 196]. When energy intake exceeds energy expenditure over a prolonged period of time, the result is a positive energy balance, which leads to the development of obesity.

Adequate levels of regular physical activity appear to be important for prevention of weight gain and treatment of obesity. Physical activity also appears to have an independent, advantageous effect on health, suggesting that adequate levels of physical exercise may also counteract the negative influence of excessive body weight on health outcomes [197]. Health advantage of regular physical activity is equivocal and exercise plays pivotal role in the prevention of breast cancer both in obese and lean women [198-200].

Sufficient estrogen exposure advantageously improves cellular glucose uptake through the regulation of insulin receptor signaling and by the promotion of expression and intracellular translocation of glucose transporters [201, 202]. During estrogen loss in both perimenopausal and postmenopausal periods, muscle strength exhibits a striking decline that can be reversed by hormone replacement therapy (HRT), suggesting that estrogens are important players in muscle physiology [203, 204].

Nevertheless, there are controversial literary data concerning the correlations between health improving physical exercise and estrogen level in women. The traditional concept supports a role of estrogens in the development and growth of breast cancer. Lowered estrogen exposure associated with physical activity was erroneously presumed to reduce breast cancer recurrence and new diagnoses in high-risk women [205, 206]. Further study supplied evidences for an inverse association between physical activity and breast cancer risk, which was stronger for mammary carcinogenesis in postmenopausal than in premenopausal women [198]. This valuable observation suggests that physical activity rather increases estrogen levels, which exhibits higher defense for estrogen deficient older women as compared with young cases.

Recently, physical activity seems to be a potential intervention for treating women with reduced estrogen function [207]. Weight loss alone did not improve glucose utilization and insulin sensitivity in postmenopausal women; however, when weight loss was coupled with exercise training, it resulted in a significant improvement in both outcomes [208]. Healthy diet alone was not effective at reducing circulating inflammatory markers in obese postmenopausal women; however, when coupled with exercise training, there was a significant reduction in these same cytokines [209].

GENDER RELATED DIFFERENCES IN THE PREVALENCE OF OBESITY ASSOCIATED CARDIOVASCULAR DISEASES

Recent data have shown that physical activity improves not only the metabolic dysfunctions but also the survival rates of postmenopausal women with breast cancer [210]. These data suggest that exercise training is an advantageous intervention that is critical to women who clinically are experiencing reductions in estrogen function.

Prevalence of cardiovascular diseases (CVDs) is strongly associated to sexual steroid equilibrium. In healthy premenopausal women female sexual steroid hormones ensure a strong defense against hypertension, CVD and cerebrovascular events as compared with age matched men. This striking difference has been hypothesized to be because of the protective effects of estrogens [18]. However, even a moderate decrease in the bioavailable estradiol level associated with obesity, type-2 diabetes or polycystic ovarian syndrome; markedly increases the risk for arteriosclerotic morbidities in young women [69, 211]. After menopause, women become estrogen deficient due to ovarian senescence resulting in reduced level of circulating estrogens. Obese postmenopausal women have more male-like fatty tissue deposition concentrated in the abdominal, visceral location attributed to the increased male to female sexual steroid ratio [9].

The health implications of obesity derive from its correlations with the development and progression of several health derangements and diseases. Cardiovascular morbidity, which is the preponderant killer of women and men, is strongly influenced by obesity [212]. The Society for Women's Health Research convened a workshop for obesity and cardiovascular disease experts in November 2005 to identify the gaps in scientific knowledge and crucial next steps in research related to sex differences in obesity and cardiovascular disease [212].

Obesity is associated with increased cardiovascular disease risk factors in some, but not all, individuals, and blood pressure responses to weight loss are also heterogeneous. There is an increasing recognition of a metabolically healthy but obese phenotype, observed in 9% of obese men and 16% of obese women [213]. The low rate of cardiometabolic abnormalities in these metabolically healthy obese individuals is not explained by diet composition or the level of physical activity, highlighting the importance of genetic predisposition to obesity associated co-morbidities [214]. The higher prevalence of metabolically healthy women than men among obese cases may partially be explained by the predominance of protective estrogen over androgen in healthy premenopausal cases. Estrogens maintain and control the ideal fat deposition and in the majority of obese premenopausal cases the metabolically inert subcutaneous fat accumulation is characteristic [88].

Conversely, in severely insulin resistant young obese women with type-2 diabetes, or polycystic ovarian syndrome (PCOS) the concomitant central adiposity and increased cardiometabolic risk may be attributed to a decreased level of circulating estrogens [20, 70].

The polycystic ovarium syndrome (PCOS) in young, premenopausal women is an important pathologic example of the correlations between the imbalance of sexual steroid synthesis and insulin resistance [23, 143]. The cardinal symptoms are anovulation, infertility, hirsutism and obesity. In the background, hyperinsulinism, hyperandrogenism and defective estrogen synthesis are the main laboratory findings [58].

PCOS is not only an infertility disease but is also a systemic health risk with long-term consequences. In young women PCOS may predict an increased risk of both metabolic syndrome and type-2 diabetes [215, 216]. Similarly, among premenopausal women with type-2 diabetes, an increased prevalence of PCOS could be observed [217]. Increased prevalence of diabetes mellitus, hypertension and cardiac complications were observed in a follow up study of a Dutch population of women with PCOS [215]. Close associations between PCOS and premature coronary and aortic atherosclerosis were revealed in middle-aged women [218]. Increased incidence of coronary artery disease and of cerebrovascular events are directly related to androgen excess in women with PCOS [211].

A study was undertaken on 155 consecutive obese male and female patients enrolled in a weight loss programme in West Virginia [219]. The purposes of this study were to assess associations between cardiovascular disease risk factors in obese individuals and to determine the clinical predictors of a hypotensive response to weight loss in men and women. Before weight loss, obese men exhibited higher cardiovascular disease risk factors (body mass indices, systolic and diastolic blood pressures, serum glucose, and lower HDL cholesterol) than did women. Among women, but not men, cardiovascular disease risk factors preferentially clustered in individuals with higher waist-to-hip ratios. Furthermore, in response to weight loss, a high original waist-to-hip ratio in women was associated with a greater reduction in systolic blood pressure in contrast to men.

Central adiposity as reflected in waist-to-hip ratios, proved to be a more robust risk factor for cardiovascular diseases in female than in male obese patients [219]. Considering the higher estrogen demand of cardiovascular system in women compared to man, androgen excess and hyperinsulinemia associated with abdominal obesity means stronger cardiometabolic risk in women than in men [21, 69].

In the Nurses' Health Study, high body mass index was strongly associated with death due to cardio-hypertensive diseases (CHD). The risk of CHD was over three times higher among women with a body mass index of 29 or higher. Much of this increased risk could be attributed to the harmful influences of obesity on blood pressure, glucose tolerance and lipid levels [220]. A report from the Framingham offspring study suggests that the prevalence of risk factors for CHD rises rapidly at body mass index levels of over $20kg/m^2$ [221].

OBESITY RELATED CANCER RISK AMONG WOMEN AS COMPARED WITH MEN

As estrogen is the predominant sexual steroid in women, maintenance of the integrity and physiologic functions of female organs require much higher estrogen level compared to male organs [144]. The defensive effect of estrogen against cardiovascular diseases and malignancies in the reproductive period of healthy women is highly reflected by their lower morbidity as compared with men at the same age period. This preventive effect is marked even in the majority of obese young cases when the fat deposition is predominantly subcutaneous and metabolically indifferent [20]. Conversely, in obese postmenopausal women with predominance of central adiposity or with concomitant type-2 diabetes the reduced aromatase activity mediates defective estrogen synthesis [20], and both CVD and cancer morbidity increases [9, 18, 77]. High estrogen demand of female organs may explain why in insulin resistant states the associated estrogen deficiency means higher overall cancer risk factor among women in comparison to men [21, 222, 223].

Gender related overall cancer risk of obesity exhibits great differences, depending on the included malignancies, on the ratio of pre- and postmenopausal women and on the geographic location of the performed studies.

In Canada, a population based case-control study was conducted on 21,022 incident cases of 19 types of malignancies and on 5,039 controls aged 20-76 years, to examine the association between obesity and the risks of various cancers [224]. Compared with people with normal weight (≤ 25 kg/m^2) obese men and women (≥ 30 kg/m^2) had an increased risk of overall cancer (OR: 1.34). In general, excessive body mass accounted for 7.7% of all malignancies in Canada; 9.7% among men and 5.9% among women. This study provided further evidences that obesity increases the risk of overall malignancy, different lymphoid tumors and many types of cancers. The higher prevalence of obesity associated malignancies among men as compared with women may be attributed to the wide age range of included cases (20-76 yrs) with many premenopausal women having a relatively protected status against cancer. Close correlation between postmenopausal status and increased obesity associated cancer risk was stressed only in breast tumor cases.

Quite inversely, a population based cohort study in Northern Sweden provided evidences that women are highly endangered by obesity related cancer risk, whereas men were not markedly affected. [225]. Effect of body mass index (BMI) on overall cancer risk and on the risk of several common cancer types was analyzed. Women with BMI $\geq$ 27.1 had a 29% higher risk of developing any malignancy as compared with women within normal weight range. In northern Sweden, up to 7% of all cancers were attributable to overweight and obesity in women. Individual cancer sites most strongly related to obesity in women were the highly estrogen dependent endometrium and ovary as well as the colon. In men, there was no significant association of BMI with overall cancer risk; however, obese men were at increased risk of developing kidney and colon cancer.

Geographic differences may have a great role in the contradictory correlations between obesity and gender related cancer morbidity. Among European countries marching at the head in the rank of female overall cancer morbidity and mortality, northern regions are conspicuously highly represented, such as; Denmark, Iceland, Norway and Sweden [226]. By contrast, countries with highest male cancer incidence and mortality do not exhibit accumulation in special geographic location. This excessive female risk for overall cancer morbidity and mortality in Northern countries suggests that women have peculiar susceptibility to certain cancerogenic agents in Northern regions owing to their special hormonal features [227].

A recent study revealed that poor light exposure in northern countries may provoke deleterious metabolic and hormonal alterations through increased melatonin secretion, such as; insulin resistance and deficiencies of estrogen, thyroxin and vitamin D [228]. Each of these disorders confers excessive cancer risk and the darkness associated decrease in estrogen levels might preferentially endanger the obese dysmetabolic women in Northern Sweden.

Based on these findings, studies on obesity associated cancer morbidity should be concentrated for the inhabitants of restricted regions with the similar geographic longitude. Large European or American cohort studies assembling the cases and controls from several centers may lead to deceiving results attributed to the diversity of cancer risks in different geographic locations. Further important aspect is the separated investigation of the cancer risk among Caucasian and African-American people as the dark skinned immigrants suffer of deficient light exposure and associated hormonal deficiencies in northern countries [228].

GENDER RELATED DIFFERENCES IN THE OBESITY ASSOCIATED RISK FOR INDIVIDUAL CANCER SITES

Excess bodyweight, expressed as increased body-mass index (BMI), is associated with the risk of several common adult cancers. Systematic review and meta-analysis of literary data help to assess the strength of associations between BMI and different sites of cancer and to investigate differences in these associations between male and female groups [229].

Cancers of the moderately estrogen dependent organs occur in both genders and typically in older cases among women as compared with men [230]. Women suffering of cancer are predominantly postmenopausal, suggestive of a profound estrogen loss in association with development of these tumors [144]. Though cancer initiation is multicausal, estrogen deficiency and the concomitant insulin resistance in obese postmenopausal women seems to be crucial cancer risk at several sites [21].

The risk for *kidney cancer* is 1.5-2.5 fold higher in overweight and obese persons than in normal weight cases. In several studies, the risk is higher in women than in men with increasing BMI [13, 231]. Obesity associated chronic hyperinsulinemia and type-2 diabetes may also contribute to the high prevalence of kidney cancer risk [232].

Increased prevalence of obesity related *salivary gland tumors* suggests that obesity and the associated metabolic and hormonal alterations have important role in their development [233]. Close correlations between obesity, insulin resistance and risk for salivary gland tumors proved to be stronger among women as compared with men. Among women with malignant salivary gland tumors, the postmenopausal status was predominant and a high prevalence of insulin resistance and obesity were characteristic concomitants [234].

There are controversial correlations concerning the gender differences in *colorectal cancer.* Obese men are more likely to develop colorectal cancer than obese women, which has been observed in the majority of studies [1]. As a speculative reason central adiposity emerged as it has higher prevalence in men than in women. By contrast, according to a new study high waist circumference was associated with slightly lower increase in colorectal cancer incidence in men (RR:1.68) as compared with women (RR:1.75) [235]. These inconsistent results may be associated with the differences in the age distribution of obese colon cancer cases. Central obesity is prevalent in aged, postmenopausal women; consequently, the older the examined group of obese cases with colon cancer the higher the ratio of female cases in relation to males.

CONCLUSIONS

Visceral obesity and the associated metabolic and hormonal imbalances provoke severe, life threatening diseases in pre- and postmenopausal women, as well as in men. Overwhelming literary data suggest that estrogens have advantageous impact against obesity and the associated dysmetabolism and hyperandrogenism, which have essential role in the development of obesity related co-morbidities; CVD and malignancies.

Healthy premenopausal women are typically protected from CVD, hypertension and cancers of the moderately estrogen dependent organs as compared with men supposedly because of the predominance of protective estrogens over androgens. By contrast, in obese young women, even a moderate estrogen loss and androgen excess might provoke premature cardiovascular diseases and cancers preferentially in the highly estrogen dependent female organs. After menopause, the health advantage of women disappears with a deepening estrogen loss and inclination to insulin resistance and the prevalence of obesity associated life threatening diseases becomes similar like in men.

Estrogen administration seems to be a realistic perspective for the prevention and treatment of obesity and obesity related pathologies.

ACKNOWLEDGEMENTS

Declared none.

CONFLICT OF INTEREST

The author confirms that this chapter contents have no conflict of interest.

REFERENCES

[1]   Calle EE, Kaaks R. Overweight, obesity and cancer: epidemiological evidence and proposed mechanisms. Nat Rev Cancer. 2004; 4: 579-91.
[2]   Davis SR, Castelo-Branco C, Chedraui P *et al*; Writing Group of the International Menopause Society for World Menopause Day 2012. Understanding weight gain at menopause. Climacteric. 2012; 15(5): 419-29.
[3]   Bianchini F, Kaaks R, Vainio H. Overweight, obesity, and cancer risk. Lancet Oncol. 2002; 3(9): 565-74.
[4]   Flegal KM, Carroll MD, Ogden CL *et al*. Prevalence and trends in obesity among US adults, 1999-2000. JAMA. 2002; 288(14): 1723-7.
[5]   Mokdad AH, Ford ES, Bowman BA, *et al*. Prevalence of obesity, diabetes, and obesity-related health risk factors, 2001. JAMA 2003; 289(1): 76-9.
[6]   Seidell J, Rissanen A. Etiology and Pathophysiology. In: Bray G, Bouchard C Eds. Handbook of Obesity. New York: Marcel Dekker, 2004; pp. 93-107
[7]   Björntorp P. Obesity. Lancet. 1997; 350(9075): 423-6.
[8]   Flegal KM, Carroll MD, Ogden CL, *et al*. Prevalence and trends in obesity among US adults, 1999-2008. JAMA. 2010; 303(3): 235-41.
[9]   Donohoe CL, Doyle SL, Reynolds JV. Visceral adiposity, insulin resistance and cancer risk. Diabetol Metab Syndr. 2011; 3:12.
[10]   Suba Z, Ujpál M. Correlations of insulin resistance and neoplasms. Magy Onkol. 2006; 50(2):127-35. [Hungarian].
[11]   Jee SH, Kim HJ, Lee J. Obesity, insulin resistance and cancer risk. Yonsei Med J. 2005; 46(4): 449-55.
[12]   Jerant A, Franks P. Body mass index, diabetes, hypertension, and short-term mortality: a population-based observational study, 2000-2006. J Am Board Fam Med. 2012; 25(4): 422-31.
[13]   Calle EE, Rodriguez C, Walker-Thurmond K, *et al*. Overweight, obesity, and mortality from cancer in a prospectively studied cohort of U. S. adults. N Engl J Med. 2003; 348: 1625-38.
[14]   Allison DB, Fontaine KR, Manson JE, *et al*. Annual deaths attributable to obesity in the United States. JAMA. 1999; 282(16): 1530-8.

[15] Banegas JR, López-García E, Gutiérrez-Fisac JL, *et al.* A simple estimate of mortality attributable to excess weight in the European Union. Eur J Clin Nutr. 2003; 57: 201-8.

[16] Mokdad AH, Marks JS, Stroup DF, *et al.* Actual causes of death in the United States, 2000. JAMA. 2004; 291(10): 1238-45.

[17] Pallottini V, Bulzomi P, Galluzzo P, *et al.* Estrogen regulation of adipose tissue functions: involvement of estrogen receptor isoforms. Infect Disord Drug Targets. 2008; 8(1): 52-60.

[18] Reckelhoff JF. Sex steroids, cardiovascular disease, and hypertension: unanswered questions and some speculations. Hypertension. 2005; 45: 170-4.

[19] Rose DP, Vona-Davis L. Interaction between menopausal status and obesity in affecting breast cancer risk. Maturitas 2010; 66(1): 33-8.

[20] Suba Z. Circulatory Estrogen Level Protects Against Breast Cancer in Obese Women. Recent Pat Anticancer Drug Discov 2013; 8(2): 154-67.

[21] Suba Z. Interplay between insulin resistance and estrogen deficiency as co- activators in carcinogenesis. Pathol Oncol Res. 2012; 18(2): 123-33.

[22] Reaven GM. Banting lecture 1988: Role of insulin resistance in human disease. Diabetes 1988; 37(12): 1595-607.

[23] Bloomgarden ZT. Second World Congress on the Insulin Resistance Syndrome: Mediators, pediatric insulin resistance, the polycystic ovary syndrome, and malignancy. Diabetes Care 2005; 28(7): 1821-30.

[24] Gupta K, Krishnaswamy G, Karnad A, *et al.* Insulin: A novel factor in carcinogenesis. Am J Med Sci 2002; 323(3): 140-5.

[25] Yu H, Rohan T. Role of insulin-like growth factor family in cancer development and progression. J Natl Cancer Inst 2000; 92(18): 1472-89.

[26] Smith GD, Gunnell D, Holly J. Cancer and insulin-like growth factor-I. A potential mechanism linking the environment with cancer risk. BMJ. 2000; 321(7265): 847-8.

[27] Kleinberg, D. L. Somatostatin analogs and IGF-I inhibition for breast cancer prevention. *US20090325863 (2009)*.

[28] Reaven GM. Insulin resistance, cardiovascular disease, and the metabolic syndrome: How well do the emperor's clothes fit? Diabetes Care 2004; 27(4): 1011-1012.

[29] Cowey S, Hardy RW. The metabolic syndrome. A high risk state for cancer? Am J Pathol 2006; 169(5): 1505-22.

[30] Doyle SL, Donohoe CL, Lysaght J, *et al.* Visceral obesity, metabolic syndrome, insulin resistance and cancer. Proc Nutr Soc. 2012; 71(1):181-9.

[31] Baynes JW, Thorpe SR. Role of oxidative stress in diabetic complications: a new perspective on an old paradigm. Diabetes 1999; 48(1): 1-9.

[32] Dang CV, Semenza GL. Oncogenic alterations of metabolism. Trends Biochem Sci 1999; 24(2): 68-72.

[33] Brownlee M. Lilly Lecture 1993. Glycation and diabetic complications. Diabetes 1994; 43(6): 836-41.

[34] Dandona P, Aljada A, Chaudhuri A, Mohanty P, Garg R. Metabolic syndrome: a comprehensive perspective based on interactions between obesity, diabetes, and inflammation. Circulation. 2005; 111:1448-54.

[35] Sieri S, Muti P, Claudia A, Berrino F, Pala V, Grioni S, *et al.* Prospective study on the role of glucose metabolism in breast cancer occurrence. Int J Cancer 2012; 130(4): 921-9.

[36] Reaven GM. Role of insulin resistance in human disease (syndrome X): an expanded definition. Annu Rev 1993; 44: 121-131.

[37] Taskinen MR. Diabetic dyslipidaemia: from basic research to clinical practice. Diabetologia. 2003; 46(6): 733-49.

[38]   McKeown-Eyssen G. Epidemiology of colorectal cancer revisited: are serum triglycerides and plasma glucose associated with risk? Cancer Epidemiol Biomarkers Prev 1994; 3: 687-695.

[39]   Welsch CW. Relationship between dietary fat and experimental mammary tumorigenesis: a review and critique. Cancer Res. 1992; 52(7 Suppl): 2040s-8s.

[40]   Muti P, Quattrin T, Grant BJ, *et al*. Fasting glucose is a risk factor for breast cancer: a prospective study. Cancer Epidemiol Biomarkers Prev 2002; 11: 1361-1368.

[41]   Landsberg L. Insulin mediated sympathetic stimulation: role in the pathogenesis of obesity related hypertension (or how insulin affects blood pressure and why). Hypertension 2001; 19(3): 523-528.

[42]   Goff DC Jr, Zaccaro DJ, Haffner SM, *et al*. Insulin sensitivity and risk the risk of incident hypertension: insights from the Insulin Resistance Atherosclerosis Study. Diabetes Care 2003; 26(3): 805-9.

[43]   Takatori S, Zamami Y, Mio M, *et al*. Chronic hyperinsulinemia enhances adrenergic vasoconstriction and decreases calcitonin gene-related peptide-containing nerve-mediated vasodilation in pithed rats. Hypertens Res 2006; 29: 361-8.

[44]   Cooper SA, Whaley-Connell A, Habibi J, *et al*. Renin-angiotensin-aldosterone system and oxidative stress in cardiovascular insulin resistance . Am J Physiol Heart Circ Physiol 2007; 293: H2009-23.

[45]   Soler M, Chatenoud L, Negri E, *et al*. Hypertension and hormone-related neoplasms in women. Hypertension. 1999; 34: 320-5.

[46]   Schneider JG, Tompkins C, Blumenthal RS, *et al*. The metabolic syndrome in women. Cardiol Rev. 2006; 14(6): 286-91.

[47]   Rosato V, Bosetti C, Talamini R, *et al*. Metabolic syndrome and the risk of breast cancer. Recenti Prog Med 2011; 102(12): 476-8.

[48]   Healy LA, Ryan AM, Carroll P, *et al*. Metabolic syndrome, central obesity and insulin resistance are associated with adverse pathological features in postmenopausal breast cancer. Clin Oncol (R Coll Radiol) 2010; 22(4): 281-8.

[49]   Kabat GC, Kim M, Chlebowski RT, *et al*. A longitudinal study of the metabolic syndrome and risk of postmenopausal breast cancer. Cancer Epidemiol Biomarkers Prev 2009; 18: 2046-53.

[50]   Altomare E, Vendemiale G, Chicco D, *et al*. Increased lipid peroxidation in type 2 poorly controlled diabetic patients. Diabetes Metab 1992; 18(4): 264-71.

[51]   Pennathur S, Heinecke JW. Mechanisms for oxidative stress in diabetic cardiovascular disease. Antioxid Redox Signal. 2007; 9(7): 955-69.

[52]   Tsuji S, Kawai N, Tsujii M, *et al*. Review article: inflammation-related promotion of gastrointestinal carcinogenesis--a perigenetic pathway. Aliment Pharmacol Ther 2003; 18(Suppl 1): 82-9.

[53]   Munkholm P. Review article: the incidence and prevalence of colorectal cancer in inflammatory bowel disease. Aliment Pharmacol Ther 2003; 18(Suppl 2): 1-5.

[54]   Grote VA, Becker S, Kaaks R. Diabetes mellitus type 2 - an independent risk factor for cancer? Exp Clin Endocrinol Diabetes 2010; 118(1): 4-8.

[55]   La Vecchia C, Giordano SH, Hortobagyi GN, *et al*. Overweight, obesity, diabetes, and risk of breast cancer: interlocking pieces of the puzzle. Oncologist. 2011; 16(6): 726-9.

[56]   Arif JM, Al-Saif AM, Al-Karrawi MA, *et al*. Causative relationship between diabetes mellitus and breast cancer in various regions of Saudi Arabia: an overview. Asian Pac J Cancer Prev. 2011; 12: 589-92.

[57]   Sartor BM, Dickey RP. Polycystic ovarian syndrome and the metabolic syndrome. Am J Med Sci. 2005; 330(6): 336-42.

[58]   Nestler JE. Obesity, insulin, sex steroids and ovulation. Int J Obes Relat Metab Disord. 2000; 24(Suppl 2): S71-3.

[59]   Cara JF, Rosenfield RL. Insulin-like growth factor I and insulin potentiate luteinizing hormone-induced androgen synthesis by rat ovarian thecal-interstitial cells. Endocrinology. 1988; 123(2): 733-9.

[60]   Nestler JE, Jakubowicz DJ, deVargas AF, *et al*. Insulin stimulates testosterone biosynthesis by human thecal cells from women polycystic ovary syndrome by activating its own receptor and using inositolglycan mediators as the signal transduction system. J Clin Endocrinol Metab 1998; 83(6): 2001-5.

[61]   Attia GR, Rainey WE, Carr BR. Metformin directly inhibits androgen production in human thecal cells. Fertil Steril. 2001; 76(3): 517-24.

[62]   Kim SW, Jun SS, Jo YG, *et al*. N, N-Dimethyl imidodicarbonimidic diamide acetate method for producing the same and pharmaceutical composition comprising the same. US20120010287 (2011).

[63]   Moghetti P, Castello R, Negri C, *et al*. Insulin infusion amplifies 17 alpha-hydroxycorticosteroid intermediates response to adrenocorticotropin in hyperandrogenic women: apparent relative impairment of 17, 20-lyase activity. J Clin Endocrinol Metab. 1996; 81(3): 881-6.

[64]   Cara JF, Fan J, Azzarello J, *et al*. Insulin-like growth factor-I enhances luteinizing hormone binding to rat ovarian theca-interstitial cells. J Clin Invest. 1990; 86(2): 560-5.

[65]   Kaaks R. Nutrition, hormones, and breast cancer: Is insulin the missing link?Cancer Causes Control 1996; 7(6): 605-25.

[66]   Secreto G, Zumoff B. Abnormal production of androgens in women with breast cancer. Anticancer Res 1994; 14(5B): 2113-7.

[67]   Micheli A, Muti P, Secreto G, *et al*. Endogenous sex hormones and subsequent breast cancer in premenopausal women. Int J Cancer. 2004; 112(2): 312-8.

[68]   Simpson ER. Sources of estrogen and their importance. J Steroid Biochem Mol Biol 2003; 86(3-5): 225-30.

[69]   Suba Z. The role of estrogen in health and disease. In: Suba Z. Ed. Estrogen *versus* Cancer. New York: Nova Science Publishers Inc, 2009; pp. 59-84.

[70]   Stamataki KE, Spina J, Rangou DB, *et al*. Ovarian function in women with non-insulin dependent diabetes mellitus. Clin Endocrinol (Oxf) 1996; 45(5): 615-21.

[71]   MacGillivray MH, Morishima A, Conte F, *et al*. Pediatric endocrinology update: an overview. The essential roles of estrogens in pubertal growth, epiphyseal fusion and bone turnover: lessons from mutations in the genes for aromatase and the estrogen receptor. Horm Res 1998; 49(Suppl 1): 2-8.

[72]   Alemany M. Do the interactions between glucocorticoids and sex hormones regulate the development of the metabolic syndrome? Front Endocrinol (Lausanne) 2012; 3: 27.

[73]   Jacobi D, Stanya KJ, Lee CH. Adipose tissue signaling by nuclear receptors in metabolic complications of obesity. Adipocyte 2012; 1(1): 4-12.

[74] Kershaw EE, Flier JS. Adipose tissue as an endocrine organ. J Clin Endocrinol Metab 2004; 89(6): 2548-56.

[75] Paoletti R, Bolego C, Poli A, Cignarella A. Metabolic syndrome, inflammation and atherosclerosis. Vasc Health Risk Manag. 2006; 2(2): 145-52.

[76] Heemskerk VH, Daemen MA, Buurman WA. Insulin-like growth factor-1 (IGF-1) and growth hormone (GH) in immunity and inflammation. Cytokine Growth Factor Rev. 1999; 10(1): 5-14.

[77] Arcidiacono B, Iiritano S, Nocera A, Possidente K, Nevolo MT, Ventura V. Insulin resistance and cancer risk: an overview of the pathogenetic mechanisms. Exp Diabetes Res. 2012; ID 789174, doi:10. 1155/2012/789174

[78] Guzik TJ, Mangalat D, Korbut R. Adipocytokines - novel link between inflammation and vascular function?J Physiol Pharmacol. 2006; 57(4): 505-28.

[79] Fantuzzi G. Adipose tissue, adipokines, and inflammation. J Allergy Clin Immunol 2005; 115(5): 911-9.

[80] Cirillo D, Rachiglio AM, la Montagna R, *et al*. Leptin signaling in breast cancer: an overview. J Cell Biochem 2008; 105(4): 956-64.

[81] Schäffler A, Schölmerich J, Buechler C. Mechanisms of disease: adipokines and breast cancer - endocrine and paracrine mechanisms that connect adiposity and breast cancer. Nat Clin Pract Endocrinol Metab. 2007; 3(4): 345-54.

[82] Grossmann ME, Cleary MP. The balance between leptin and adiponectin in the control of carcinogenesis - focus on mammary tumorigenesis. Biochimie 2012; 94(10): 2164-7.

[83] DeFronzo RA, Ferrannini E. Insulin resistance: a multifaceted syndrome responsible for NIDDM, obesity, hypertension, dyslipidemia and atherosclerotic cardiovascular disease. Diabetes Care 1991; 14(3): 173-194.

[84] Celis JE, Moreira JM, Cabezón T, Gromov P, Friis E, Rank F, *et al*. Identification of extracellular and intracellular signaling components of the mammary adipose tissue and its interstitial fluid in high risk breast cancer patients: toward dissecting the molecular circuitry of epithelial-adipocyte stromal cell interactions. Mol Cell Proteomics. 2005; 4(4): 492-522.

[85] Goldberg JE, Schwertfeger KL. Proinflammatory cytokines in breast cancer: mechanisms of action and potential targets for therapeutics. Curr Drug Targets. 2010; 11(9): 1133-46.

[86] Pallottini V, Bulzomi P, Galluzzo P, *et al*. Estrogen regulation of adipose tissue functions: involvement of estrogen receptor isoforms. Infect Disord Drug Targets. 2008; 8(1): 52-60.

[87] Macotela Y, Boucher J, Tran TT, *et al*. Sex and depot differences in adipocyte insulin sensitivity and glucose metabolism. Diabetes. 2009; 58(4): 803-12.

[88] Poehlman ET, Toth MJ, Gardner AW. Changes in energy balance and body composition at menopause: a controlled longitudinal study. Ann Intern Med. 1995; 123(9): 673-5.

[89] Choi SB, Jang JS, Park S. Estrogen and exercise may enhance beta-cell function and mass *via* insulin receptor substrate 2 induction in ovariectomized diabetic rats. Endocrinology. 2005; 146(11): 4786-94.

[90] Tagawa N, Yuda R, Kubota S, *et al*. 17Beta-estradiol inhibits 11beta-hydroxysteroid dehydrogenase type 1 activity in rodent adipocytes. J Endocrinol. 2009; 202(1): 131-9.

[91] Baghaei F, Rosmond R, Westberg L, *et al*. The CYP19 gene and associations with androgens and abdominal obesity in premenopausal women. Obes Res. 2003; 11(4): 578-85.

[92] Björntorp P. The regulation of adipose tissue distribution in humans. Int J Obes Relat Metab Disord 1996; 20(4): 291-302.

[93]   Diamanti-Kandarakis E, Baillargeon JP, Iuorno MJ, *et al*. A modern medical quandary: polycystic ovary syndrome, insulin resistance, and oral contraceptive pills. J Clin Endocrinol Metab. 2003; 88(5): 1927-32.

[94]   Salpeter SR, Walsh JM, Ormiston TM, *et al*. Meta-analysis: effect of hormone-replacement therapy on components of the metabolic syndrome in postmenopausal women. Diabetes Obes Metab 2006; 8(5): 538-54.

[95]   Morimoto LM, White E, Chen Z, *et al*. Obesity, body size and risk of postmenopausal breast cancer: the Women's Health Initiative (United States). Cancer Causes Control 2002; 13(8): 41-51.

[96]   Jensen J, Nilas L, Christiansen C. Influence of menopause on serum lipids and lipoproteins. Maturitas. 1990; 12(4): 321-31.

[97]   Walsh BW, Schiff I, Rosner B, *et al*. Effects of postmenopausal estrogen replacement on the concentrations and metabolism of plasma lipoproteins. N Engl J Med. 1991; 325(17): 1196-204.

[98]   Hamden K, Carreau S, Ellouz F, *et al*. Protective effect of 17beta-estradiol on oxidative stress and liver dysfunction in aged male rats. J Physiol Biochem. 2007; 63(3): 195-201.

[99]   Harrison-Bernard LM, Schulman IH, Raij L. Postovariectomy hypertension is linked to increased renal AT1 receptor and salt sensitivity. Hypertension 2003; 42(6): 1157-63.

[100]   Gallagher PE, Li P, Lenhart JR, *et al*. Estrogen regulation of angiotensin-converting enzyme mRNA. Hypertension. 1999; 33(1 Pt 2): 323-8.

[101]   Widder J, Pelzer T, von Poser-Klein C, *et al*. Improvement of endothelial dysfunction by selective estrogen receptor-alpha stimulation in ovariectomized SHR. Hypertension 2003; 42(5): 991-6.

[102]   Yanes LL, Reckelhoff JF. Postmenopausal hypertension. Am J Hypertens 2011; 24(7): 740-9.

[103]   Dantas AP, Tostes RC, Fortes ZB, *et al*. *In vivo* evidence for antioxidant potential of estrogen in microvessels of female spontaneously hypertensive rats. Hypertension. 2002; 39(2 Pt 2): 405-11.

[104]   Viña J, Sastre J, Pallardó FV, *et al*. Role of mitochondrial oxidative stress to explain the different longevity between genders: protective effect of estrogens. Free Radic Res. 2006; 40(12): 1359-65.

[105]   Barros RP, Machado UF, Gustafsson JA. Estrogen receptors: new players in diabetes mellitus. Trends Mol Med. 2006; 12(9): 425-31.

[106]   Tiano JP, Mauvais-Jarvis F. Importance of oestrogen receptors to preserve functional β-cell mass in diabetes. Nat Rev Endocrinol 2012; 8(6): 342-51.

[107]   Bryzgalova G, Gao H, Ahren B, *et al*. Evidence that oestrogen receptor-alpha plays an important role in the regulation of glucose homeostasis in mice: insulin sensitivity in the liver. Diabetologia. 2006; 49(3): 588-97.

[108]   Nagira K, Sasaoka T, Wada T, *et al*. Altered subcellular distribution of estrogen receptor alpha is implicated in estradiol-induced dual regulation of insulin signaling in 3T3-L1 adipocytes. Endocrinology. 2006; 147(2): 1020-8.

[109]   Welch RD, Gorski J. Regulation of glucose transporters by estradiol in the immature rat uterus. Endocrinology. 1999; 140(8): 3602-8.

[110]   Rosenbaum D, Haber RS, Dunaif A. Insulin resistance in polycystic ovary syndrome: decreased expression of GLUT-4 glucose transporters in adipocytes. Am J Physiol. 1993; 264(2 Pt 1): E197-202.

[111] Leung KC, Johannsson G, Leong GM, *et al*. Estrogen regulation of growth hormone action. Endocr Rev. 2004; 25(5): 693-721.

[112] Abu-Taha M, Rius C, Hermenegildo C, *et al*. Menopause and ovariectomy cause a low grade of systemic inflammation that may be prevented by chronic treatment with low doses of estrogen or losartan. J Immunol 2009; 183(2): 1393-402.

[113] Geraldes P, Sirois MG, Tanguay JF. Specific contribution of estrogen receptors on mitogen-activated protein kinase pathways and vascular cell activation. Circ Res 2003; 93(5): 399-405.

[114] Llaneza P, González C, Fernandez-Iñarrea J, *et al*. Soy isoflavones, diet and physical exercise modify serum cytokines in healthy obese postmenopausal women. Phytomedicine 2011; 18(4): 245-50.

[115] Adlercreutz HJ. Phytoestrogens and breast cancer. Steroid Biochem Mol Biol 2002; 83(1-5): 113-8.

[116] Veldhuis JD, Frystyk J, Iranmanesh A, *et al*. Testosterone and estradiol regulate free insulin-like growth factor I (IGF-I), IGF binding protein 1 (IGFBP-1), and dimeric IGF-I/IGFBP-1 concentrations. J Clin Endocrinol Metab. 2005; 90(5): 2941-7.

[117] Smith CL. Cross-talk between peptide growth factor and estrogen receptor signaling pathways. Biol Reprod. 1998; 58(3): 627-32.

[118] Xu J, Xiang Q, Lin G, *et al*. Estrogen improved metabolic syndrome through down-regulation of VEGF and HIF-1α to inhibit hypoxia of periaortic and intra-abdominal fat in ovariectomized female rats. Mol Biol Rep 2012; 39(8): 8177-85.

[119] Driggers PH, Segars JH. Estrogen action and cytoplasmic signaling pathways. Part II: the role of growth factors and phosphorylation in estrogen signaling. Trends Endocrinol Metab. 2002; 13(10): 422-7.

[120] Massarweh S, Schiff R. Resistance to endocrine therapy in breast cancer: exploiting estrogen receptor/growth factor signaling crosstalk. Endocr Relat Cancer. 2006; 13 (Suppl 1):S15-24.

[121] Stoica A, Saceda M, Doraiswamy VL, *et al*. Regulation of estrogen receptor-alpha gene expression by epidermal growth factor. J Endocrinol. 2000; 165(2): 371-8.

[122] Nedungadi TP, Clegg DJ. Sexual dimorphism in body fat distribution and risk for cardiovascular diseases. J Cardiovasc Transl Res. 2009; 2(3): 321-7.

[123] Suzuki R, Iwasaki M, Inoue M, *et al*. Body weight at age 20 years, subsequent weight change and breast cancer risk defined by estrogen and progesterone receptor status – the Japan public health center-based study. Int J Cancer 2011; 129(5): 1214-24.

[124] Baer HJ, Tworoger SS, Hankinson SE, *et al*. Body fatness at young ages and risk of breast cancer throughout life. Am J Epidemiol 2010; 171(11): 1183-94.

[125] Michels KB, Terry KL, Willett WC. Longitudinal study on the role of body size in premenopausal breast cancer. Arch Intern Med. 2006; 166(21): 2395-402.

[126] Huang Z, Willett WC, Colditz GA, *et al*. Waist circumference, waist:hip ratio, and risk of breast cancer in the Nurses' Health Study. Am J Epidemiol 1999; 150(12): 1316-24.

[127] Harris HR, Willett WC, Terry KL, *et al*. Body fat distribution and risk of premenopausal breast cancer in the Nurses' Health Study II. J Natl Cancer Inst. 2011; 103(3): 273-8.

[128] Sonnenschein E, Toniolo P, Terry MB, *et al*. Body fat distribution and obesity in pre- and postmenopausal breast cancer. Int J Epidemiol. 1999; 28(6): 1026-31.

[129] Page JH, Rexrode KM, Hu F, *et al*. Waist-height ratio as a predictor of coronary heart disease among women. Epidemiology. 2009; 20(3): 361-6.

[130] Caprio S, Hyman LD, Limb C, *et al.* Central adiposity and its metabolic correlates in obese adolescent girls. Am J Physiol 1995; 269(1 Pt 1): E118-26.

[131] Gurtcheff SE, Klein NA. Diminished ovarian reserve and infertility. Clin Obstet Gynecol. 2011; 54(4): 666-74.

[132] Tobisch B, Blatniczky L, Barkai L. Correlation between insulin resistance and puberty in children with increased cardiometabolic risk. Orv Hetil 2011; 152(27): 1068-74.

[133] Theintz G. From obesity to type-2 diabetes in children and adolescents. Rev Med Suisse. 2005; 1(7): 477-80.

[134] Berkey CS, Frazier AL, Gardner JD, *et al.* Adolescence and breast carcinoma risk. Cancer. 1999; 85(11): 2400-9.

[135] Colditz GA, Frazier AL. Models of breast cancer show that risk is set by events of early life: prevention efforts must shift focus. Cancer Epidemiol Biomarkers Prev. 1995; 4(5): 567-71.

[136] Pilia S, Casini MR, Foschini ML, *et al.* The effect of puberty on insulin resistance in obese children. J Endocrinol Invest. 2009; 32(5): 401-5.

[137] Vanhala MJ, Vanhala PT, Keinänen-Kiukaanniemi SM, *et al.* Relative weight gain and obesity as a child predict metabolic syndrome as an adult. Int J Obes Relat Metab Disord. 1999; 23(6): 656-9.

[138] Stoll BA. Teenage obesity in relation to breast cancer risk. Int J Obes Relat Metab Disord. 1998; 22(11): 1035-40.

[139] Apter D, Vihko R. Endocrine determinants of fertility: serum androgen concentrations during follow-up of adolescents into the third decade of life. J Clin Endocrinol Metab. 1990; 71(4): 970-4.

[140] Baer HJ, Colditz GA, Willett WC, *et al.* Adiposity and sex hormones in girls. Cancer Epidemiol Biomarkers Prev. 2007; 16(9): 1880-8.

[141] Althuis MD, Brogan DD, Coates RJ, *etal.* Breast cancers among very young premenopausal women (United States). Cancer Causes Control 2003; 14(2): 151-60.

[142] Velentgas P, Daling JR. Risk factors for breast cancer in younger women. J Natl Cancer Inst Monogr. 1994; 16: 15-24.

[143] Suba Z. Insulin resistance, estrogen deficiency and cancer risk. In: Suba Z. Ed. Estrogen *versus* Cancer. New York: Nova Science Publishers Inc., 2009; pp. 127-46.

[144] Suba Z. Common soil of smoking-associated and hormone-related cancers: estrogen deficiency. Oncol Rev 2010; 4(2): 73-87.

[145] Suba Z, Kásler M. Interactions of insulin and estrogen in the regulation of cell proliferation and carcinogenesis. Orv Hetil. 2012; 153(4): 125-36.

[146] Opdahl S, Alsaker MD, Janszky I, *et al.* Joint effect of nulliparity and other breast cancer risk factors. Br J Cancer 2011; 105(5): 731-6.

[147] Newcomb PA, Trentham-Dietz A, Hampton JM, *et al.* Late age at full term birth is strongly associated with lobular breast cancer. Cancer 2011; 117(9): 1946-56.

[148] Key TJ. Hormones and cancer in humans. Mutat Res 1995; 333(1-2): 59-67.

[149] Britt K, Ashworth A, Smalley M. Pregnancy and the risk of breast cancer. Endocrine-Related Cancer 2007; 14(4): 907-33.

[150] Källén B, Finnström O, Lindam A, *et al.* Malignancies among women who gave birth after *in vitro* fertilization. Hum Reprod. 2011; 26(1): 253-8.

[151] Polson DW, Wadsworth J, Adams J, *et al.* Polycystic ovaries: a common finding in normal women. Lancet 1988; 1(8590): 870-872.

[152] Carmina E, Lobo RA. Polycystic ovaries in hirsute women with normal menses. Am J Med 2001; 111(8):602-606.

[153] Soliman PT, Oh JC, Schmeler KM, *et al*. Risk factors for young premenopausal women with endometrial cancer. Obstet Gynecol 2005; 105(3): 575-80.

[154] Uccella S, Cha SS, Melton LJ 3rd, Bergstralh EJ, Boardman LA, Keeney GL, *et al*. Risk factors for developing multiple malignancies in patients with endometrial cancer. Int J Gynecol Cancer. 2011; 21(5): 896-90.

[155] Gadducci A, Gargini A, Palla E, *et al*. Polycystic ovary syndrome and gynecological cancers: is there a link? Gynecol Endocrinol, 2005; 20(4):200-208.

[156] Nelson VL, Legro RS, Strauss JF 3rd, *et al*. Augmented androgen production is a stable steroidogenic phenotype of propagated theca cells from polycystic ovaries. Mol Endocrinol. 1999; 13(6): 946-57.

[157] ESHRE Capri Workshop Group. Ovarian and endometrial function during hormonal contraception. Hum Reprod 2001; 16(7): 1527-35.

[158] Deligeoroglou E, Michailidis E, Creatsas G. Oral contraceptives and reproductive system cancer. Ann NY Acad Sci 2003; 997: 199-208.

[159] Tejura, B. Methods of treating hyperandrogenism and conditions associated therewith by administering a fatty acid ester of an estrogen or an estrogen derivative. *US20100286105*(2010).

[160] Shibli-Rahhal A, Schlechte J. The effects of hyperprolactinemia on bone and fat. Pituitary. 2009; 12(2): 96-104.

[161] Berinder K, Akre O, Granath F, *et al*. Cancer risk in hyperprolactinemia patients: a population-based cohort study. Eur J Endocrinol 2011; 165(2): 209-15.

[162] Ostberg JE, Thomas EL, Hamilton G, *et al*. Excess visceral and hepatic adipose tissue in Turner syndrome determined by magnetic resonance imaging: estrogen deficiency associated with hepatic adipose content. J Clin Endocrinol Metab 2005; 90(5): 2631-5.

[163] Sutton-Tyrrell K, Zhao X, Santoro N, *et al*. Reproductive hormones and obesity: 9 years of observation from the Study of Women's Health Across the Nation (SWAN). Am J Epidemiol 2010; 171(11): 1203-13.

[164] Guthrie JR, Dennerstein L, Dudley EC. Weight gain and the menopause: a 5-year prospective study. Climacteric1999; 2(3): 205-11.

[165] Rogers NH, Perfield JW 2nd, Strissel KJ, *et al*. Reduced energy expenditure and increased inflammation are early events in the development of ovariectomy-induced obesity. Endocrinology2009; 150(5): 2161-8.

[166] Stubbins RE, Najjar K, Holcomb VB, *et al*. Oestrogen alters adipocyte biology and protects female mice from adipocyte inflammation and insulin resistance. DiabetesObes Metab2012; 14(1): 58-66.

[167] Misso M, Murata Y, Boon W, *et al*. Cellular and molecular characterization of the adipose phenotype of the aromatase-deficient mouse. Endocrinology2003; 144(4): 1474-80.

[168] Ho SC, Wu S, Chan SG, *et al*. Menopausal transition and changes of body composition: a prospective study in Chinese perimenopausal women. Int J Obes. 2010; 34(8): 1265-74.

[169] Thurston RC, Sowers MR, Sternfeld B, *et al*. Gains in body fat and vasomotor symptom reporting over the menopausal transition: the Study of Women's Health across the Nation. Am J Epidemiol. 2009; 170(6): 766-74.

[170] Morris DH, Jones ME, Schoemaker MJ, *et al.* Body mass index, exercise, and other lifestyle factors in relation to age at natural menopause: analyses from the Breakthrough Generations Study. Am JEpidemiol. 2012; 175(10): 998-1005.

[171] McCarthy AM, Menke A, Ouyang P, *et al.* Bilateral oophorectomy, body mass index, and mortality in U. S. women aged 40 years and older. Cancer Prev Res (Phila). 2012; 5(6):847-54.

[172] Davis SR, Walker KZ, Strauss BJ. Effects of estradiol with and without testosterone on body composition and relationships with lipids in post-menopausal women. Menopause 2000; 7(6): 395-401.

[173] Chen Z, Bassford T, Green SB, *et al.* Postmenopausal hormonetherapy and body composition – a substudy of the estrogen plus progestin trial of the Women's Health Initiative. Am J Clin Nutr 2005; 82(3): 651-6.

[174] Sites CK, L'Hommedieu GD, Toth MJ, *et al.* The effect of hormone replacement therapy on body composition, body fat distribution, and insulin sensitivity in menopausal women: a randomized, double-blind, placebocontrolled trial. J Clin Endocrinol Metab. 2005; 90(5): 2701-7.

[175] Bonds DE, Lasser N, Qi L, *et al.* The effect of conjugated equineoestrogen on diabetes incidence: the Women's Health Initiativerandomised trial. Diabetologia. 2006; 49(3): 459-68.

[176] Rossouw JE, Anderson GL, Prentice RL, *et al.* Wrighting Group for the Women's Health Initiative Investigators. Risks and benefits of estrogen plus progestin in healthy postmenopausal women: principal results from the Women's Health Initiative randomized controlled trial. JAMA 2002; 288(3): 321-33.

[177] Ragaz J, Shakeraneh S. Estrogen prevention of breast cancer: A critical review. In: Suba Z. Ed. Estrogen Prevention for Breast Cancer. New York; Nova Science Publishers Inc. 2013; pp. 93-104.

[178] LaCroix AZ, Chlebowski RT, Manson JE, *et al.* Health outcomes after stopping conjugated equine estrogens among postmenopausal women with prior hysterectomy. A randomized controlled trial. JAMA 2011; 305(13): 1305-14.

[179] Chlebowski RT, Anderson GL. Changing concepts: Menopausal hormone therapy and breast cancer. J Natl Cancer Inst 2012; 104(7):517-27.

[180] de Villiers TJ, Gass ML, Haines CJ, *et al.* Global consensus statement on menopausal hormone therapy. Climacteric 2013; 16(2):203-4.

[181] Ogden CL, Carroll MD, Curtin LR, *et al.* Prevalence of overweight and obesity in the United States, 1999-2004. JAMA. 2007; 295(13):1549–1555.

[182] Popkin BM. The nutrition transition and its health implications in lower income countries. Public Health Nutr. 1988; 1(1):5–21.

[183] Suba Zs:Beneficial role of estrogen signaling in glucose homeostasis and energy metabolism. In: Johnson CC, Williams DB. Eds. Glucose Uptake: Regulation, Signaling Pathways and Health Implications. New York: Nova Science Publishers Inc. 2013; pp. 169-192.

[184] Morton GJ, Cummings DE, Baskin DG, *et al.* Central nervous system control of food intake and body weight. Nature. 2006; 443(7109):289-95.

[185] Thammacharoen S, Geary N, Lutz TA, *et al.* Divergent effects of estradiol and the estrogen receptor-alpha agonist PPT on eating and activation of PVN CRH neurons in ovariectomized rats and mice. Brain Res. 2009; 1268:88-96.

[186] Musatov S, Chen W, Pfaff DW, *et al*. Silencing of estrogen receptor alpha in the ventromedial nucleus of hypothalamus leads to metabolic syndrome. Proc Natl Acad Sci USA 2007; 104(7):2501–2506.

[187] Ørgaard A, Jensen L. The Effects of Soy Isoflavones on Obesity. Exp Biol Med (Maywood) 2008; 233(9):1066-1080.

[188] Bhathena SJ, Velasquez MT. Beneficial role of dietary phytoestrogens in obesity and diabetes. Am J Clin Nutr. 2002; 76(6):1191-1201.

[189] Velasquez MT, Bhathena SJ. Role of Dietary Soy Protein in Obesity. Int J Med Sci 2007; 4(2):72-82.

[190] *Wagner JD, Cefalu WT, Anthony MS, et al. Dietary soy protein and estrogen replacement therapy improve cardiovascular risk factors and decrease aortic cholesteryl ester content in ovariectomized cynomolgous monkeys.* Metabolism. 1997; 46(6):698-705.

[191] Cabanes A, Wang M, Olivo S, *et al*. Prepubertal estradiol and genistein exposures up-regulate BRCA1 mRNA and reduce mammary tumorigenesis. Carcinogenesis. 2004; 25(5): 741-8.

[192] Qin LQ, Xu JY, Wang PY, *et al*. Soyfood intake in the prevention of breast cancer risk in women: a meta-analysis of observational epidemiological studies. J Nutr Sci Vitaminol (Tokyo). 2006; 52(6): 428-36.

[193] *Kotake Y,* Nlijima J, Fukuda Y, *et al.* Novel physiologically active substances. US20080275059 (2007).

[194] Barros RP, Gustafsson JÅ. Estrogen receptors and the metabolic network. Cell Metab 2011; 14(3):289-99.

[195] Balkau B, Mhamdi L, Oppert J-M *et al*. Physical Activity and Insulin Sensitivity the RISC Study. Diabetes 2008; 57(10):2613-2618.

[196] Borghouts LB, Keizer HA. Exercise and insulin sensitivity: a review. Int J Sports Med 2000; 21(1): 1-12.

[197] Jakicic JM, Otto AD. Physical activity considerations for the treatment and prevention of obesity. Am J Clin Nutr. 2005; 82(Suppl 1): 226S-229S.

[198] Monninkhof EM, Elias SG, Vlems FA *et al*. Physical activity and breast cancer: a systematic review. Epidemiology. 2007; 18(1): 137-57.

[199] Pronk A, Ji BT, Shu XO, *et al*. Physical activity and breast cancer risk in Chinese women. Br J Cancer. 2011; 105(9): 1443-50.

[200] Dieli-Conwright CM, Sullivan-Halley J, Patel A *et al*. Does hormone therapy counter the beneficial effects of physical activity on breast cancer risk in postmenopausal women?Cancer Causes Control. 2011; 22(3): 515-22.

[201] Muraki K, Okuya S, Tanizawa Y. Estrogen receptor alpha regulates insulin sensitivity trough IRS-1 thyrosin phosphorylation in mature 3T3-L1 adipocytes. Endocr J 2006; 53(6):841-851.

[202] Moreno M, Ordoñez P, Alonso A, *et al*. Chronic 17beta-estradiol treatment improves skeletal muscle insulin signaling pathway components in insulin resistance associated with aging. Age (Dordr.) 2010; 32(1):1–13.

[203] Phillips SK, Rook KM, Siddle NC, *et al*. Muscle weakness in women occurs at an earlier age than in men, but strength is preserved by hormone replacement therapy. Clin Sci 1993; 84(1):95–98.

[204] Greising SM, Baltgalvis KA, Lowe DA, *et al*. Hormone therapy and skeletal muscle strength: a meta-analysis. J Gerontol A Biol Sci Med Sci 2009; 64(10):1071–1081.

[205] Kossman DA, Williams NI, Domchek*et al.* SM, Exercise lowers estrogen and progesterone levels in premenopausal women at high risk of breast cancer. J Appl Physiol 2011; 111(6): 1687-93.

[206] van Gils CH, Peeters PHM, Schoenmakers MCJ, *et al.* Physical Activity and Endogenous Sex Hormone Levels in Postmenopausal Women: a Cross-Sectional Study in the Prospect-EPIC Cohort. Cancer Epidemiol Biomarkers Prev 2009; 18(2):377-383.

[207] Spangenburg EE, Wohlers LM, Valencia AP. Metabolic dysfunction under reduced estrogen levels. Looking to exercise for prevention disclosures. Exerc Sport Sci Rev. 2012; 40(4): 195-203.

[208] Ryan AS, Nicklas BJ, Berman DM. Aerobic exercise is necessary to improve glucose utilization with moderate weight loss in women. Obesity (Silver Spring). 2006; 14(6):1064–72.

[209] You T, Berman DM, Ryan AS, *et al.* Effects of hypocaloric diet and exercise training on inflammation and adipocyte lipolysis in obese postmenopausal women. J Clin Endocrinol Metab 2004; 89(4): 1739–46.

[210] McTiernan A, Kooperberg C, White E, *et al.* Recreational physical activity and the risk of breast cancer in postmenopausal women: the Women's Health Initiative Cohort Study. JAMA 2003; 290(10): 1331–6.

[211] Christakou CD, Diamanti-Kandarakis E. Role of androgen excess on metabolic aberrations and cardiovascular risk in women with polycystic ovary syndrome. Womens Health (Lond Engl) 2008; 4(6): 583-94.

[212] Resnick EM, Simon VR, Iskikian SO, *et al*; Society for Women's Health Research. Future research in sex differences in obesity and cardiovascular disease: report by the Society for Women's Health Research. J Investig Med. 2007; 55(2): 75-85.

[213] Pajunen P, Kotronen A, Korpi-Hyövälti E, *et al.* Metabolically healthy and unhealthy obesity phenotypes in the general population: the FIN-D2D Survey. BMC Public Health. 2011; 11: 754.

[214] Hankinson AL, Daviglus ML, Van Horn L, *et al.* Diet composition and activity level of at risk and metabolically healthy obese American adults. Obesity (Silver Spring)2013; 21(3):637-43.

[215] Elting MW, Dorsen TJM, Bezemer PD, *et al.* Prevalence of diabetes mellitus, hypertension and cardiac complaints in a follow-up study of a Dutch PCOS population. Hum Reprod 2001; 16(3): 556-60.

[216] Glueck CJ, Papanna R, Wang P, *et al.* Incidence and treatment of metabolic syndrome in newly referred women with confirmed polycystic ovarian syndrome. Metabolism 2003; 52(7): 908-15.

[217] Peppard HR, Marfori J, Luorno MJ, *et al.* Prevalence of polycystic ovary syndrome among premenopausal women with type 2 diabetes. Diabetes Care 2001; 24(6): 1050-52

[218] Talbott EO, Zborowski JV, Rager JR, *et al.* Evidence for an association between metabolic cardiovascular syndrome and coronary and aortic calcification among women with polycystic ovary syndrome. J Clin Endocrinol Metab 2004; 89(11): 5454-61

[219] Kotchen JM, Cox-Ganser J, Wright CJ, *et al.* Gender differences in obesity-related cardiovasculardisease risk factors among participants in a weight loss program. Int J Obes Relat Metab Disord 1993; 17(3): 145-51.

[220] Manson JE, Willett WC, Stampfer MJ, *et al.* Body weight and mortality among women. N Engl J Med. 1995; 333(11): 677-85.

[221] Garrison RJ, Kannel WB. A new approach for estimating healthy body weights. Int J Obes Relat Metab Disord 1993; 17(7): 417-23.

[222] Takács D, Koppány F, Mihályi S, Suba Z. Decreased oral cancer risk by moderate alcohol consumption in non-smoker postmenopausal women. Oral Oncol. 2011; 47(6): 537-40.

[223] Suba Z. Gender-related hormonal risk factors for oral cancer. Pathol Oncol Res. 2007; 13(3):195-202.

[224] Pan SY, Johnson KC, Ugnat AM, *et al.* Canadian Cancer Registries Epidemiology Research Group. Association of obesity and cancer risk in Canada. Am J Epidemiol. 2004; 159(3): 259-68.

[225] Lukanova A, Björ O, Kaaks R, *et al.* Body mass index and cancer: results from the Northern Sweden Health and Disease Cohort. Int J Cancer. 2006; 118(2): 458-66.

[226] Otto Sz. Cancer epidemiology in Hungary and the Béla Johan National Program for the Decade of Health. PatholOncol Res 2003; 9(2): 126-130.

[227] Suba Z. Newly recognized player in breast cancer risk: light deficiency. In: Suba Z. Ed. Estrogen prevention for breast cancer. New York: Nova Science Publishers Inc. 2013; pp. 77-92.

[228] Suba Z. Light deficiency confers breast cancer risk by endocrine disorders. Recent Pat Anticancer Drug Discov 2012; 7(3): 337-44.

[229] Renehan AG, Tyson M, Egger M, *et al.* Body-mass index and incidence of cancer: a systematic review and meta-analysis of prospective observational studies. Lancet 2008; 371(9612): 569-78.

[230] Kumar V, Abbas AK, Fausto N, Mitchell RN. Robbins basic pathology. 8th edn. Philadelphia:Saunders Elsevier. 2007.

[231] Chow WH, McLaughlin JK, Mandel JS, *et al.* Obesity and risk of renal cell cancer. Cancer Epidemiol Biomarkers Prev. 1996; 5(1): 17-21.

[232] Lindblad P, Chow WH, Chan J, *et al.* The role of diabetes mellitus in the aetiology of renal cell cancer. Diabetologia. 1999; 42(1): 107-12.

[233] Suba Z, Barabás J, Szabó G, *et al.* Increased prevalence of diabetes and obesity in patients with salivary gland tumors. Diabetes Care. 2005; 28(1): 228.

[234] Suba Zs. Obesity and risk for salivary gland tumors. In:Watanabe HS Ed. Horizons in Cancer Research. New York: Nova Science Publishers Inc. 2011; pp. 45-58.

[235] Wang Y, Jacobs EJ, Patel AV, *et al.* A prospective study of waist circumference and body mass index in relation to colorectal cancer incidence. Cancer Causes Control. 2008; 19(7): 783-92.

Send Orders for Reprints to reprints@benthamscience.net

CHAPTER 3

Herbal and Microbial Products for the Management of Obesity

Essam Abdel-Sattar[*], Soheir M. El Zalabani and Maha M. Salama

Pharmacognosy Department, College of Pharmacy, Cairo University, 11562, Cairo, Egypt

Abstract: Obesity is a global epidemic and one of the major health burdens of modern times. The prevalence of obesity is increasing worldwide; it constitutes a serious problem in developed as well as developing countries. Beside adults, the number of obese teenagers and children in particular has dramatically increased. Obesity is characterized by accumulation of excess fat in adipose tissues in an extent to produce adverse effects on health, leading to a reduction in life expectancy and/or a raise in health hazards. People are classified as overweight (pre-obese) and obese on the basis of the Body Mass Index (BMI), crude measure which compares weight to height. Obesity is usually associated with and can lead to many disease conditions, mainly type-2 diabetes, cardiac diseases, hypertension, sleep apnea, cerebrovascular incidents, osteoarthritis and certain types of cancers. The tremendously increasing number of reviews on the subject of obesity obviously reflects the amount of investigations currently dedicated to this field. The core of obesity treatment is dieting and physical exercise. The consumption of energy-dense food is reduced *versus* an increase in that of dietary fibers. Conventional medication relies mainly on drugs which either reduce appetite or inhibit fat absorption. However, drug treatment of obesity despite short-term benefits, is often associated with undesirable harmful side effects, rebound weight gain after discontinuation of drug intake, and the incidence of drug abuse. If diet, exercise and pharmacological therapy are ineffective; surgical intervention may be useful. The anti-obesity potential of natural products if accurately explored might provide an excellent alternative strategy for the scientifically-based development of safe and effective drugs. Especially that, they are actually widespread for this purpose as nutritional supplements. OTC anti-obesity natural products are mostly complex in terms of chemical composition and may exert a variety of pharmacological actions leading to weight loss. These include: inhibition of lipases activity, suppression of appetite, stimulation of energy expenditure, inhibition of adipocyte differentiation and regulation of lipid metabolism. A variety of natural products, including crude extracts and isolated compounds induce body weight reduction and prevent diet-induced obesity. Examples of these constituents are polyphenols, triterpenoidal and steroidal saponins, pregnane glycosides, alkaloids, abietane diterpenes and carotenoids amongst others. In addition, a number of lipase inhibitors are obtained from microbial sources.

*****Address correspondence to Essam Abdel-Sattar:** Pharmacognosy Department, College of Pharmacy, Cairo University, 11562 Cairo, Egypt; Tel: +201065847211; Fax: +20225321900; E-mail: abdelsattar@yahoo.com

The present chapter is intended to survey the vast array of natural products from plant and microbial origin currently suggested as conventional drug alternatives for management of obesity. This will cover the natural sources, extracts, safety assessment and structures of bioactive compounds, as well as the biochemical markers used to evaluate the anti-obese effect and/or determine the mechanism of action. New drug targets that may play a role in the regulation of body weight will also be considered.

Keywords: Anti-obesity, herbal medicine, micro-organisms, mechanisms, natural products, phytochemicals, plants.

INTRODUCTION

Obesity, which was once regarded as a cosmetic problem prevalent in high income countries, has been formally recognized by the World Health Organization as a global epidemic in 1997 [1]. Currently, the incidence of overweight and obesity is dramatically rising in low- and middle-income countries due to adoption of western life-style characterized by decreased physical activity and overconsumption of high energy-yielding foods [2]. Together with underweight, malnutrition, and infectious diseases, overweight and obesity are now considered as major health problems threatening the developing world [2, 3]. There is also strong evidence that obesity is associated with morbidity and mortality [4].

Definition

The World Health Organization [5, 6] defines obesity as abnormal or excessive fat accumulation that represents a risk to health. Obesity has also been described as an increased adipose tissue mass, which is the result of an enlargement in fat cells and/or an increase in their number [7] resulting in hypertrophic and/or hyperplasic obesity [8]. A crude measure of underweight, overweight and obesity is the body mass index (BMI) that is a person's weight (in kilograms) divided by the square of his/or her height (in meters) [5, 6].

Prevalence

The 2010 IASO/IOTF analysis (International Association for the Study of Obesity/International Obesity Task Force, 2010) estimates that approximately 1.0 billion adults are currently overweight and a further 475 million are obese. In addition, when Asian-specific thresholds for the definition of overweight (BMI > 23 kg/m^2) and obesity (BMI > 28 kg/m^2) are taken into consideration, to adjust for ethnic differences, 1.7 billion people could be classified as overweight worldwide, and the number of adults considered as obese exceeds 600 million [9-11]. About 65% of the world's populations live in countries where overweight and obesity kill more people than underweight (at least 2.8 million adults die each year as a result of being overweight or obese). More than 40 million children under the age of five were overweight in 2011 [12]. Moreover, the most recent WHO fact sheet (2013) recorded that more than 1.4 billion adults (20 years old and older) are overweight (BMI 25-29.9 kg/m²) of these over 200 million men and nearly 300 million women were obese, 312 million were clinically obese (BMI > 30 kg/m^2) [12].

Causes and Complications

Obesity is a multifactorial disease characterized by a chronic imbalance between energy intake and energy expenditure [13-16] together with enlarged fat deposition in adipose tissue [17]. The high calorie intake is often ascribed to change in lifestyle and inadequate dietary habits [2, 13]. Meanwhile, decreased energy expenditure is often associated with an inherited low basal metabolic rate, reduced physical activity and low capacity for fat oxidation [18]. To maintain the energy balance, the energy input in the form of food should be equal to the energy expenditure through exercise, basal metabolism, thermogenesis and fat biosynthesis [8].

Obesity is generally linked with an increased risk of excessive fat-related metabolic disorders and chronic diseases such as type-2 diabetes mellitus, hypertension, dyslipidemia, cardiovascular diseases and certain types of cancer [4, 19-21]. These obesity-associated serious complications are forcing research towards long-term safe solutions for weight management and control [22, 23]. Drugs that prevent weight regain appear necessary in obesity treatment [24].

STRATEGIES FOR MANAGEMENT OF OVERWEIGHT AND OBESITY

Overview

The key strategy to combat overweight and obesity is to prevent chronic positive impairments in the energy equation [17]. A change in lifestyle is still the crucial cornerstone [24]; in this respect, physical activity appears to be helpful by elevating average daily metabolic rate and increasing energy expenditure [13], yet this approach is short-term lasting and weight regain is usually observed [24].

Management of obesity usually necessitates a combination of lifestyle modification and pharmacological therapy. Surgical interventions, although effective in some circumstances, are not always appropriate [25, 26]. An alternative strategy to surgery is to develop therapeutic agents that can reduce body weight by decreasing the consumption or absorption of food, and/or by increasing energy expenditure [27, 28]. The ideal anti-obesity drug would produce sustained weight loss with minimal side effects [26]. Unfortunately, drug treatment of obesity despite short-term benefits, is often associated with rebound weight gain after cessation of drug use and side effects from the medication.

Modern Pharmacotherapy: Present and Future

Pharmacologic options for treatment of obesity include the use of synthetic drugs such as sibutramine, phentermine, diethylpropion, celistat and fluoxetine. Among these phentermine and diethylpropion have potential for abuse [29].

Currently, two approved drugs are available on the market, orlistat and sibutramine [26, 30, 31]. Orlistat (Xenical) reduces intestinal fat absorption through inhibition of pancreatic lipase [32-35]; while sibutramine (Reductil) is an anorectic, or appetite suppressant [36-38]. Both drugs have hazardous side-effects, including increased blood pressure, dry mouth, constipation, headache, and insomnia [35, 39-41].

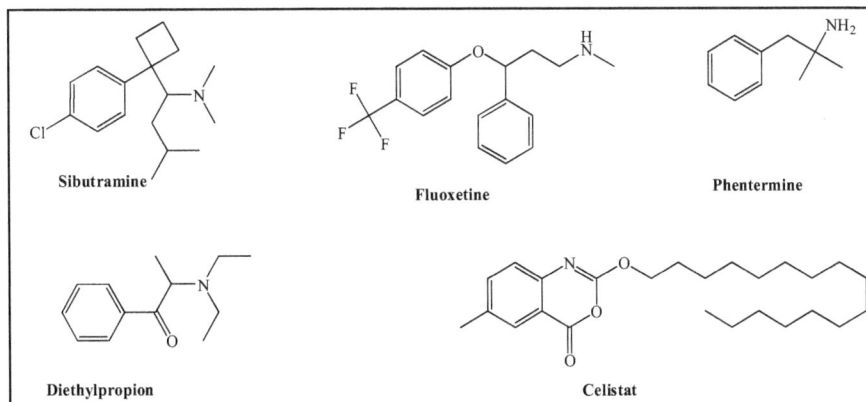

Moreover, a number of anti-obesity drugs are undergoing clinical development [26, 42, 43] including:

a.　Centrally-acting drugs, such as the noradrenergic and dopaminergic reuptake inhibitor radafaxine, the selective serotonin 5-HT$_2$c agonist APD-356, and oleoyl-estrone.

b.　Drugs that target peripheral intermittent satiety signals, such as glucagon-like peptide-1 (*e.g.* exenatide, exenatide-LAR and liraglutide), peptide YY (*e.g.* intranasal PYY3-36 and AC-162325) and amylin (*e.g.* pramlintide).

c.　Drugs that block fat absorption, such as the novel lipase inhibitors cetilistat and GT-389255; and a human growth hormone fragment (AOD-9604) that increases adipose tissue breakdown [42].

However, even for those agents that meet the preliminary requisites for selectivity of action and potential safety profile, extensive testing is still needed, to demonstrate efficacy in terms of weight loss sustainability, as well as long-term benefits for diabetes prevention and treatment, cardiovascular disease, and psychiatric safety [26].

The role of modern medication in weight loss is, thus, controversial and its effectiveness appears too limited. The Food and Drug Administration (FDA) has approved no weight loss drug for use for more than five years. Hence drugs represent a short-term solution for a long-term problem with only modest benefits and unclear risk(s) [44].

Naturotherapy: A Prospective Solution

Plants have been used as traditional natural medicines for healing many diseases since antiquity [16]. Many medicinal plants may provide safe, natural, and cost-effective alternatives to synthetic drugs [45, 46].

The potential of natural products for management of overweight and obesity is currently under extensive exploration to overcome high manufacture costs of synthetic drugs, the rebound of weight gain after stopping medication and the hazardous side effects. Naturotherapy seems, thus, an outstanding alternative strategy for developing future effective, long-term safe drugs for weight management and control [22, 23, 47-49].

A variety of natural products (including crude extracts and isolated compounds from plant and microbial sources) that induce body weight reduction and prevent diet-induced obesity, are widely used in management of these metabolic disorders [50-52]. However, the development of anti-obesity natural drugs appears as a challenging task, which can be launched faster and cheaper than conventional single-entity pharmaceuticals [53].

NATURAL PRODUCTS AND MANAGEMENT OF OVERWEIGHT AND OBESITY

Anti-obesity natural products are supplied in different forms including: comminuted whole plants or plant parts either in the form of teas or encapsulated, in addition to aqueous or alcoholic extracts dispensed in suitable formulations. Extraction and purification are intended to ensure concentration of the bioactive components. Further isolation and formulation of this (these) constituent(s) will possibly enhance the bioavailability of the drug, although in certain cases the synergistic effect of the whole extractives is favored.

The wide variety of anti-obesity natural agents harbored by plants, microbes or their extracts act through various mechanisms to either prevent weight gain or induce weight loss [54-56]. The inhibition of key enzymes involved in lipid and carbohydrate metabolism, disruption of adipogenesis and modulation of the adipocyte life-cycle, as well as, appetite suppression are among the major targeted approaches for development of efficient anti-obesity medications.

On the basis of the mechanisms of action through which they exert their activity, natural anti-obesity products are categorized as follows:

Nutrient Digestion and Absorption Inhibitors

Strategies based on the use of nutrient digestion and/or absorption inhibitors appear the most promising in terms of safety, efficacy and sustainability for management of overweight and obesity. This approach involves reduction of energy intake through gastrointestinal rather than central mechanisms [45, 57]. The most reputed are the lipase and amylase inhibitors.

Lipase Inhibitors

Dietary fat is absorbed by the intestine only after being subjected to the action of pancreatic lipase (PL) that is a key enzyme in dietary triacylglycerol absorption. Pancreatic lipase hydrolyzes triacylglycerols to monoacylglycerols and fatty acids. The potential of natural products as anti-obesity agents is commonly evaluated through monitoring their pancreatic lipase-inhibitory effect [45].

Orlistat, the clinically approved anti-obesity drug, is the tetrahydroderivative of the naturally-occurring lipase inhibitor, lipstatin, a metabolite of *Streptomyces toxytricini* [32]. It acts through irreversible covalent bonding to serine, the active site of PL and thus inactivating the enzyme [58-61]. The unpleasant gastrointestinal side-effects of this drug, such as oily spotting, liquid stools, fecal urgency or incontinence, flatulence, and abdominal cramping [35, 36, 41], directed research towards screening novel natural sources for PL inhibitors derived from either plants or microorganisms [45]. Several biomass-derived extracts and metabolites are claimed to exert PL inhibitory effects. The lipase inhibitory mechanisms of these natural products (extracts and pure isolates) are either reversible or irreversible reaction inhibitor like Orlistat [45, 61].

Among higher plant extracts are those of: *Panax japonicus* (T. Nees) C. A. Mey [62], Platycodi radix (roots of *Platycodon grandiflorum* (Jacq.) A. DC.) [63]; *Salacia reticulata* Wight [64]; and *Nelumbo nucifera* Gaertn [65]. Lower plants including fungi and algae have been also screened in this respect; certain fruiting bodies or mycelia of macrofungi [66, 67] and a number of algae are reported to possess lipase inhibitory activity [60]. However, since crude extracts include both active and inactive components, their lipase inhibitory potencies are usually significantly weak compared to orlistat [68].

Phytochemicals reported as lipase inhibitors comprise saponins, polyphenols, flavonoids, and certain alkaloids such as caffeine [68-71]. Tea leaves polyphenols (L-epicatechin, ECG, EGG, and EGCG) showed strong inhibitory activity against

PL [72-75]. The PL inhibitory activity of polyphenols is enhanced by the presence of galloyl moieties within their chemical structures and/or polymerization of flavan-3-ols [73]. Several carbohydrates are claimed to possess PL inhibitory effects [76]. For example, chitin/chitosan mixtures increase fat excretion in the feces of experimental animals resulting in reduction in body weight [51]. However, the effects of these carbohydrates are said to be controversial in humans [77-85].

Furthermore, various lower plant and microbial metabolites demonstrated PL inhibitory activity. Representatives of lower plant metabolites include: caulerpenyne from the alga, *Caulerpa taxifolia* [86]; vibralactone from the Basidomycete, *Boreostereum virans* [87]; and percyquinin from the Basidiomycete, *Stereum complicatum* [88]. Among microbial metabolites are: the aforementioned lipstatin isolated from *Streptomyces toxytricini* [89]; the panclicins from *Streptomyces* sp. NR0619 [90, 91]; valilactone and ebelactones from *Streptomyces albolongus* [92, 93]; and esterastin from *Streptomyces lavendulae* [94].

Amylase Inhibitors

Drugs which interfere with the digestion of carbohydrates are called starch blockers. These act mainly through inhibition of the activity of salivary and pancreatic amylases. Theoretically, when amylase activity is blocked, ingested starch escapes digestion in the small intestine, thus contributing no calories. Certain plants extracts or herbal supplements can promote weight loss through interfering with the breakdown of complex carbohydrates (amylase inhibitors) or by providing resistant or inaccessible starches (the third type of dietary fibers) to the lower gastrointestinal tract [95]. On the other hand, some plants'extracts *e.g. Phaseolus vulgaris* (white kidney beans), and whole grains extract of *Triticum aestivum* (wheat) inhibit the activity of salivary and pancreatic amylases [96]. Starch blockers demonstrate potential activity in the treatment of obesity, but further studies are necessary to decisively establish their efficacy.

Appetite Suppressants and/or Satiety Inducers

Generally, regulation of the quantity of food intake (appetite control) may be:

a. Short-term regulation, which is concerned primarily with preventing overeating at each meal.

b. Long term regulation, which is primarily related with the maintenance of normal quantities of energy stores in the form of fat in the body [8] (Fig. **1**):

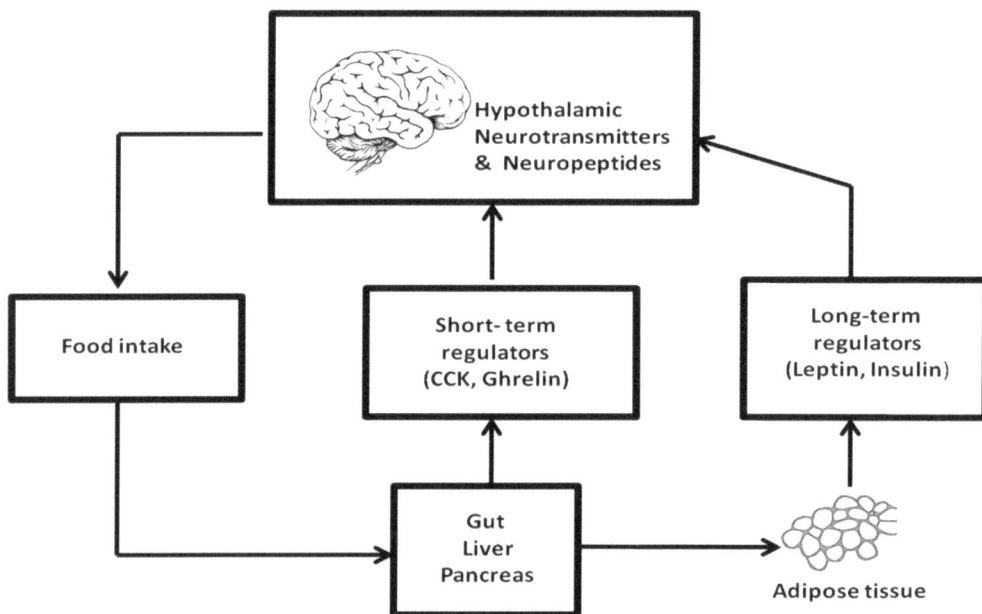

Figure 1: Schematic presentation of the short- and long-term regulation in appetite and food intake (Through reference [8]).

Factors Influencing Appetite Control

Regulation of body weight through appetite control is influenced by neurological and hormonal interrelated factors. The neuromodulators serotonin, histamine and dopamine, and their related receptor activities are closely linked with satiety regulation and constitute suitable targets in searching for drugs that could manage obesity through energy intake reduction [97]. In addition, appetite suppression may be induced by acting on the peripheral satiety peptide systems. Bioactive products may, in this respect, act by altering either the CNS levels of various hypothalamic neuropeptides, or the levels of the key CNS appetite monoamine neurotransmitters [98, 99].

Natural Appetite Suppressants

The first synthetic appetite suppressant to be approved by the FDA within the past 30 years is Sibutramine [38]. The increase in satiety sensation induced by the drug is through controlling noradrenaline, serotonin, 5-hydroxytryptamine, and dopamine levels [36, 37]. The major adverse side effects observed are dry mouth, constipation, and insomnia [30].

Natural appetite suppressants are usually dietary supplements that control appetite typically through affecting hunger control centers in the brain, resulting in a feeling of satiety. The secretion of the peptide hormone, ghrelin, in human and animal stomach increases with decreased food intake thus stimulating hunger sensation and increased food intake; therefore, development of ghrelin antagonists could provide suitable appetite suppressant candidates for treatment of obesity [100]. Melanin-concentrating hormone (MCH) receptor antagonism may also constitute an important target for appetite control and management of obesity.

Among reputed plant appetite suppressants is *Hoodia gordonii* (Masson) Sweet ex Decne., a succulent plant growing in South African countries. Although, there is still inadequate clinical information to prove its efficacy, yet, the plant extract has been found effective in appetite control resulting in significant reduction of calorie intake and enhancement of weight loss [101-105]. The extract was found to regulate food intake in rats through increasing adenosine triphosphate (ATP) level in the hypothalamic neurons [101]. Another natural appetite depressant available on the drug market is the extract of *Cissus quadrangularis* L. [105].

Other plant extracts and herbal supplements reported as appetite suppressants are derived from *Panax ginseng* C. A. Meyer (Korean red ginseng) [106], *Camellia sinensis* (L.) Kuntze [107-110], *Caralluma fimbriata* Wall. [111], *Ephedra sinica* Stapf. [112], *Citrus aurantium* L. [113], *Phaseolus vulgaris* L. [114, 95] and *Robinia pseudoaccacia* L. [114]; as well as the oil of the seeds of *Helianthus annuus* L. (sunflower oil) [115-118]. The mechanisms of appetite regulation reported for these herbal products are different. These mechanisms will be discussed individually in "plant and microbial sources with multi-functional anti-obesity activity" section.

Several active metabolites derived from the aforementioned plants were found to possess appetite-suppressive properties including saponins, flavonoids and other polyphenols. However, in most cases, the exact mechanism of action of these constituents is still unclear; they are thought to intensify signaling in the basal energy-sensing function of the hypothalamus.

The most famous among these metabolites is (-)-hydroxycitric acid (HCA), isolated from the fruits of *Garcinia cambogia* Desr., which is a potential natural appetite suppressant; it acts by increasing the release of serotonin, a neurotransmitter involved in regulation of eating behavior and appetite control [119]. Central metabolism of glucose suppresses food intake, mediated by the hypothalamic adenosine monophosphate-activated protein kinase (AMPK)/malonyl-CoA signaling system [120]. In fact, glucose administration increases hypothalamic malonyl-CoA resulting in a decrease in orexigenic neuropeptide expression and suppression of food intake [120, 121]. Certain natural appetite suppressants induce a decrease in expression of either neuropeptide Y (NPY) in the hypothalamus or of serum leptin levels [106, 122], such as the crude saponin mixture isolated from Korean ginseng [106]. The oxypregnane steroidal glycoside P57, reported as major active constituent from Hoodia, was found responsible for ATP level increase in hypothalamic neurons [123].

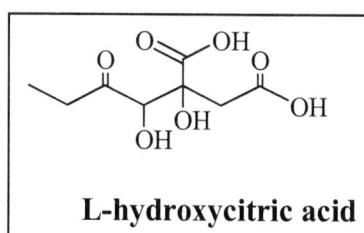

L-hydroxycitric acid

The alkaloid ephedrine has also been associated with significant weight loss, by either enhancing thermogenesis or inducing anorexia [124-129]. As anorexic it acts by inhibiting gastric emptying, which may result in a feeling of satiety and thereby aiding weight loss [130]. Its effects have been enhanced by combination with aspirin and/or methyl xanthines (caffeine or theophylline) [131-136].

Certain dietary fats (*e.g.* conjugated linoleic acid, lauric acid, and salatrim) have suppressive effects on energy intake; yet, significant body weight reduction was not recorded [137-139].

Stimulators of Energy Expenditure

The influence of reduced energy expenditure in the development of human obesity is still not obvious, despite its evidence in many rodent models. Adiposity is a consequence of imbalance in energy homeostasis where food intake is not balanced by energy expenditure [140, 141]. Energy is usually expended through [142]:

a.   Physical activity.

b.   Obligatory energy expenditure.

c.   Adaptive thermogenesis.

Mammalian brown adipose tissue (BAT) plays an important role in obesity management by controlling energy balance through dissipation of excess energy as heat to establish non-shivering thermogenesis [143]. The major participant in this process is the proton-carrier mitochondrial uncoupling protein 1 (UCP1), which discharges the proton gradient generated in oxidative phosphorylation, thus dissipating energy as heat. Therefore, the search for upregulators of UCP1 gene expression may constitute a valuable approach for achieving obesity control through increased energy expenditure [144]. UCP3, an analogue of UCP1 is, as well, an effective anti-obesity agent, which mediates thyroid hormone-regulated thermogenesis β_3-adrenergic agonists, and/or leptin levels in some organs [145]. The ethanol extract of *Solanum tuberosum* L. was found to activate the expression of UCP3 in BAT and liver rats fed with high fat diet (HFD) and consequently appreciable reduction in weight or fat mass was observed [54].

On the other hand, BAT can be recruited under certain conditions; thus searching for natural compounds that can recruit BAT within white adipose tissue (WAT) may provide another helpful anti-obesity strategy [142], this on the basis that the remodeling of mature WAT into mitochondria-rich cells with a high capacity for fatty acid oxidation has been reported [146, 147]. Several natural products, including ϖ-3 polyunsaturated fatty acids and fucoxanthin, a marine-derived xanthophyll, stimulate thermogenesis in BAT and promote the *in vivo* acquisition of WAT deposits BAT features in rodents [148-151].

In addition, numerous naturally-occurring compounds have been proposed for enhancement of weight loss *via* increased energy expenditure, mainly due to their thermogenic capacities. These include the alkaloids caffeine [136, 152], ephedrine [136] and capsaicin [52, 153] Caffeine increases energy expenditure by inhibiting the phosphodiesterase (PDE)-induced degradation of intracellular cyclic adenosine monophosphate (cAMP) [146] and decreases energy intake through reduction of food intake [152]. Although, the effect of ephedrine was shown to be markedly potentiated by caffeine [132] owing to adverse cardiovascular side effects, the FDA has prohibited the sale of ephedra-containing dietary supplements [154].

The most reputed thermogenics are green tea, its extract and component catechins *viz.*, epigallocatechin (EGC) and epigallocatechin gallate (EGCG) [109, 110]. EGCG was also reported to stimulate thermogenesis through inhibition of the catechol-*O*-methyltransferase involved in degradation of norepinephrine [52, 75, 97, 155, 156]. Other extracts such as those of *Pinellia ternata* (Thunb.) Makino [157] and *Panax ginseng* (berry) [158] also boosted energy expenditure.

Moreover, the ethanol extract of *Ilex paraguariensis* A. St-Hil improved high fat diet-induced obesity through enhancing β-oxidation of fatty acids, increasing adenosine monophosphate protein kinase (AMPK) activation in visceral adipose tissue, and reducing Acetyl-CoA carboxylase (ACC) activity [159]. Activated AMPK phosphorylates (inactivates) ACC and lowers levels of intracellular malonyl-CoA, which is the fatty acid synthesis substrate. Simultaneously, malonyl-CoA inhibits Carnitine palmitoyltransferase 1 (CPT-1), the rate-limiting enzyme in mitochondrial fatty acid oxidation and metabolism. Hence, these combined processes lead to promotion of fatty acid oxidation [159].

Modulators of Adipocyte Life-Cycle

The adipocyte life cycle (Fig. **2**) includes alteration of cell shape and growth arrest, clonal expansion and a complex sequence of changes in gene expression leading to storage of lipid and finally cell death [52, 160].

Adipocytes play a central role in the maintenance of lipid homeostasis and energy balance, by storing triglycerides and releasing free fatty acids in response to changing energy demands [142]. Since the growth of adipose tissue involves both hyperplasia (proliferation) and hypertrophy (enlargement) of adipocytes, the search for anti-obesity materials largely focused on their modulating behavior towards the processes of adipocyte proliferation and differentiation [161]. Adipose tissue mass can thus be reduced by both inhibiting adipogenesis and inducing apoptosis of adipocytes and natural products that specifically target both these pathways will, therefore, have better potential for treatment and prevention of obesity.

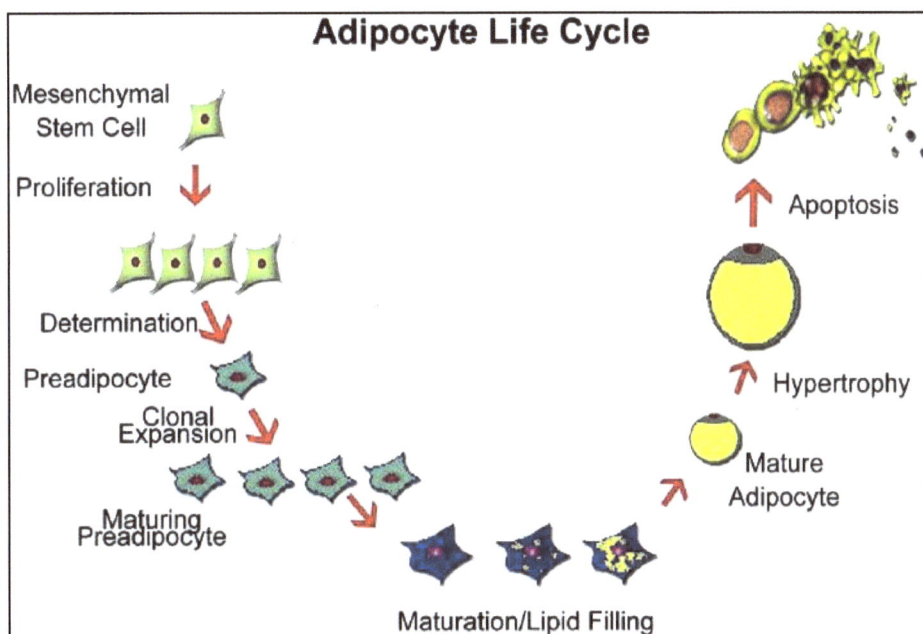

Figure 2: Adipocyte life-cycle: Mesenchymal stem cells are the precursors of several different types of cells, including myoblasts, chondroblasts, osteoblasts and preadipocytes. Once preadipocytes are triggered to mature, they begin to change shape and undergo a round of cell division known as clonal expansion, followed by initiation of the genetic program that allows them to synthesize and store triglycerides. Mature adipocytes can continue storing lipid when energy intake exceeds output, and they can mobilize and oxidize lipid when energy output exceeds input. Mature adipocytes can also undergo apoptotic cell death under certain conditions (Through reference [8]).

Usually, 3T3-L1 pre-adipocytes cells are used as an *in vitro* cell-culture model to elucidate the molecular mechanisms involved in modulation of adipogenesis, because they accumulate triglycerides upon differentiation [162, 163] due to the expression of adipocyte specific genes, such as the transcription factor peroxisome proliferator-activated receptor-gamma (PPARγ) and the CCAAT/enhancer-binding protein (C/EBPα) [164, 165]. Consequently, natural products that target adipogenesis inhibition, in particular, could be effective in management of overweight and obesity [166]. Still, the inhibition of adipogenesis or adipose tissue expansion was reported to be unhealthy, inducing a number of metabolic diseases, such as type-2 diabetes and atherosclerosis [165].

Fatty acids, particularly polyunsaturated fatty acids (PUFA), act as signal transducing molecules in adipocyte differentiation. In adipocyte tissue, saturated and monounsaturated fatty acids are more readily acylated into triglycerides than PUFA are [167-169]. Thus, PUFA play a central role in suppressing fatty acid synthesis and regulating adipocyte differentiation through suppression of late-phase adipocyte differentiation [20, 167]. Recent reports have demonstrated another interesting mechanism, in the extract of the mycelia of the macrofungus *Cordyceps militaris* (L.: Fr.) Link., which suppressed 3T3-L1 adipocyte differentiation through activation of the aryl hydrocarbon receptor [170].

On the other hand, numerous natural compounds have demonstrated apoptotic activies on maturing pre-adipocytes and could thus be considered as suitable candidates for treatment of obesity [142]. These include phenolics such as: esculetin, resveratrol, quercetin, genistein and EGCG; capsaicin alkaloid; as well as conjugated linoleic acids. These compounds were found to induce apoptosis of maturing 3T3-L1 pre-adipocytes through a number of mechanisms including suppressing the phosphorylation of the extracellular-signal-regulated kinase ERK1/2, activation of the mitochondrial pathway, AMPK activation, or anti-oxidant activity [171-175].

Other herbal and dietary inhibitors of adipose differentiation identified include isorhamnetin [166], (-)-epigallocatechin-3-gallate (EGCG) [176], silibinin [177] retinoic acid [178] and 1, 25(OH) 2D3 (1, 25-dihydroxy vitamin D3, calcitriol) [179].

A number of phenolics were found to interfere with 3T3-L1 adipocyte differentiation by arresting the adipocyte cell cycle at the G1 phase [180]. Meanwhile, others efficiently induce apoptosis in 3T3-L1 adipocytes through

AMPK activation [181, 182]. Piceatannol, a natural polyphenolic stilbene, inhibits adipogenesis *via* modulation of mitotic clonal expansion and insulin receptor-dependent insulin signaling in early phase of differentiation [183].

A combination of ajoene, the unsaturated sulfide of *Allium sativum* L. (garlic), with conjugated linoleic acid, has significantly enhanced apoptosis in mature 3T3-L1 adipocytes through a synergistic increase of expression in several proapototic factors [52].

The NAD-dependent deacetylase, Sirtuin 1 (SIRT1), is an enzyme that deacylates proteins; it contributes to cellular regulation and could be targeted in anti-obesity management. Resveratrol, a phenolic stilbenoid, was found to decrease adipogenesis; its effect was indicated to be associated with increased expression of SIRT1, which promotes fat mobilization by repressing the peroxisome proliferator-activated receptor c (PPARc) [52, 184].

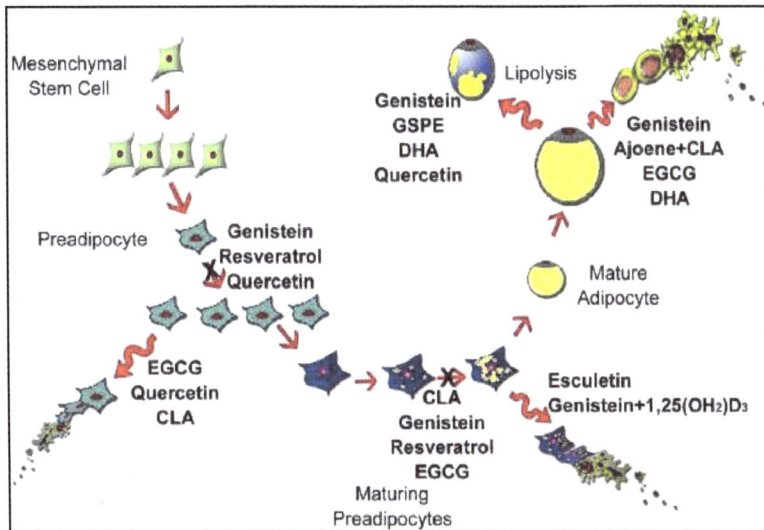

Figure 3: Effect of selected natural compounds on the different stages of the adipocyte life-cycle: Genistein inhibits preadipocyte proliferation and suppresses lipid accumulation in maturing preadipocytes. It also triggers lipolysis and induces apoptosis in mature adipocytes, and in combination with 1, 25(OH)$_2$D$_3$, it can induce apoptosis in maturing preadipocytes. EGCG induces apoptosis in both preadipocytes and mature adipocytes, and it can inhibit lipid accumulation in maturing preadipocytes. Quercetin also has multiple effects: it can inhibit preadipocyte proliferation, induce preadipocyte apoptosis and stimulate lipolysis in mature adipocytes. Ajoene+CLA are especially potent in inducing apoptosis in mature adipocytes (Through reference [52]).

The modulator effects of selected natural compounds, used single or in combination, on the adipocyte life-cycle are illustrated in Fig. **3** [52].

Regulators of Lipid Metabolism

Lipolysis could be achieved by stimulating triglyceride hydrolysis in order to diminish fat stores and thereby controlling overweight and obesity. This alternative mechanism of action is associated with oxidation of the recently released fatty acids and led to the development of the β_3-adrenergic agonists [185]. Yet, extreme lipolysis results in high circulating fatty acid levels and development of dyslipidemia; therefore, blocking of fatty acid release may be of therapeutic interest [185]. Among, natural products involved in β-adrenergic receptor activation are the flavonoid constituents of the extract of the leaves of *Nelumbo nucifera* Gaertn. (Lotus leaves) [186].

Peroxisome proliferator-activated receptor gamma (PPARγ), the transcription factor chiefly expressed in adipose tissue activates adipocyte differentiation both *in vivo* and *in vitro* [187]; when this factor is overexpressed, 3T3-L1 pre-adipocyte induction starts. This suggests that PPARγ suppression blocks adipogenesis and lipogenesis [165]. As a matter of fact, PPARγ agonists were found to improve dyslipidemia and insulin resistance. Beside, PPARγ agonists prevented increased adiposity and body weight without any reduction in food intake [188]. PPARα is another enzyme responsible for fatty acid β-oxidation.

The aqueous extract of the root of *Salacia oblonga* Wall., having the phenolic xanthonoid magniferin as major component, has demonstrated PPARα activator effect. This extract improved postprandial (after meal) hyperlipidermic and hepatic steatosis (fatty degeneration) in animal model [181].

Caffeine, a major component of oolong tea, helps in obesity control through a different structure-related mechanism. Caffeine molecule, similar to adrenaline, possesses both a positive charge and a hydrophobic moiety. Its lipolytic effect might be exerted through binding to the phospholipid phosphate groups and subsequent interactions between the lipase and triglyceride portions of lipid droplets, thus eliciting lipolysis [72].

A number of lipid metabolism inhibitors were discovered from microbial sources [86]. These mainly affect fatty acid and cholesterol metabolic pathways by acting as fatty acid synthase inhibitors (*e.g.* cerulenin), acyl-CoA synthetase inhibitors (*e.g.* triacsin C) or HMG-CoA synthase inhibitors (*e.g.* hymeglusin). Others comprise thiotetromycin, chlorogentisylquinone, as well as the beauverolides, pyripyropenes, terpendoles, and ferroverdins [86].

Natural Products with Multi-Functional Anti-Obesity Activity

The previous survey reveals that a large number of natural products manage overweight and anti-obesity through variable mechanisms. A promising approach to efficiently fulfill this purpose is to use single products having multiple activities or to combine the synergistic effects of several products [52].

The most reputed natural products with possible multi-functional anti-obesity activity are green tea (*Camellia sinensis*) [72] and *Garcina cambogia* [189]. Although other examples such as roselle (*Hibiscus sabdariffa*) [190], pomegranate (*Punica granatum*) [191], peanut (*Arachis hypogaea*) [70] and lotus (*Nelumbo nucifera*) [65] can be also cited.

Green tea was reported to possess a more pronounced anti-oxidant than anti-obesity activity, this due to its high catechin content, namely epicatechin, ECG, and EGCG. Later on, catechins were found to exert an antiobesity activity through a complex pharmacological action including: appetite suppression, increased lipolysis and energy expenditure, and decreased lipogenesis and adipocyte differentiation [74, 75, 97, 107-109, 156, 173, 176,192]. Thus, green tea extracts exert anti-obesity activities mainly through lipase inhibition and thermogenesis stimulation [97].

The commercially-available dried fruit extract of *Garcina cambogia* tree is widely used to control obesity owing to its main active constituent, (-)-hydroxycitric acid [193]. *Garcina cambogia* reduces lipogenesis by preventing the metabolism of carbohydrates into fats; moreover, it enhances excess fats burning, and suppresses appetite [193]. Its ability to inhibit adipocyte differentiation and to reduce fatty acid synthesis, lipogenesis as well as epididymal fat accumulation was established to be *via* reduction of ATP-citrate lyase activity [193, 194].

The aqueous extract of *Hibiscus sabdariffa* calyx and epicalyx (major constituents, anthocyanins) exert a potential anti-obesity effect through a number of mechanisms including anti-hyperglycemic activity, reduction of plasma cholesterol level, inhibition of gastric and pancreatic lipases, stimulation of thermogenesis, inhibition of lipid droplet accumulation in adipocytes, and inhibition of fatty acid synthase [190].

Pomegranate leaf extract (major components, ellagic and tannic acids) acts through a dual anti-obesity mechanism; it was reported as PL inhibitor, in addition to energy intake suppressant closely resembling sibutramine in this respect but acting through a different mechanism [191].

Extracts of peanut (*Arachis hypogaea)* shell were also reported to aid in obesity control by inhibiting fat absorption in the digestive tract, activating lipid metabolism in the liver, and reducing adipocyte lipolysis [70].

The lotus (*Nelumbo nucifera*) leaf extract possesses multiple anti-obesity activities, including inhibition of lipid and carbohydrate absorption and acceleration of lipid metabolism and energy expenditure [65].

Salacia reticulata stem extract met multiple obesity-reduction targets by both inhibition of α-glucosidase and PL and modulation of PPARα-mediated lipogenic gene transcription and angiotensin II type 1 receptor signaling [195].

Among isolated metabolites, raspberry ketone (rheosmin, a natural phenolic isolated from *Rubus* spp.) and numerous polyunsaturated fatty acids aid in obesity control *via* combined mechanisms of action. Raspberry ketone increases norepinephrine-induced lipolysis in WAT and enhances thermogenesis in BAT [196, 197]. Polyunsaturated fatty acids upregulate mitochondrial biogenesis and suppress adipocyte lipogenesis [150].

Taken together, combination therapies employing natural products that target different obesity genes and/or different stages of the adipocyte life cycle might prove beneficial in treating obesity.

PLANT AND MICROBIAL SOURCES WITH MULTI-FUNCTIONAL ANTI-OBESITY ACTIVITY

Higher Plants

Aesculus turbinata

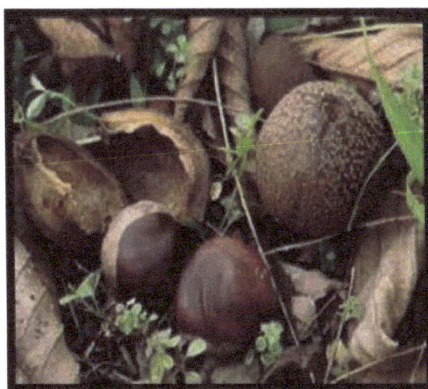

Name: *Aesculus turbinata* Blume, Sapindaceae (Hippocastanaceae).

Common name: Japanese horse chest nut.

Part used: Seeds.

Main active constituents: Saponins; escins.

Pharmacological action: The total escins (1 mg/ml) inhibit pancreatic lipase (PL) activity. *In vivo*, total escins suppress the increase in body weight, parametrial adipose tissue weight, TG (triglyceride) and TC (total cholesterol) contents in mice's liver, with an increase TG level in the feces [198]. Also, anti-obesity effects of the polymerized proanthocyanidins from seed shells in mice are reported. Highly polymerized proanthocyanidins suppress the elevation of blood glucose, by preferential inhibition of the digestive enzymes of carbohydrates. Their anti-obesity effects is more evident after 9 weeks by the attenuation of the elevation in body weight, the mass of peritoneal adipose tissues, and the plasma levels of total cholesterol and leptin. Furthermore, a dietary supplement of the total proanthocyanidin fraction normalizes the increased size of hepatocytes and the generation of steatosis with micro- and macrovesicles in liver [199].

Allium victoralis

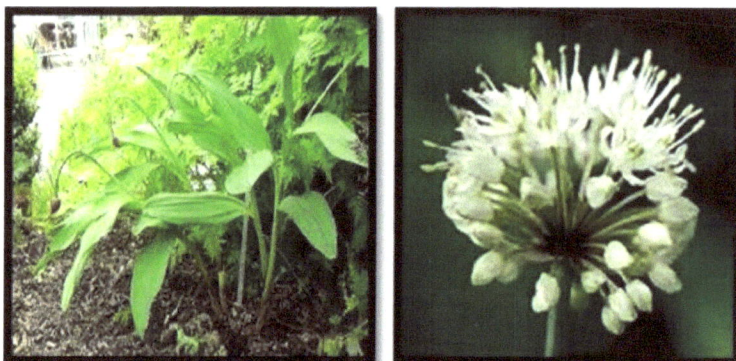

Name: *Allium victoralis* var. *platyphyllum* Makino, Alliaceae (Liliaceae).

Common name: Korean long-rooted garlic.

Part used: Leaves.

Main active constituents: Polyphenols.

Pharmacological action: The ethanolic extract decreases body weight gain, liver triglyceride content and liver size in association with an increase fecal lipid excretion, suggesting an inhibitory mechanism on lipid absorption [200]. The extract also causes considerable reduction of retroperitoneal, epididymal and total abdominal fat weight [29].

Arachis hypogea

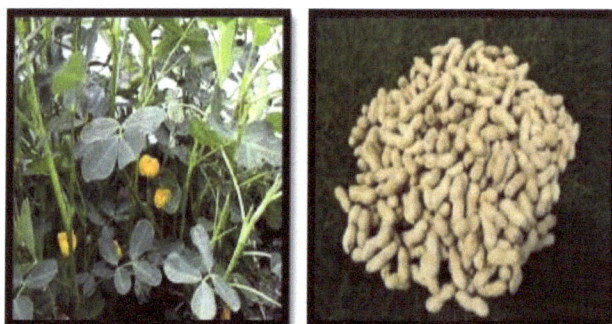

Name: *Arachis hypogea* L., Fabaceae.

Common name: Peanut, Groundnut.

Part used: Seed shell, nut shell.

Main active constituents: Phytoalexins, stilbenoids.

Pharmacological action: An ethanolic extract of peanut shell PS (peanut shell extract) inhibits a number of lipases, including PL, LPL and, possibly, hormone sensitive lipase (HSL) [70]. Body weight and body weight gain, and liver size are decreased in rats fed the high-fat diet and 1% of PSE (w:w diet). Also, TG content in the liver, as well as the serum glucose and insulin are lowered. It also reduces intracellular lipolytic activity of cultured adipocytes which may reduce the levels of circulating free fatty acids. These effects are likely induced by more than one bioactive component of PSE. The PSE actions may, at least in part, be attributed to the inhibition of fat absorption in the digestive tract and the reduction of the adipocyte lipolysis [70].

Aralia elata

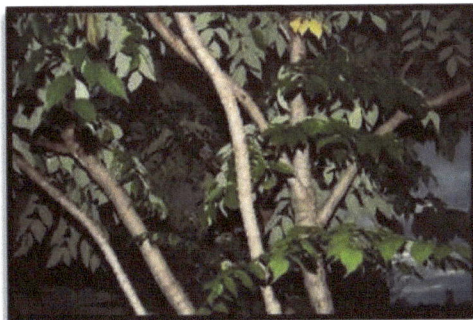

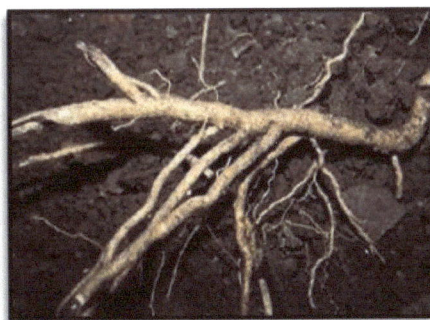

Name: *Aralia mandshurica, Aralia elata* Miq. var. *mandshurica*, Arialaceae.

Common name: Japanese Angelica tree and Manchurian thorn.

Part used: Root and stem barks.

Main active constituents: Triterpenoid saponins, aralosides. Root and stem barks contain oleanolic acid, oleanolic acid derivatives and glucopyranoside, araloside A, C, and G. Tarasaponin I-VIIl; stigmasterol; sitosterol.

Pharmacological action: Stimulation of hormone-sensitive lipase [201].

Asparagus officinalis

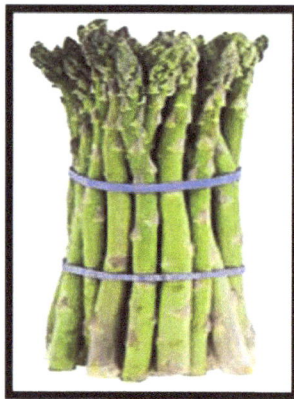

Name: *Asparagus officinalis L.* (DC), Asparagaceae.

Common name: Asparagus or garden asparagus.

Part used: Stems.

Main active constituents: Steroidal saponins; sarsasapogenin.

Pharmacological action: Ethanolic and aqueous extracts of asparagus significantly decrease the levels of body weight gain; serum total cholesterol and serum low-density lipoprotein cholesterol in hyperlipidaemic mice when administered at a daily dose of 200 mg kg^{-1} for 8 weeks. Also, serum high-density lipoprotein cholesterol levels are evidently increased. Moreover, both extracts dramatically decrease the activities of alanine and aspartate transaminases in serum [202]. Clinical studies revealed improvement of blood pressure, physical and emotional well-being and quality of life [203].

Camellia sinensis

Name: *Camellia sinensis* L. (Kuntze), Theaceae.

Common name: White tea, green tea, oolong and black tea.

Part used: Leaves.

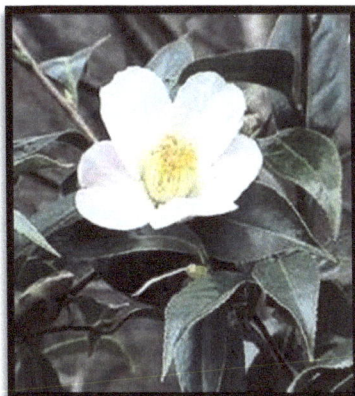

Main active constituents: Polyphenols, caffeine, acylated oleanane triterpene saponins, floratheasaponins.

Pharmacological action: *In vitro*, green tea extract (hydro-alcoholoic extract) exerts a direct inhibition of gastric and pancreatic lipases, inhibition of triglycerides lipolysis and a stimulation of thermogenesis [97]. The extract significantly, decreases hepatic steatosis and serum ALT and AST activities are lowered [204]. **Oolong tea** (Black dragon tea) extract enhances noradrenaline induced lypolysis and inhibits pancreatic lipase activity [72].

Caralluma fimbriata

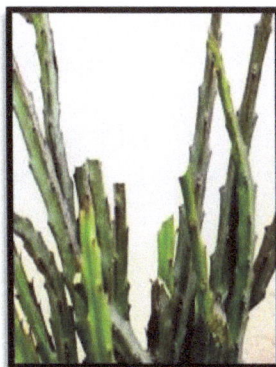

Name: *Caralluma fimbriata* Wall., Asclepiadiaceae (Apocyanaceae).

Common name: Cactus, Kalli Mooliyan, Kallimudayan (Tamil), Karallamu (Telegu) (Sanskrit), Ranshabar, Makad Shenguli, Shindala Makadi.

Part used: Aerial parts (edible cactus).

Main active constituents: Flavonoids, tannins proanthocyanidins and pregnane glycosides.

Pharmacological action: Pregnane glycosides or its related molecules suppress appetite, by amplifying the signaling sensing function in the basal hypothalamus [101, 111]. Clinical studies evidence a significant decrease in waist circumference, hunger levels, body weight, BMI (body mass index), hip circumference and body fat in over weight volunteers fed with *Caralluma* extract [111].

Cissus quadrangularis

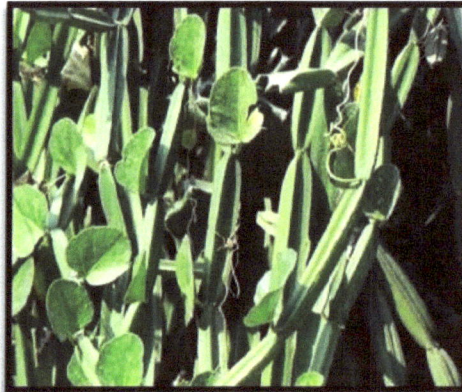

Name: *Cissus quadrangularis* L. = Vitis quadrangularis L., Vitaceae.

Common name: Veldt Grape, Devil's Backbone.

Part used: Aerial parts.

Main active constituents: Flavonols, isoflavones, resveratrol and its stilbene glycosides.

Pharmacological action: A standardized extract of *C. quadrangularis* containing 2.5% keto-steroids and 15% soluble plant fiber significantly reduces plasma TBARS (Thiobarbituric acid reactive substance- byproduct of lipid peroxidation) and carbonyls, as well as body weight, body fat, total cholesterol, LDL-cholesterol, triglycerides, and fasting blood glucose levels. This decrease in serum lipids improves cardiovascular risk factors. While the increase in plasma 5-HT and creatinine hypothesizes a mechanism of controlling appetite and promoting the increase of lean muscle mass by *Cissus quadrangularis*, thereby supporting the clinical data for weight loss and improving cardiovascular health [205].

Citrus auriantium

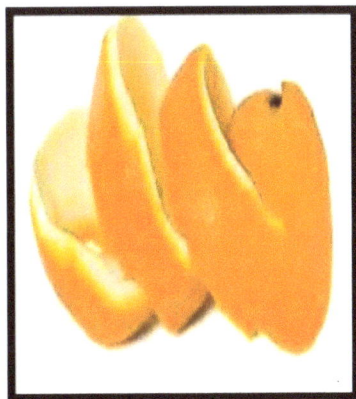

Name: *Citrus auriantium* L., Rutaceae.

Common name: Bitter orange, Seville orange.

Part used: Peels.

Main active constituents: Tyramine derivative; synephrine.

Pharmacological action: Bitter orange peel works in a similar way to ephedrine, stimulating the release of catecholamines. Bitter orange peel extract raises the metabolic rate. Synephrine, which has thermogenic properties, is structurally related to ephedrine. The extract of bitter orange peel contains tyramine and octopamine. Studies show that octopamine gives the feeling of fullness on fewer calories. This makes bitter orange peel very popular with dieters who struggle to control their food cravings [206, 207].

Commiphora mukul

Name: *Commiphora mukul* (Stocks) Hook. = *Commiphora wightii* (Arn.) Bhandari, Burseracea.

Common name: Guggal, guggul or mukul, myrrh tree.

Part used: Gum, gummy resin.

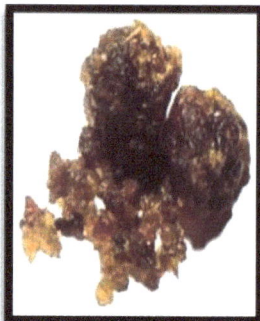

Main active constituents: Extract of gugul gum (gugulipid), pregnane derivative, guggulsterone; 20(S), 21-epoxy-3-oxocholest 4-ene, 8β-hydroxy-3, 20-dioxopregn-4,6-diene, and 5-(13' Z-nonadecenyl) resorcinol.

Pharmacological action: The extract inhibits NO formation in lipopolysaccharide (LPS)-activated murine macrophages J774 [208]. Guggulsterone inhibits the differentiation of preadipocytes, induces apoptosis and promotes lipolysis of mature adipocytes [175].

Dimocarpus longan

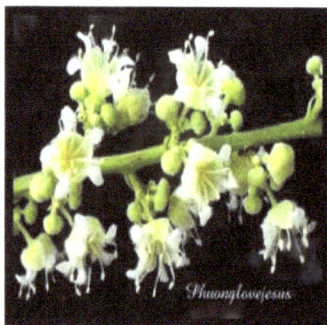

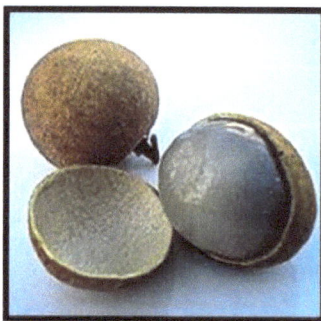

Name: *Dimocarpus longan* Lour. = *Euphoria longan* Steud., Sapindaceae.

Common name: Longan or dragon eye (as it resembles an eyeball when its fruit is shelled, the black seed shows through the translucent flesh-like a pupil/iris).

Part used: Flower and fruit.

Main active constituents: Polyphenolic compounds; phenolic acids and flavonoids.

Pharmacological action: Longan flower water extract inhibits pancreatic lipase activity, sterol regulatory element binding protein-1c (SREBP-1c) and fatty acid synthase (FAS) gene expressions, and increases fecal triglyceride excretion. This results in a decrease in, body weight, size of epididymal fat, serum triglyceride level and atherogenic index, and hepatic lipids [209].

Ephedra sinica

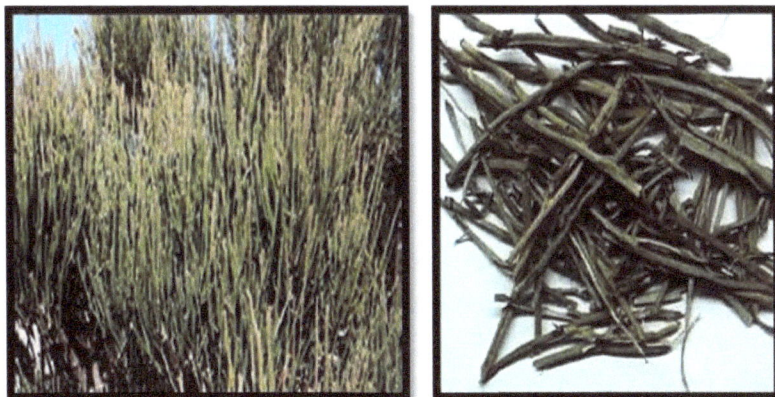

Name: *Ephedra sinica S*tapf, Ephedraceae.

Common name: Ma Huang, Chinese ephedra.

Part used: Stems.

Main active constituents: Phenyl alkylamine alkaloids, ephedrine.

Pharmacological action: Ma Huang (*Ephedra sinica*) significantly decrease food intake and body weight in animals treated with the aqueous herb extract (25 and 50 mg/100 g bw/day). However, the fluid intake increases, even above the levels of control animals and tests, in Ma Huang treated groups, 100 mg/100 mg/100 g bw/day, indicating that Ma Huang effects on adipogenesis are dose-dependent [210]. Clinically, ephedra extract significantly decreases serum cholesterol, triglycerides, glucose, fasting insulin and leptin levels in obese and over-weight women [211].

Garcinia cambogia

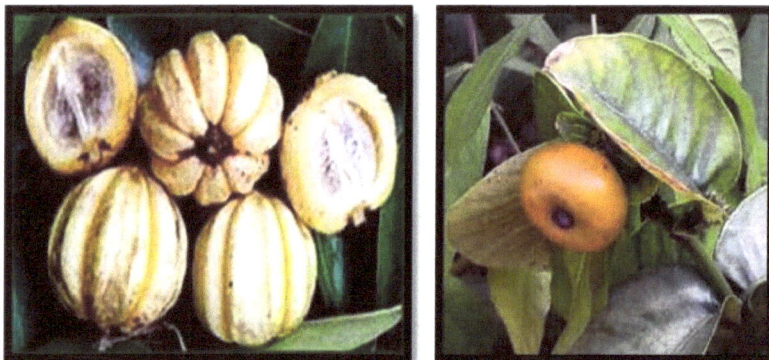

Name: *Garcinia cambogia* L., *Garcinia gummi-gutta* (L.) N. Robson, *G.quaestia, Mangostana cambogia* (Gaern.) Clusiaceae (Guttifereae).

Common name: Gambooge, brindleberry, bitter cola, brindall berry, Malabar tamarind or Essam fruit. Commonly, the plants in this genus are called saptrees, mangosteens (which may refer specifically to the purple mangosteen, *G. mangostana*), garcinias or, ambiguously, "monkey fruit".

Part used: Fruits, rind and seed.

Main active constituents: Hydroxy-citric acid.

Pharmacological action: Administration of *Garcinia cambogia* (powder) containing HCA suppresses body fat accumulation in obese rats at different doses of HCA. The highest dose of HCA-containing *Garcinia cambogia* (154 mmol HCA/kg diet) causes significant suppression of epididymal fat accumulation in male obese rats. Fifty-one mmol HCA/kg diet (389 mg HCA/kg BW/d) is the chosen dose with no observed adverse effect level (NOAEL) [194]. *Garcinia cambogia* seed (220 and 400 mg/kg) fed for 5 weeks in rats decreases triglyceride pool of adipose tissue and liver, with a significant increase in HDL and decrease in LDL [189].

Glycyrrhiza glabra

Name: *Glycyrrhiza glabra L.,* European licorice, *Glycyrrhiza uralensis,* Chinese licorice, *Glycyrrhiza lepidota* American licorice, Fabaceae

Common name: Liquorice or licorice.

Part used: Rhizomes and roots.

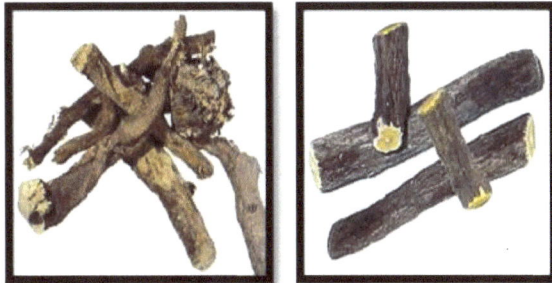

Main active constituents: Triterpenoidal saponins and flavonoids.

Pharmacological action: Licorice flavonoids decrease abdominal WAT and body weight gain (at concentrations of 1% and 2%) with a decrease in adipocyte size in obese mouse. Moreover, at concentration 2% it improves fatty degeneration of hepatocytes and changes in genes implicating regulation of lipid metabolism [212]. Clinical studies on obese women, with impaired glucose tolerance, taking an herbal medicine containing licorice, show a significant decrease in body weight and abdominal visceral fats with significant improvement in insulin resistance [213].

Gymnema sylvestra

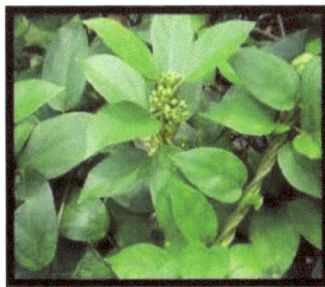

Name: *Gymnema sylvestre* R. Br., Asclepiadaceae.

Common name: Gurmar (sugar destroyer), miracle fruit.

Part used: Leaves.

Main active constituents: Oleanane saponins, gymnemic acids (saponins), flavones and anthraquinones.

Pharmacological action: Gymnemic acids stimulate the pancreas and thus increase insulin release. These compounds have also been found to increase fecal excretion of cholesterol. There are some possible mechanisms by which the leaves extract of *G. sylvester* or (gymnemic acid) exerts its hypoglycemic acid effects including: [214, 215].

a.   Promotion for the regeneration of islet cells.

b.   Enhancement of insulin secretion.

c.   Inhibition of glucose absorption from intestine.

d.   Enhancement of glucose utilization due to an increase in the enzyme activity responsible for utilization of glucose by insulin-dependent pathways, an increase in phosphorylase activity, decrease in gluconeogenic enzymes and sorbitol dehydrogenase.

Hibiscus sabdariffa

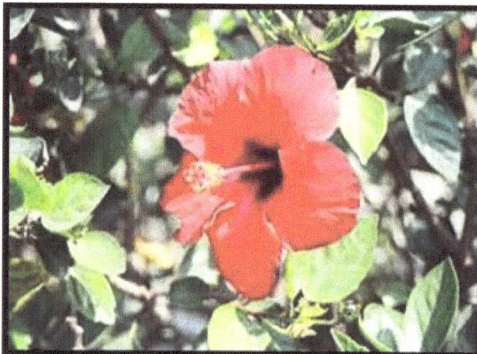

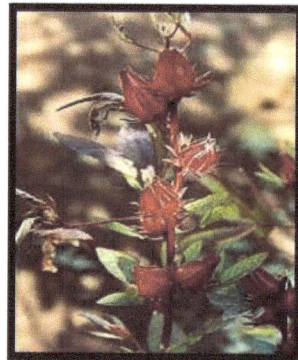

Name: *Hibiscus sabdariffa* L., Malvaceae.

Common name: Roselle.

Part used: Calyx and epicalyx.

Main active constituents: Anthocyanins.

Pharmacological action: *Hibiscus sabdariffa* aqueous extract (33.64 mg of total anthocyanins/120 mg of extract) significantly reduces body weight gain in obese mice and increases liquid intake in healthy and obese mice. ALT levels are significantly increased in obese mice, but AST levels are not affected. Triglycerides and cholesterol levels are not affected as well [190].

Hoodia gordonii

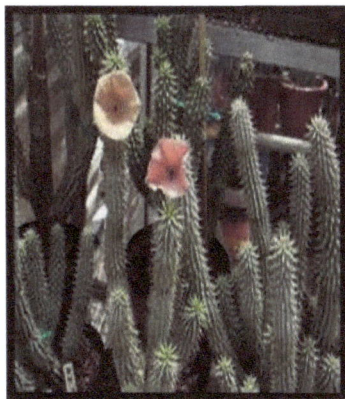

Name: *Hoodia gordonii* (Masson) Sweet ex Decne. *Opuntia dillenii* (Ker Gawl.) Haw., *Stapelia gordon* (Masson), Asclepiadaceae (Cactaceae).

Common name: Hoodia.

Part used: Stem.

Main active constituents: Pregnane glycosides (calogenin glycoside)

Pharmacological action: It acts as an appetite suppressant and reduces food intake [216]. Methylene chloride extract of *Hoodia gordonii* and two isolated pregnane glycosides (tested orally at doses 6.25-50 mg/kg) decrease food consumption and food intake [103].

Hordeum vulgare

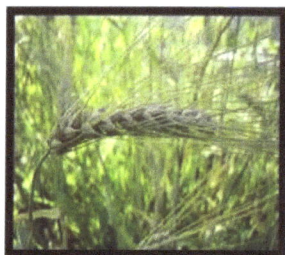

Name: *Hordeum vulgare* L., Poaceae.

Common name: Barley.

Part used: Seeds.

Main active constituents: Polysaccharides and saponins.

Pharmacological action: Plasma lipid-lowering effects of barley have been attributed to its high content of β-glucan, a water-soluble fiber [217-219]. The β-glucan component of barley slows down the gastric emptying time, prolonging the feeling of fullness, and hence stabilizes blood sugars. Other contributory factors may be d-α-tocotrienol, which has the ability to affect lipid controlling enzymes and lower cholesterol. Barley contains fermentable carbohydrates; fermentation of undigested carbohydrate produces short chain fatty acids, some of which may reduce hepatic glucose production and affect postprandial glycemia. The β-glucan significantly decreases glycemic and insulinemic responses on food [220].

Ilex paraguariensis

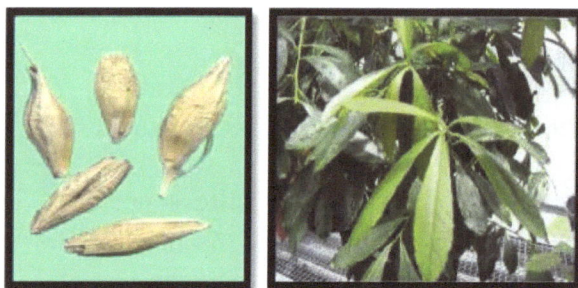

Name: *Ilex paraguariensis* A. St. Hil., Aquifoliaceae.

Common name: Yerba mate.

Part used: Leaves.

Main active constituents: Polyphenols, caffeine and saponins.

Pharmacological action: The effect of mate on weight loss is due to both its caffeine content, contributing to lipolytic activity and saponin content, interfering with cholesterol metabolism and delaying intestinal absorption of dietary fat [221]. Mate tea also affects other aspects of lipid metabolism; it has the ability to inhibit atherosclerosis (in rabbits) when fed with a high cholesterol diet and an aqueous extract of Mate tea [222]. Giving Mate extracts to hypercholesterolemic-diet fed rats reduces serum concentrations of cholesterol and triglycerides [223]. Mate is a potential digestive aid due to a choleretic effect and through increasing the rate of bile flow [224].

Irvingia gabonensis

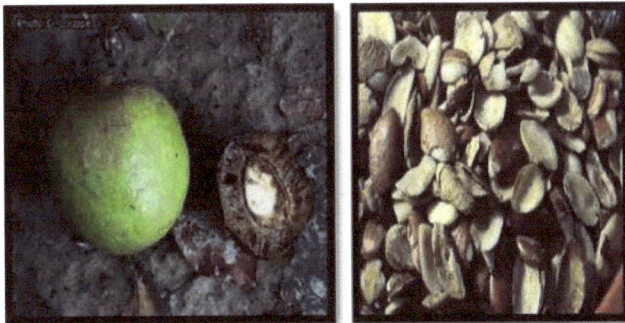

Name: *Irvingia gabonensis*, (Aubry-Lecomte ex O'Rorke) Baill., Irvingiaceae.

Common name: African mango.

Part used: Seeds.

Main active constituents: Ascorbic acid, polyphenols and carotenoids.

Pharmacological action: *Irvingia gabonensis* seed extract decreases body weight. The obese patients under *Irvingia gabonensis* treatment show a significant decrease of total cholesterol, LDL-cholesterol, triglycerides, and an increase of HDL-cholesterol [225]. The soluble fibre of the seed of *I. gabonensis* like other forms of water-soluble dietary fibres, are "bulk-forming" laxatives. *Irvingia gabonensis* seeds delay stomach emptying, leading to a more gradual absorption of dietary sugar. This effect can reduce the elevation of blood sugar levels that is typical after a meal [226]. The soluble fibers of *I. gabonensis* seed can bind to bile acids in the gut and carry them out of the body in the feces, which requires the body to convert more cholesterol into bile acids. This can result in lowering blood cholesterol as well as other blood lipids [227].

Kochia scoparia

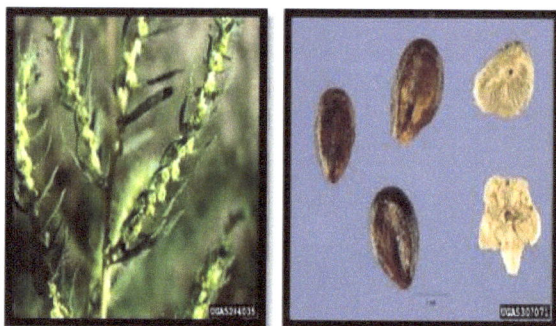

Name: *Kochia scoparia* (L.) Schrad. = *Bassia scoparia*, (L.) A.J. Scott, *Chenopodium scoparia* L., Chenopodiceae.

Common name: Mock cypress, kochia, fireweed, summer cypress.

Part used: Fruits.

Main active constituents: Saponins; scoparianosides, momordin Ic, IIc and its 2'-O-ß-D- glucopyranoside.

Pharmacological action: Momordin and its 2'-O-ß-D-glucopyranoside (principal saponin constituents) potently inhibit glucose and ethanol absorption [228]. The ethanol extract of *K. scoparia* fruit prevents the increase in body weight and parametrial adipose tissue weight induced by the high-fat diet. Furthermore, consumption of a high-fat diet containing 1% or 3% *K. scoparia* extract significantly increase the fecal content and the fecal triacylglycerol level. The ethanol extract (250 mg/kg) and total saponins (100 mg/kg) of *K. scoparia* inhibit the elevation of the plasma triacylglyccerol level. Total saponins and momordin isolated from *K. scoparia* fruit inhibit the PL activity (*in vitro*). Therefore, the anti-obesity actions of *K. scoparia* extract in a high-fat diet may be partly mediated through delaying the intestinal absorption of dietary fat by inhibiting PL activity [229].

Ligusticum sinense

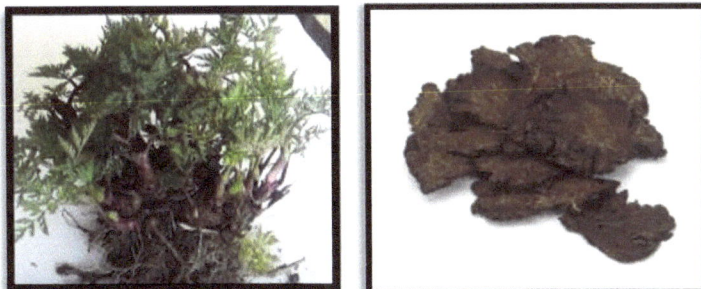

Name: *Ligusticum sinense* (Lour.) Oliv. *(= Ligusticum chuanxiong* S. H.), Oleaceae.

Common name: Chinese privet, gaoben, lovage root.

Part used: Roots.

Main active constituents: Volatile oil and phenolic acids.

Pharmacological action: An herbal preparation (Slimax) containing *Ligusticum sinense* decreases body weight, waist and hip circumference and Body Mass Index (BMI). The basis of its anti-obesity effect is through modification of lipid metabolism, with significant impact on both the accumulation and the release of lipid from adipose tissue [230].

Lilium brownii

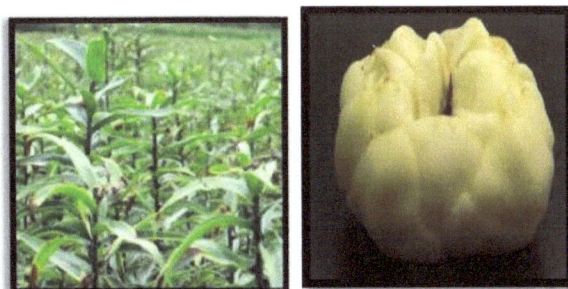

Name *Lilium brownii* F. E. Brown var. *viridulum* Baker, Liliaceae.

Common name: Lily bulb.

Part used: Dried fleshy scale leaf.

Main active constituents: Steroidal saponins, phenolic compounds and alkaloids.

Pharmacological action: An herbal preparation (Slimax) containing Lilly bulb extract decreases body weight, waist and hip circumference and body mass index (BMI), by modification of lipid metabolism affecting accumulation and release of lipid from adipose tissue [230].

Momordica charantia

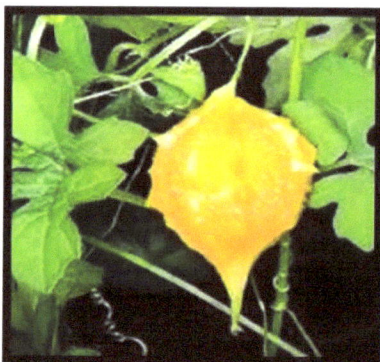

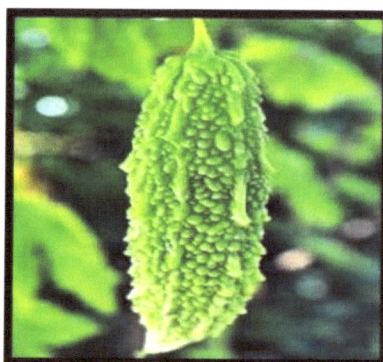

Name: *Momordica charantia* L., Cucurbitaceae,

Common name: Bitter melon, bitter gourd or bitter squash.

Part used: Fruit.

Main active constituents: Terpenoid compounds; momordicin I and II, and cucurbitacin.

Pharmacological action: The fruit water extract significantly decreases the epididymal WAT weight and visceral fat weight. Also, it improves blood glucose level and leptin [231]. In other studies, the treatment of rats with high fat diet (HFD) with the fruit extract causes a significant decrease in the number of large adipocytes and also a decrease in adipose tissue mass with a decrease in weight gain without affecting food consumption [4].

Panax ginseng

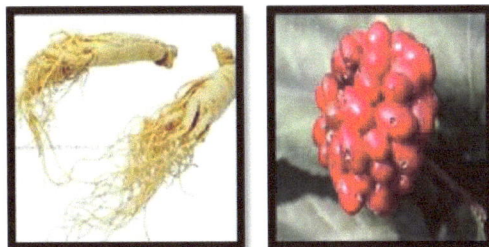

Name: *Panax ginseng* C.A. Meyer (*P. schinseng* Nees) (the most widely used), Araliaceae. *Panax japonicum* C.A. Meyer (Japanese ginseng).

Common name: Panax, Korean ginseng, Asian ginseng, Chinese ginseng, Oriental ginseng, true ginseng, Racine de ginseng.

Part used: Root and berries.

Main active constituents: Dammarane-type saponins; ginsenosides (panaxosides), steroidal and pentacyclic triterpenoid saponins.

Pharmacological action: The crude saponin of Korean red ginseng reduces body weight, food intake and fat content in (HFD) rats by reduction of hypothalamic NPY (Neuropeptide Y) expression and serum leptin [106]. On the other hand, wild ginseng ethanolic extracts exhibit significant inhibition of body weight gain (dose-dependent) with a decrease of white and brown adipoycte diameters. There is also significant inhibition of fasting blood glucose and triglyceride levels (dose-dependently) and improvement of insulin resistance [232]. Ginseng berries decrease body weight with significant increase in glucose tolerance but no significant decrease in FBG (fasting blood glucose) [233].

Phaseolus vulgaris

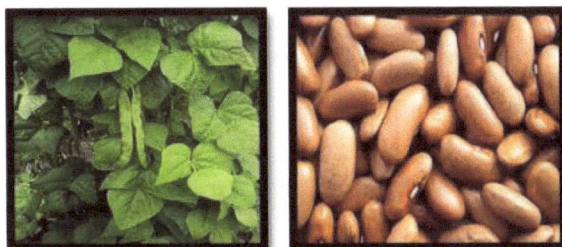

Name: *Phaseolus vulgaris* L., Fabaceae.

Common name: Kidney bean, the green bean, or common bean.

Part used: Seeds.

Main active constituents: Carbohydrates and lipids.

Pharmacological action: Reduction of body weight, BMI, fat mass, adipose tissue thickness, and waist/hip/thigh circumferences [95]. Seeds of *P. vulgaris* (300 g/kg bw) show maximal blood glucose lowering effect in diabetic rats. The combination of seeds (300 mg/kg bw) and glibenclamide (0.20 g/kg bw) are safer and potent hypoglycemics as well as antihyperglycemics, without creating severe hypoglycemia in normal rats [234]. *P. vulgaris* extract acts as α-amylase inhibitor starch blockers. Consumption of the α-amylase inhibitor causes marginal intraluminal α-amylase activity facilitated by the inhibitor's appropriate structural, physico-chemical and functional properties. As a result there is decrease in postprandial plasma hyperglycaemia and insulin levels, increase resistance of starch to digestion and an increase in the activity of colorectal bacteria. The extracts are potential ingredients in foods for increased carbohydrate tolerance in diabetics, decreased energy intake for reducing obesity and for increased resistant starch [235].

Punica granatum

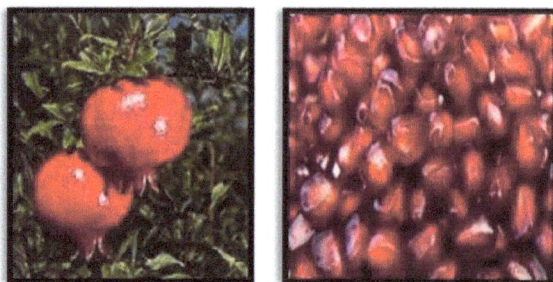

Name: *Punica granatum* L., Punicaceae

Common name: Pomegranate, Anar.

Part used: Seeds and flowers.

Main active constituents: Phenolic constituents; hydrolyzable tannins: pomegranate ellagitannins (punicalagins).

Pharmacological action: The aqueous extract of pomegranate leaves (AEP) and its isolated compounds (ellagic and tannic acid) show a significant decrease in body weight, energy intake and various adipose pad weight percent and serum, TC (total cholesterol), TG (triglycerides), glucose levels and TC/HDL-C ratio on mice fed with high fat diet (obese). Moreover, AEP significantly attenuates the raising of the serum TG level and inhibits the intestinal fat absorption, in addition to, a significant difference in decreasing the appetite of obese mice. These effects are partly mediated by inhibiting PL activity and suppressing energy intake [191].

Platycodon grandiflorum

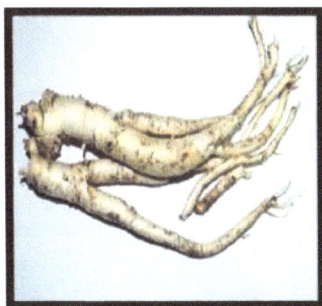

Name: *Platycodon grandiflorum* (Jacq.) A. DC., Campanulaceae.

Common name: Japanese bellflower, common balloon flower, or balloon flower.

Part used: Root.

Main active constituents: Triterpenoid saponins: sapogenins platycodigenin and polygalacic acid; platycodins A-I and polygalacins D and D2.

Pharmacological action: The aqueous *Platycodon grandiflorum* extract (150 mg/kg), when fed to obese rats, decreases significantly body weight with adipose tissues being converted to NLD (Necrobiosis lipoidica diabeticorum). In addition, it significantly decreases fat cells number and size and FABP (fatty acid binding protein) expression [236].

Rheum palmatum

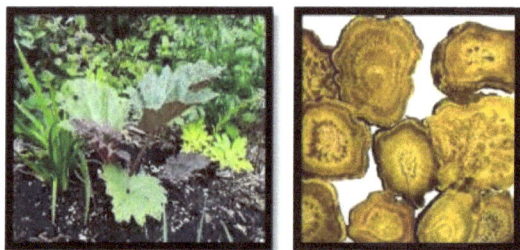

Name: *Rheum palmatum* L., Polygonaceae.

Common name: Rhubarb.

Part used: Rhizome and root.

Main Active Constituents: Anthraquinones, flavonoids; free and combined.

Pharmacological action: Methanolic extracts from *Rheum palmatum* L., at a concentration of 200 mg/mL, significantly inhibit PPL. Emodin, one of the main effective components in *R. palmatum* promotes proliferation of 3T3-L1 preadipocyte at low concentration and inhibits the proliferation at high concentration in a dose-related manner. In contrast, it inhibits cell differentiation into adipocyte at low concentration in a dose-related manner. Emodin exerts anti-lipase activity which suggests that it can be used as an anti-obesity drug [237].

Rubus coreanus

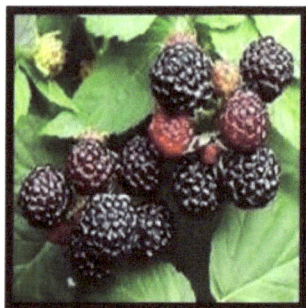

Name: *Rubus coreanus* Miq., Rosaceae.

Common name: Korean blackberry.

Part used: Berries.

Main active constituents: Anthocyanins, dimeric triterpene glucosyl ester; 23-Hydroxytormentic acid.

Pharmacological action: *Rubus coreanus* significantly reduces intracellular lipid accumulation by regulating PPARγ and C/EBPα (PPARγ and C/EBPα are critical transcription factors in adipogenesis) [238]. High content of anthocyanins attenuates the adipogenesis by inhibition of the Nrf2 binding with regions of PPARγ promoter (PPARγ is a nuclear receptor that controls lipid and glucose metabolism and exerts anti-inflammatory activities). Anthocyanins play an important role in anti-adipogenic activity by regulation of Nrf2 activation (a powerful protein that is dormant within each cell in the body, unable to move or perform until it is released by an Nrf2 activator. Once released it migrates into the cell nucleus and bonds to the DNA at the location of the Antioxidant Response Element (ARE) or also called hARE (Human Antioxidant Response Element) which is the master regulator of the entire antioxidant system that is present in all human cells) [238].

Rubus idaeus

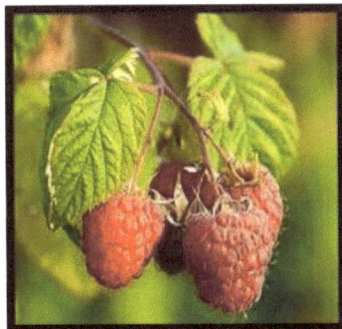

Name: *Rubus idaeus* L, Rosaceae.

Common name: Red raspberry.

Part used: Berries.

Main active constituents: Polyphenols and raspberry ketone.

Pharmacological action: RK (Raspberry ketone), administered to mice either admixed in concentrations 0.5-2% to a high-fat diet for 10 weeks or to mice fed a high-fat diet for 6 weeks and subsequently fed the same diet containing 1% RK for the next 5 weeks, reveals anti-obesity activity. RK (Raspberry ketone) prevents the high-fat-diet-induced elevations in body weight and the weights of the liver and visceral adipose tissues (epididymal, retroperitoneal, and mesenteric) in mice. RK also decreases these weights and hepatic triacylglycerol content after being increased by a high-fat diet. RK significantly increases norepinephrine-induced lipolysis associated with the translocation of hormone-sensitive lipase from the cytosol to lipid droplets in rat epididymal fat cells. In conclusion, RK prevents and improves obesity and fatty liver [196].

Salacia reticulata

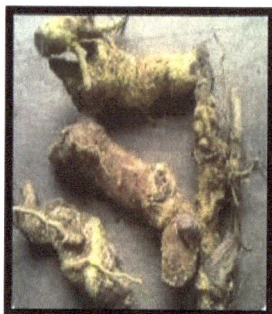

Name: *Salacia reticulata* Wight., Hippocrateaceae.

Common name: Sinhala: Kothalahimbatu.

Part used: Root bark.

Main active constituents: Polyphenols; salacinol, kotalanol, and mangiferin.

Pharmacological action: The aqueous extract of *Salacia reticulata* root (125 mg/kg) suppresses body weight and periuterine fat storage in female obese rats. Polyphenolic compounds, isolated from *Salacia reticulata*, are involved in its anti-obesity effects through inhibition of fat metabolizing enzymes (PL, LPL and GPDH (Glycerol-3-phosphate dehydrogenase; an enzyme maintaining lipid metabolism)) and enhance lipolysis [239].

Sambucus nigra

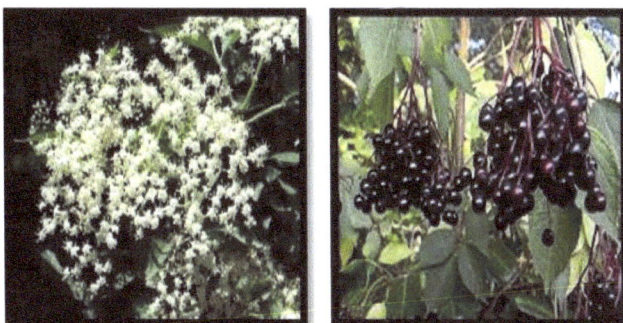

Name: *Sambucus nigra* L., Adoxaceae.

Common name: Elder, elderberry, black elder, European elder, European elderberry, European black elderberry, common elder, or elder bush.

Part used: Flower heads and berries.

Main Active Constituents: Phenolic compounds; flavonoids and anthocyanins.

Pharmacological action: The juice directly stimulates insulin secretion and glucose metabolism [240]. Powdered elder juice decreases total cholesterol and induces slight reductions in triglycerides, and HDL- and LDL-cholesterol [241]. Also, food supplements containing elderberry cause significant decrease in plasma and hepatic lipids [242].

Terminalia arjuna

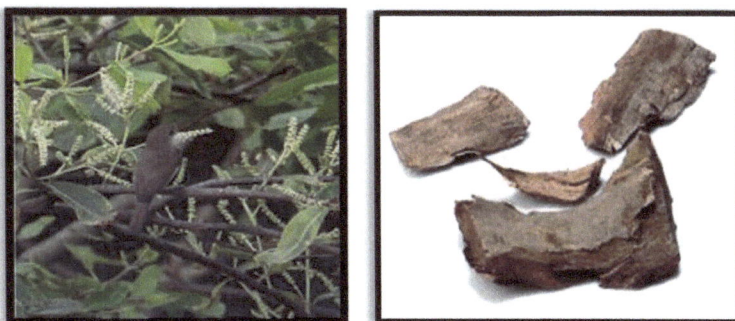

Name: *Terminalia arjuna* (Roxb.) Wight & Arn. Combretaceae.

Common name: Whitem, arjun or Koha.

Part used: Herb and bark.

Main Active Constituents: Tannins, and saponin glycosides.

Pharmacological action: The petroleum ether extract of *Terminalia arjuna* causes a significant decrease in body weight in hyperlipidemic humans, accompanied by significant decrease in serum total lipid levels [243].

Zingiber officinale

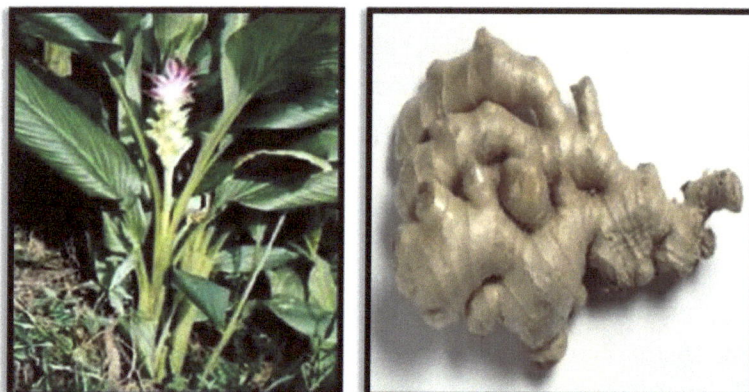

Name*: Zingiber officinale* L., Zingiberaceae.

Common name: Ginger Root.

Part used: Dried, peeled rhizome, chopped.

Main active constituents: Gingerol and shogaol (oleoresins).

Pharmacological action: Aqueous extract of *Z.officinale* at 0.4 ml/kg body weight causes significant decrease in plasma glucose and cholesterol in rats [244]. Ethanolic extract of ginger (200 mg/kg) lowers: serum triglycerides, lipoproteins, phospholipids, as well as serum and tissue cholesterol. Ginger extract consumption reduces plasma cholesterol, inhibits LDL oxidation and attenuates development of atherosclerosis in atherosclerotic, apolipoprotein E-deficient mice [245].

Lower Plants and Micro-Organisms

Algae

Brown algae

Phaeophyta, Phylum Heterokontophyta and Class Phaeophyceae; about 1800 species; examples of brown algae are the seaweeds of genus *Fucus* commonly called "rockweed," or "wracks," and members of genus *Sargassum*, which form floating mats.

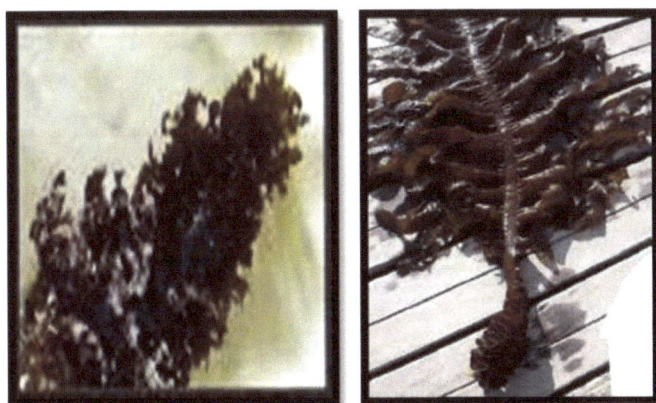

Name*: Undaria pinnatifida* (Harvey) Suringar = *Alaria pinnatifida* Harvey, Alariaceae.

Common name: Brown algae, wakame, kelp and seaweeds.

Part used: Thallus.

Main active constituents: Fucoidan (sulfated fucose containing polysaccharide, found in the fibrillar cell walls and intercellular spaces of brown seaweeds of the class Phaeophyceae) and fucoxanthin (carotenoid).

Pharmacological action: PL inhibitors; Fucoidan reduces lipid accumulation by stimulating lipolysis. Treatment with fucoidan reduces lipid accumulation in cells in a dose-dependent manner suggesting that it can be useful for prevention or treatment of obesity [246]. Fucoxanthin, isolated from wakame significantly suppresses body weight and white adipose tissues (WAT). A dietary of wakame may ameliorate alterations in lipid metabolism and insulin resistance induced by a HFD (high fat diet) [247]. The anti-obesity effect of fucoxanthin is likely linked to its structural characteristic- an allene bond and an additional hydroxyl substituent on the side group of the fucoxanthin metabolites, fucoxanthinol and amarouciaxanthin A [248].

Green algae

Phyllum chlorophyta includes about 4300 species of green algae.

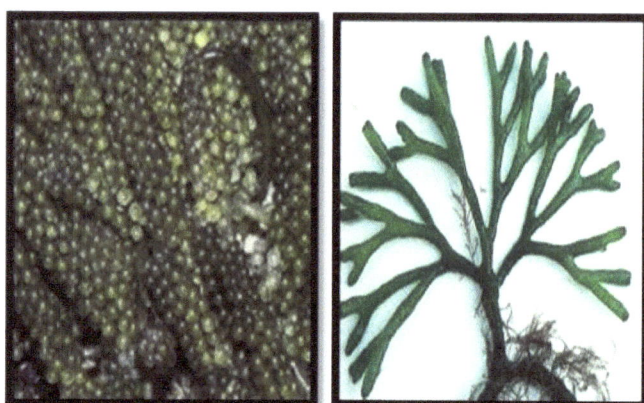

Name: *Caulerpa lentillifera* J. Agardh, class: Bryopsidophyceae, order: Bryopsidale F. Caulerpaceae; and *Codium fragile* (suringar) Hariot, class: Bryopsidophyceae, order: Bryopsidales F. Codiaceae.

Common name: *Caulerpa lentillifera* is known as sea grapes, green caviar and *Codium fragile* as Green sea fingers, Dead man's fingers, felty fingers, felt-alga, green fleece.

Part used: Thallus.

Main active constituents: Siphonaxanthin (carotenoid).

Pharmacological action: PL inhibitor; siphonaxanthin (isolated from green algae as *Caulerpa lentillifera* and *Codium fragile*) significantly reduces lipid accumulation during differentiation to adipocytes. This suppressive effect is stronger than that of fucoxanthin [249].

Fungi

Ganoderma lucidum

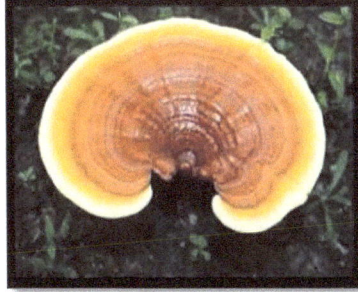

Name: *Ganoderma lucidum* (Curtis) P. Karst, Ganodermataceae.

Common name: Mushroom of immortality, lingzhi mushroom or reishi mushroom, supernatural mushroom.

Part used: Whole mushroom.

Main active constituents: Lanostane triterpenes.

Pharmacological action: Extracts from *Ganoderma* reduce glucose levels [193] Lanostane triterpenes reduce TG accumulation [250]. This suggests that *G. lucidum* may serve as a new potential natural product for the prevention of obesity.

Phellinus linteus

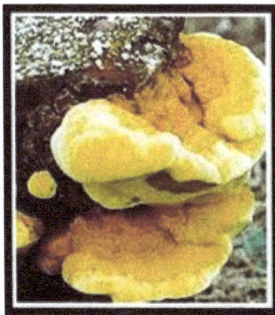

Name: *Phellinus linteus* (Berkeley & M. A. Curtis), class: Basidiomycetes, Hymenochaetaceae.

Common name: Medicinal mushroom, black hoof fungus (Japanese, "meshimakobu"; Chinese, "song gen"; Korean "sanghwang").

Part used: Whole mushroom.

Main active constituents: Polyphenolic compounds, polysaccharides [251].

Pharmacological action: Lipase inhibitor. Methanolic extract of the fruiting bodies of *Phellinus linteus* reveals anti-obesity activity by inhibition of lipase enzyme (a key enzyme for dietary fat adsorption, hydrolyzing triacylglycerols to 2-monoacylglycerols and fatty acids). A potent lipase inhibitor which could be very useful as an anti-obesity compound [252].

Sparassis crispa

Name: *Sparassis crispa* Fr., *Sparassis radicata* Weir, Sparassidaceae.

Common name: Cauliflower mushroom of immortality, lingzhi mushroom, reishi mushroom, supernatural mushroom.

Part used: Whole mushroom.

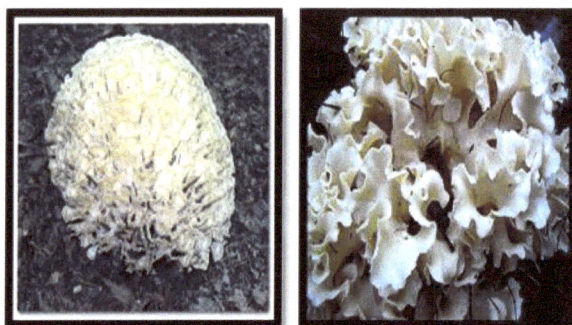

Main active constituents: Diterpenes, triterpenes and fatty acids [253].

Pharmacological action: Water-soluble extract of Cauliflower mushroom reduces weight gain of the mice. Additionally, serum level of total cholesterol, triglyceride and glucose are decreased in mice fed with CM (cauliflower mushroom). Moreover, hepatic triglyceride and total cholesterol level are also lowered. These results demonstrate that the water extract of CM improves serum and hepatic lipids and body weight reduction [254].

Micro-Organisms

Streptomyces species

(Phyllum, Actinobacteria; Order, Actinomycetales; F. Streptomycetaceae).

Name: *Streptomyces toxytricini.*

Active constituent: Lipstatin, a PL inhibitor was first isolated from this *Streptomyces* sp. [89], its saturated derivative is the popular antiobesity drug, Orlistat. The lipstatin molecule has an unusual β-lactone structure incorporated into a hydrocarbon backbone.

Pharmacological action: Lipstatin is a potent, irreversible inhibitor of pancreatic lipase. The *β*- lactone structure probably accounts for the irreversible lipase inhibition [89].

Name: *Streptomyces* sp. MTCC 5219.

Source: Isolated from a soil sample of a cow barnyard in India.

Pharmacological action: PL inhibitor. A low molecular weight molecule, (E)-4-aminostyryl acetate (belonging to the class of enol acetate of *p*-amino phenyl acetaldehyde), isolated from this *Streptomyces* sp., has shown *in vitro* lipid lowering activity in mammalian lipase inhibition assay. The small size along with the good solubility property would give this molecule a better druggability character [255].

Name: *Streptomyces* sp.

Source: Isolated from the western ghat soil samples of Agumbe, Karnataka, India.

Pharmacological action: PL inhibitor. The activity of lipase enzyme is drastically inhibited by the *n*-butanol extract of the culture broth in dose-dependent manner [256].

Bifidobacterium species

(Phyllum, Actinobacteria; Order, Bifidobacteriales; Family, Bifidobacteriaceae).

Name: *Bifidobacterium pseudocatenulatum* SPM 120, *B. longum* SPM 1205, and *B. longum* SPM 1207.

Pharmacological action: α-amylase and PL inhibitors. They significantly decrease activities of ß-glucosidase, β-glucuronidase, and tryptophanase [257].

They act through the following [257-259]:

a. Inhibition of cholesterol synthesizing enzymes and thus reducing cholesterol production.

b. Enhancement of cholesterol elimination in feces.

c. Inhibition of back absorption of cholesterol into the body by binding with it.

d. Interference with recycling of bile salt (a metabolic product of cholesterol) and enhancement of its elimination, which raises the demand for bile salt produced from cholesterol and thus results in body cholesterol consumption.

e. Reduction of levels of triglyceride, glucose, AST, and ALT in serum.

TYPES OF SECONDARY PLANT AND MICROBIAL METABOLITES WITH ANTI-OBESITY ACTIVITY

Natural products, particularly medicinal plants, are believed to harbor potential antiobesity agents that can act through various mechanisms either by preventing weight gain or promoting weight loss amongst others. New technologies such as metabolomics, which deals with the study of the whole metabolome has been identified to be a promising technique to probe the progression of diseases, elucidate their pathologies and assess the effects of natural health products on certain pathological conditions. The inhibition of key lipid and carbohydrate hydrolyzing and metabolizing enzymes, disruption of adipogenesis and modulation of its factors or appetite suppression are some approaches to probe the anti-obesity potential of medicinal plants [56]. The potential and relevance of metabolomics in obesity are discussed below:

Phenolics

Phenolics in particular polyphenols are a group of antioxidants characterized by the presence of several hydroxyl groups on an aromatic ring. Over the last decade, polyphenols have been implicated in the prevention of a number of oxidative-related diseases including cardiovascular diseases, hypertension and diabetes. They are often categorized into 4 groups depending on the number of phenol rings embodied in their structure and the elements that bind these rings together [260]. Distinction is hence made between phenolic acids, flavonoids, stilbenes and lignans [260, 261].

    a.   Phenolic acids.

    b.   Flavonoids.

    c.   Stilbenes.

    d.   Lignans.

Pharmacological Action:

- Phenolics are PL inhibitors [56, 70, 228].

- Phenolic extracts are able to decrease the blood levels of glucose, triglycerides and LDL cholesterol, increase energy expenditure and fat oxidation, and reduce body weight and adiposity [262, 263].

- Catechin acts as anti-obesic through its anti-lipase activity and by increasing thermogenesis [97].

- Epigallocatechingallate suppresses the number of adipocytes and triacylglycerols uptake [264].

- Selected examples of phenolis with reported anti-obesity activity are represented in Figs. **4, 5** and **6**.

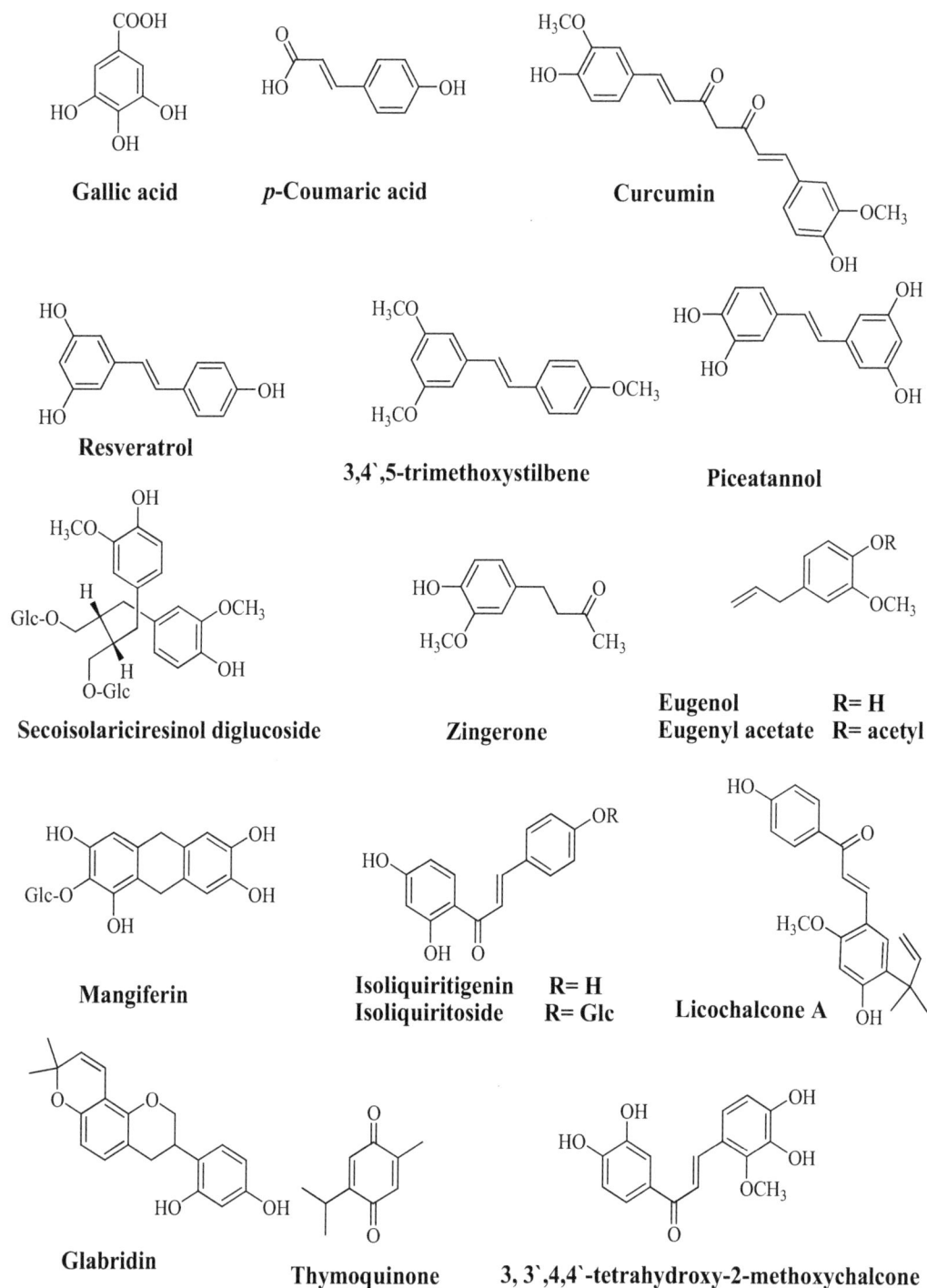

Gallic acid   *p*-**Coumaric acid**   **Curcumin**

Resveratrol

3,4`,5-trimethoxystilbene   **Piceatannol**

Secoisolariciresinol diglucoside   **Zingerone**   **Eugenol**   R= H
                                                            Eugenyl acetate   R= acetyl

Mangiferin   **Isoliquiritigenin**   R= H   **Licochalcone A**
                      Isoliquiritoside   R= Glc

Glabridin   **Thymoquinone**   **3, 3`,4,4`-tetrahydroxy-2-methoxychalcone**

Figure 4: Phenolic compounds.

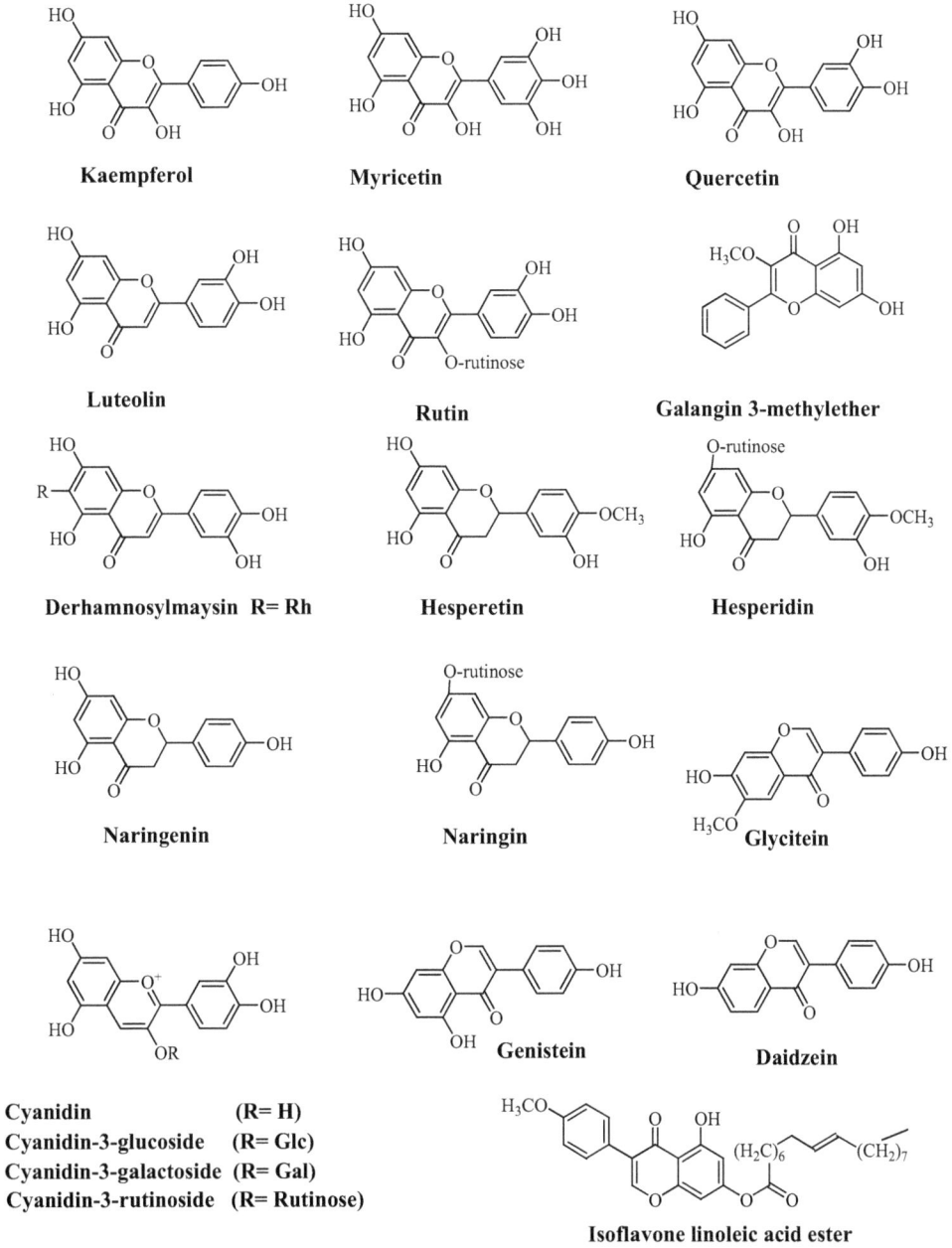

Kaempferol

Myricetin

Quercetin

Luteolin

Rutin

Galangin 3-methylether

Derhamnosylmaysin R= Rh

Hesperetin

Hesperidin

Naringenin

Naringin

Glycitein

Cyanidin   (R= H)
Cyanidin-3-glucoside   (R= Glc)
Cyanidin-3-galactoside (R= Gal)
Cyanidin-3-rutinoside   (R= Rutinose)

Genistein

Daidzein

Isoflavone linoleic acid ester

Figure 5: Flavonoidal compounds.

(-)-Catechin

(-)-Epigallocatechin gallate

(-)-Epicatechin gallate

Theaflavin

Theaflavin-3-gallate

Theaflavin-3, 3`-gallate

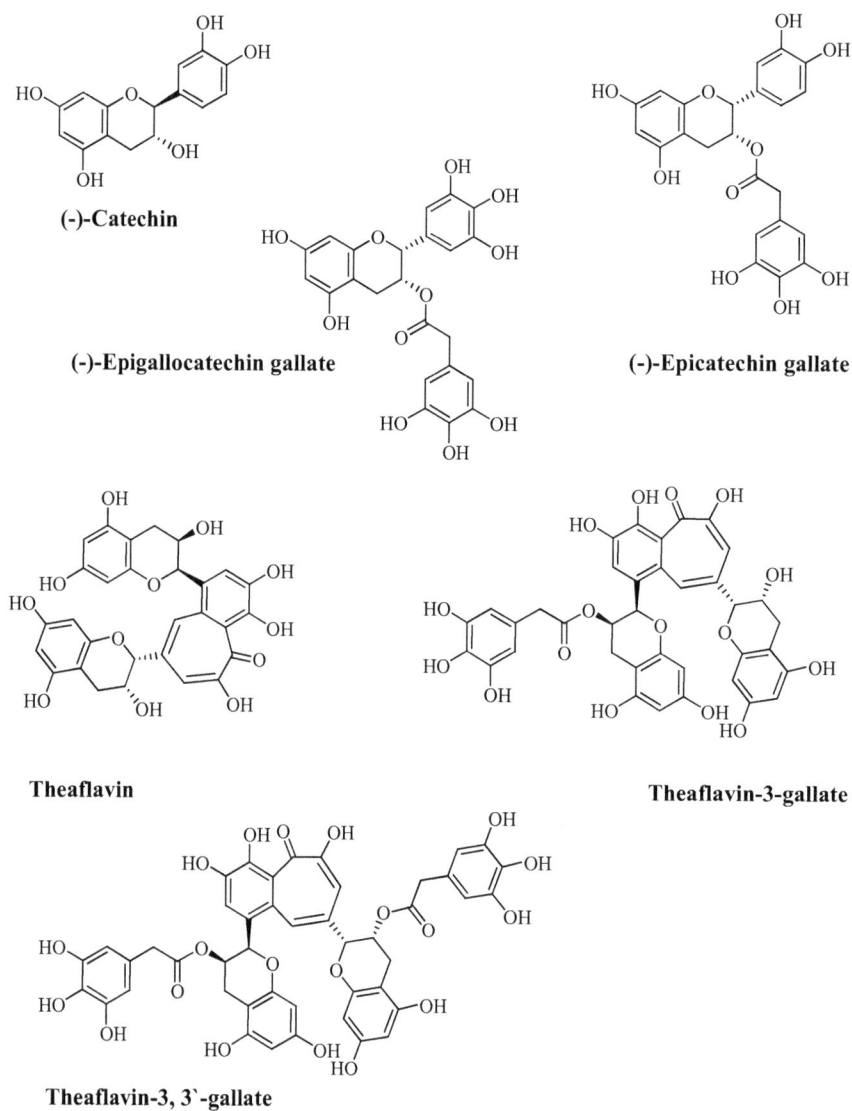

Figure 6: Catechins and theaflavins.

Pregnane Glycosides

These are steroidal compounds mostly present in the Milkweed family; *e.g.* P57 or P57A53.

Pharmacological Action

-   Pregnane glycosides are reputed for their appetite suppressant property [103, 265].

-   Pregnane glycosides act on two levels; by blocking the growth of pre-adipocytes and reducing the level of leptin. These immature cells (pre-adipocytes) are the source of adipocytes which absorb fat and produce leptin, a hormone involved in the long-term regulation of bodyweight. High levels of leptin are found in overweight and obese people. In human trials, there is a significant reduction in the feelings of hunger and body weight in overweight people [266].

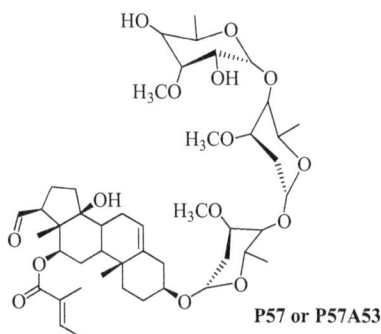

P57 or P57A53

Saponins

Saponins are a major family of secondary metabolites that occur in a wide range of plants species [267]. These compounds have been isolated from different plant parts, including roots, rhizomes, stems, bark, leaves, seeds and fruits. Occasionally, the whole plant has been used [268].

Saponins are categorized into two major classes;

   a.   Triterpenoidal saponins.

   b.   Steroidal saponins.

Both are from the 30 carbon atoms-containing precursor oxidosqualene [268, 269].

Pharmacological Action

- Saponins inhibit P enzyme.

- Escins (triterpenoidal saponins) suppress the increase in body weight, adiposity and liver fat, and the increase in triglyceride level in the feces, also they decrease plasma triglycerides [270].

- Steroidal saponins *e.g.* Ginsenosides decrease plasma triacylglycerides and cause a delay in intestinal fat absorption due to inhibition of pancreatic lipase [62, 271, 272].

- Diosgenin (steroidal saponin) decreases the plasma and hepatic total cholesterol levels, and increases the plasma high-density lipoprotein (HDL) cholesterol level [273].

- Steroidal and triterpenoidal saponins of reported anti-obesity effect are represented in Fig. **7**.

Alkaloids

Alkaloids are a group of naturally occurring chemical compounds that contain mostly basic nitrogen atoms. This group also includes some related compounds with neutral and even weakly acidic properties. Alkaloids are produced by a large variety of organisms, including bacteria, fungi, plants, and animals.

Pharmacological Action

- Berberine (isoquinoline alkaloid) reduces blood lipid levels (triglycerides and cholesterol levels) in human [274].

- Ephedrine (phenylalkylamine) and caffeine (methylxanthine alkaloid) exert their anti-obesity activity by thermogenesis (significant increase in energy expenditure) [131].

- Capsaicin (proto-alkaloid) increases thermogenesis through enhancement of catecholamine secretion from the adrenal medulla [274, 275].

Corosolic acid

Silphioside   **R= H**
Copteroside   **R= OH**

Chikusetsusaponin III

Oleanolic acid

Gymnemic acid
R= glucuronic acid

chikusetsusaponin IV R_1= Glc, R_2= H   R=R_3= Ara
28-deglucosyl-chikusetsusaponins IV R_1, R_2= H, R_3=Ara
28-deglucosyl-chikusetsusaponins V R_1, R_3= H, R_2=Glc

Dioscin R_1=R_3= Rh, R_2= H
Gracillin R_1=H, R_2=Glc, R_3= Rh

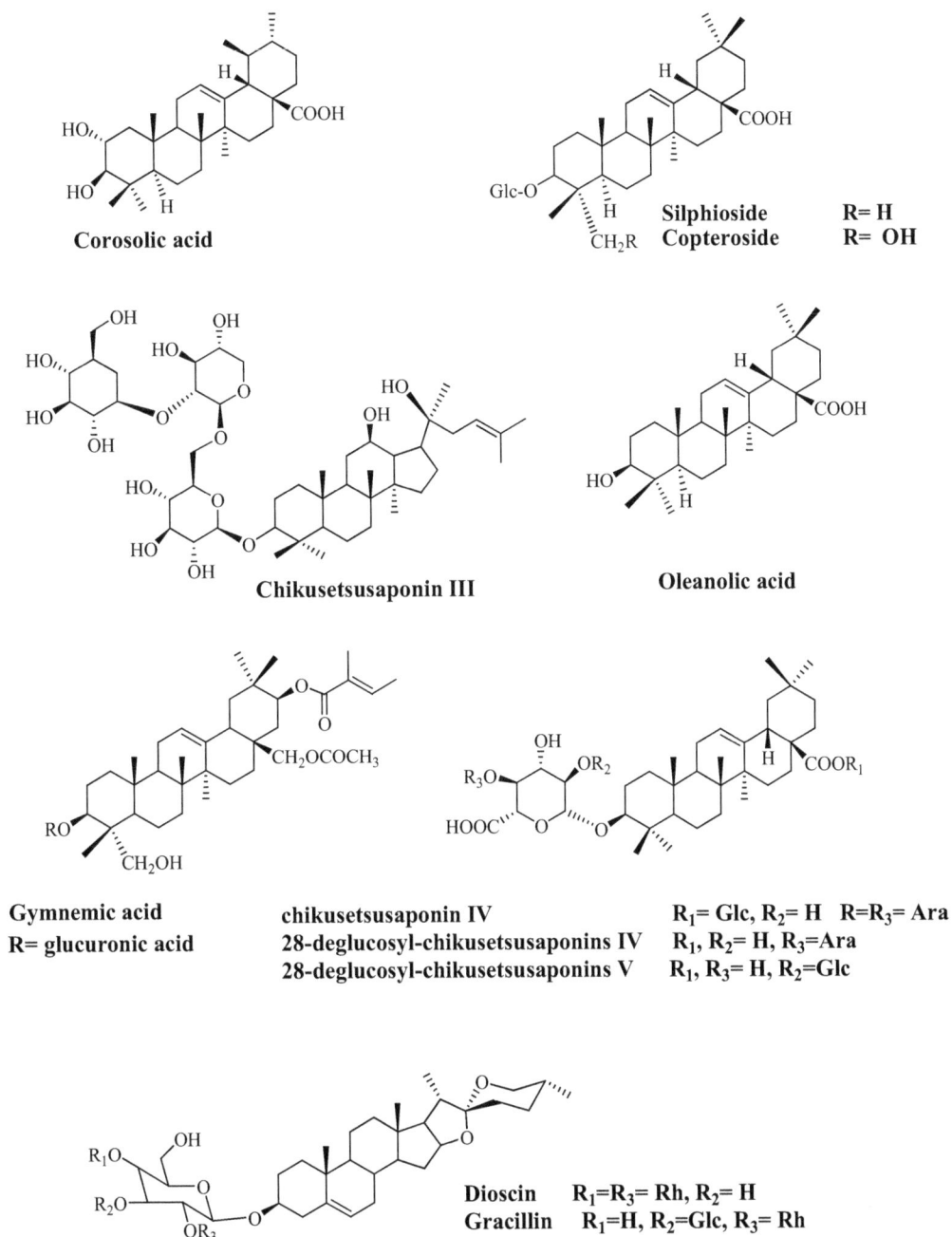

Figure 7: Steroidal and triterpenoidal saponins.

- Alkaloids reported to play a role in management of obesity are represented in Fig. **8**.

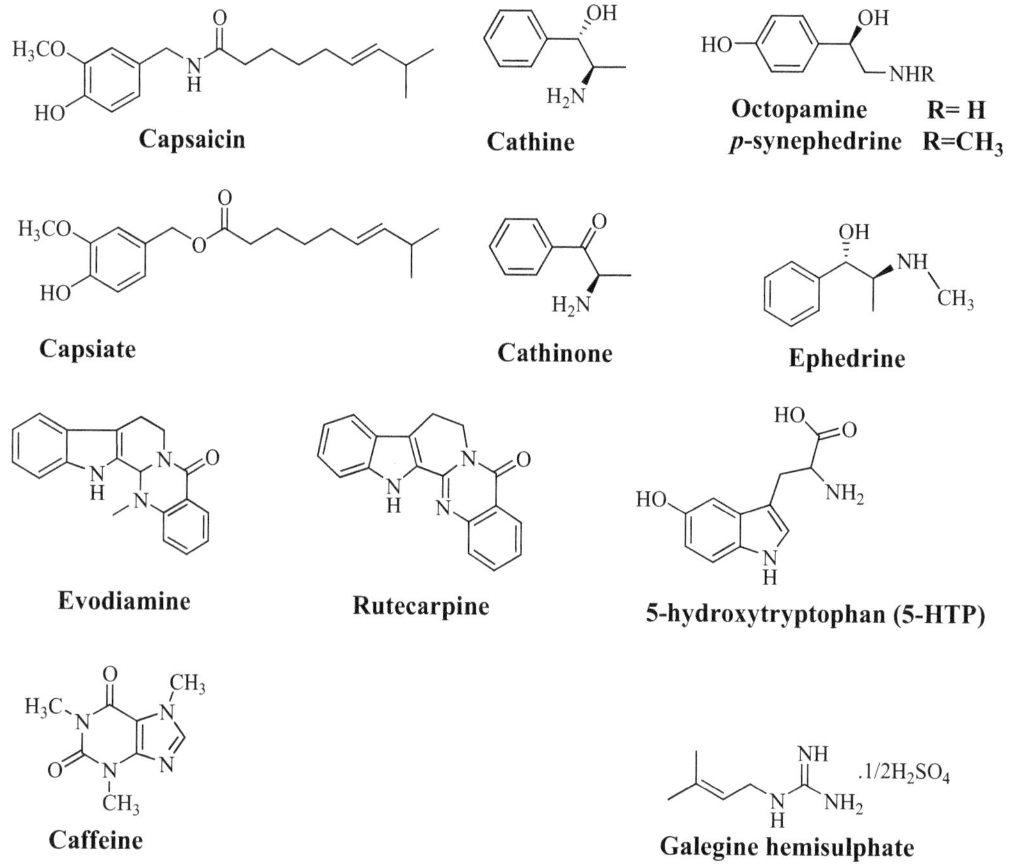

Figure 8: Alkaloids.

Diterpenes

Diterpenes are a type of terpenoids composed of four isoprene units and have the molecular formula $C_{20}H_{32}$. They derive from geranylgeranyl pyrophosphate. Abietane is a diterpene skeleton that forms the structural basis for a variety of natural compounds such as abietic acid, carnosic acid, and ferruginol which are collectively known as abietanes or abietane diterpenes.

Pharmacological Action

Carnosic acid inhibits pancreatic lipase [276], activates peroxisome proliferators-activated receptor gamma (PPARγ) [277], and prevents the differentiation of pre-adipocytes into adipocytes [278].

Selected examples of diterpenes with reported anti-obesity activity are displayed in Fig. **9**

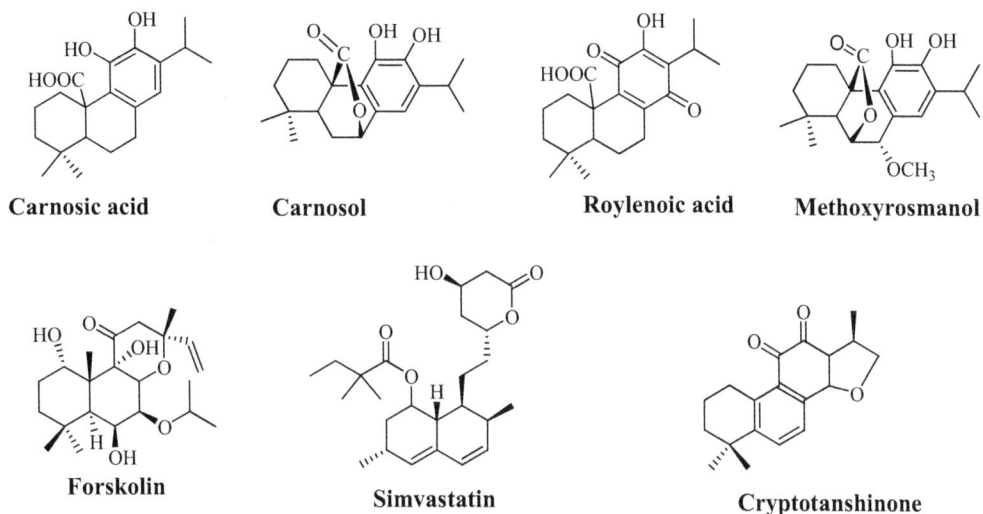

Carnosic acid   Carnosol   Roylenoic acid   Methoxyrosmanol

Forskolin   Simvastatin   Cryptotanshinone

Figure 9: Diterpenes.

Carotenoids

Carotenoids are organic pigments that are found in chloroplasts of plants and some other photosynthetic organisms like algae, and certain bacteria and fungi. Carotenoids can be produced from fats and other basic organic metabolic building blocks by all these organisms. Carotenoids generally cannot be manufactured by species in the animal kingdom so animals obtain carotenoids in their diets, and may employ them in various ways in metabolism. All carotenoids are tetraterpenoids, *i.e.* that they are produced from 8 isoprene molecules and contain 40 carbon atoms.

They are split into two classes:

a.   Xanthophylls (which contain oxygen).

b.   Carotenes (which are purely hydrocarbons, and contain no oxygen).

Pharmacological Action

-   Carotenoids containing an allene bond, such as fucoxanthin and fucoxanthinol, show anti-obesity effects by suppressing adipocyte differentiation; fucoxanthin intake leads to oxidation of fatty acids and heat production in WAT mitochondria [279].

- Carotenoids, *e.g.* fucoxanthin, exert their anti-obesity activity through protein and gene expressions of UCP1 (uncoupling-protein 1, a gene restricted to BAT, where it provides a mechanism for the enormous heat-generating capacity of the tissue) in WAT [280].

- Structural formulae of selected carotenoids with anti-obesity activity are shown in Fig. **10**.

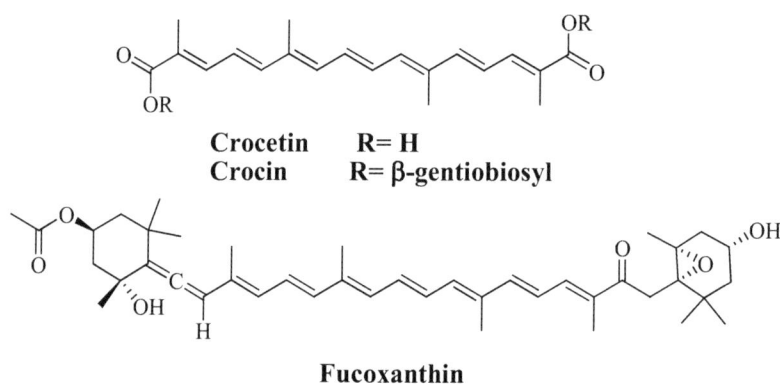

Crocetin   R= H
Crocin   R= β-gentiobiosyl

Fucoxanthin

Figure 10: Carotenoids.

Secondary Metabolites from Microbial Sources

Microbial secondary metabolites are important sources for development drugs against various human diseases such as bacterial and fungal infections, cancer, transplant rejection, high cholesterol and many others. Actinomycetes are the most economically and biotechnologically valuable prokaryotes, especially the strains of *Streptomyces* producing streptomycin. Lipstatin (Orlistat®), a very potent PL inhibitor was first isolated from *Streptomyces toxytricini*. It has an unusual β-lactone structure incorporated into a hydrocarbon backbone. Furthermore, *Streptomyces* lactic acid bacteria of genus *Bifidobacterium* showed α-amylase and PL inhibitory activity (*B. pseudocatenulatum*) [70].

Microbial metabolites with reported anti-obesity potentiality are represented in Fig. **11**.

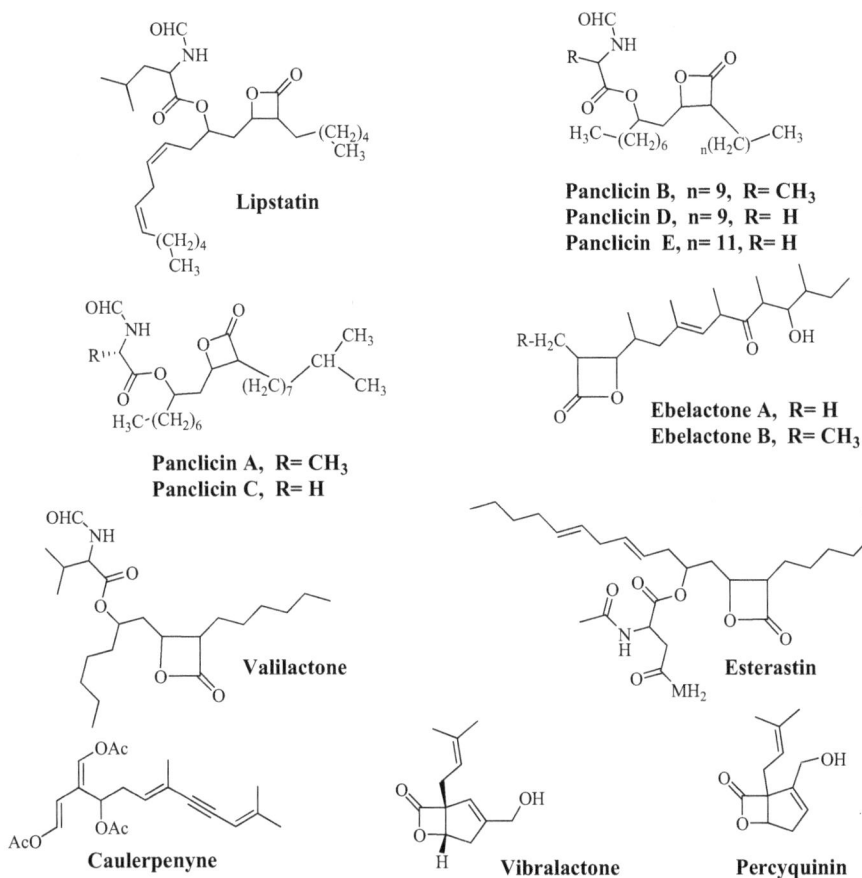

Figure 11: Secondary metabolites from microbial sources.

ADVERSE EFFECTS OF NATURAL ANTI-OBESITY PRODUCTS

Synthetic drugs designed to suppress hunger have promoted weight loss, but are often accompanied by untoward side effects. Most anorectic drugs act by central mechanisms have many side effects on the central nervous system, the development of tolerance, abuse potential, and rebound hyperphagia (over-eating) on discontinuation of treatment.

Natural products used in management of obesity experience also a number of side effects which range from mild to seriously adverse.

According to the amount of administered doses, herbal supplements containing ephedra and/or caffeine were reported to produce greatly variable results in terms of both effectiveness and experienced side effects. Minor adverse effects, such as dry mouth, insomnia, headache and nervousness, were reported at low doses and short term use. On the other hand, palpitation, increase in blood pressure and loose bowel movements were observed at higher doses and long term use. Ephedrine, a sympathomimetic alkaloid and major constituent of ephedra and stimulator of α- and β-adrenergic receptors lead to increase blood pressure and vasoconstriction which may be taxing on the hear [29]. Adverse events reported to be attributable to ephedra or ephedrine consumption exposed five deaths, five myocardial infarctions, 11 cerebrovascular accidents, four seizures, and eight psychiatric cases of an idiopathic nature. In 2004, FDA banned the sale of dietary supplements containing ephedra alkaloids because such supplements present an unreasonable risk of illness or injury [281].

The administration of *Garcinia cambogia* extract to obese male Zucker rats resulted in suppression of epididymal fat accumulation at a dose of 154 mmol hydroxyl citric acid (HCA)/kg diet, but diets containing 102 mmol/kg HCA and more caused testicular toxicity, while the no-observed-adverse-effect-level was determined to be 51 mmol HCA/kg diet [194]. A few adverse events were reported, mostly related to GIT disturbances, headache and upper respiratory tract symptoms. Toxicity studies on CitriMax, which contains a calcium/potassium-HCA complex, revealed low oral acute toxicity with mild skin and eye irritation in rats. No significant toxic effects were found in a sub-chronic toxicity study and mutagenicity has not been demonstrated. Taking all of the clinical trials and other scientific studies into consideration, consumption of HCA at 2800 mg/day was proposed as safe [194, 282].

Data on the toxicity/safety of *H. gordonii* is very limited. Acute toxicity studies were described in a patent application [283]. A plant extract administered orally to mice in doses of 100-3028.5 mg/kg revealed no clinical signs of toxicity. In animal study, a dose-related reversible histopathological liver changes in the form of moderate cloudy swelling and hydropic degeneration of hepatocytes was recorded from a dose of 200 mg/kg, but further investigation is required. But, no adverse effects were reported for the clinical study performed in humans.

Reviewing most animal and human studies, only few studies mentioned adverse effects, it should be noted that many serious adverse events which would have stopped a trial of a pharmaceutical agent would likely not have been identified by the authors' search methods. Moreover, important safety issues including significant adverse events or supplement-drug interactions relevant to many clinical populations may not be fully addressed. Therefore, the determination of a favorable risk-benefit ratio should always be kept in mind. It looks that most of the plants reported in this chapter has been not investigated comprehensively. In addition to safety, the quality and efficacy of these plants are also neglected to a large extent.

CONCLUSIONS

Obesity is no longer considered a cosmetic problem. The incidence of obesity is recently increasing at an enormous rate, becoming a worldwide health burden which could be described as the pandemic of the 21st century. Moreover, its consequences are not only detrimental to human health but are expected to inflict unpredicted financial and social burdens on global society, unless effective measures are taken to control its prevalence.

Anti-obesity pharmacological treatment should be administered only when considered safe and effective for long-term use. Despite the large number of drugs proposed over the past three decades, few have been developed or approved, while others have been discarded from the market due to serious side-effects or abuse. The currently available drugs Sibutramine® and Orlistat® are commonly indicated in combination with dietary, behavioral, and exercise therapy to produce 10% weight loss utmost. This necessitates a continuous search for anti-obesity drugs which are better tolerated and at the same time more efficient.

The popularity of alternative medicine is tremendously rising as revealed by the boost in demand of natural health products. Extensive attention is focused on the use of naturally-derived remedies to alleviate obesity due to the failure of synthetic drugs to achieve the necessary long-term results. In this respect, various plant and microbial products have been explored either *in vitro* or *in vivo* animal models. They were found effective through various mechanisms such as gastric and PL inhibitors, central or peripheral appetite suppressants and enhancers of energy expenditure. The chief disadvantage is the uncertainty to extrapolate those effects to human subjects. Other drawbacks include the unclear risk of toxicity, insufficient information on mechanisms of action, as well as poor quality control of natural herbal products.

Drugs that regulate energy balance overlap considerably with other physiological functions, and are influenced by social and psychological factors that limit their use. Drugs that target pathways in metabolic tissues, such as adipocytes, liver and skeletal muscles, were found effective in preclinical studies but none has yet reached clinical development. The prolong use of certain gut peptides seems to be rational, particularly, that the deficiency of these peptides in obese individuals has been documented. Certain treatments are designed to meet diverse molecular targets in the CNS and/or periphery and, others several targets simultaneously.

Successful discovery and development of potent and safe natural drugs for both prevention and long-term treatment of obesity will probably rely on polytherapeutic strategies and necessitate continuous improvement of the identification and characterization tools. Among the advantages of polytherapy are: the use of lower drug doses, improvement of weight loss through additive and possible synergistic effects, as well as reduction of incidence of adverse side effects and consequently of the possibility for counter-regulation and further withdrawal.

Finally, medicinal plants and other naturally-derived products are gaining more scientifically-based validity as antiobesity agents; some of the natural compounds have reached clinical trials such as the oxypregnane steroidal saponin, P57 from *H. gordonii*. However, there are still numerous unstudied plants around the world which have traditionally been used as slimming agents, thus justifying the need for deeper research in this field in view to reach a safer and more effective pharmacological treatment for obesity.

ACKNOWLEDGEMENTS

Declared none.

CONFLICT OF INTEREST

The author confirms that this chapter contents have no conflict of interest.

REFERENCES

[1]   Caballero B. The global epidemic of obesity: An overview. Epidemiol Rev 2007; 29: 1-5.

[2]   Hossain P, Kawar B, El Nahas M. Obesity and Diabetes in the Developing World- A Growing Challenge. N Engl J Med 2007; 356: 213-215.

[3]   Haslam DW, James WP. Obesity. Lancet 2005; 366:1197-1209.

[4]   Huang HL, Hong YW, Wong YH, Chen YN, Chyuan JH, Huang CJ, Chao PM. Bitter melon (*Momordica charantia* L.) inhibits adipocyte hypertrophy and down regulates lipogenic gene expression in adipose tissue of diet-induced obese rats. Br J Nutr 2008; 99: 230–239.

[5]   World Health Organization. 2006a."BMI classification". Global database on body mass index. Available from: http://www.who.int/bmi/index.

[6]   World Health Organization. 2009. Obesity and Overweight. Available from: http://www.who.int/dietphysicalactivity/publications/facts/obesity/en/

[7]   Couillard C, Mauriege P, Imbeault P, *et al*. Hyperleptinemia is more closely associated with adipose cell hypertrophy than with adipose tissue hyperplasia. Int J Obes Relat Metab Disord 2000; 24: 782-788.

[8]   Konturek PC, Konturek JW, Cześnikiewicz-Guzik M, Brzozowski T, Sito E, Konturek SJ. Neuro-hormonal control of food intake: basic mechanisms and clinical implications. J Physiol Pharmacol 2005; 56 (Suppl, 6): 5-25.

[9]   ISAO/IOTF analysis. Obesity the Global Epidemic. 2010[Cited on 17th August 2012]. Available from: http://www.iaso.org/iotf/obesity/obesitytheglobalepidemic

[10]   Abdollahi M, Afshar-Imani B. A review on obesity and weight loss measures. Mid. East Pharm. 2003; 11: 6-10.

[11]   Mamais G.The Pandemic of the 21st century. [Cited: 29th July 2012]. Available from : http://www.ensaa.eu/index.php/public-health/109-the-pandemic-of-the-21st-century

[12]   World Health Organization. 2013 Fact sheets [cited on 21st May 2013]. Available from : http://www.who.int/mediacentre/factsheets/fs311/en/

[13]   Schrauwen P, Westerterp KR. The role of high-fat diets and physical activity in the regulation of body weight. Br J Nutr 2000; 84: 417-427.

[14]   Voshol P, Rensen PCN, van Dijk K, Romijn J, Havekes L. Effect of plasma triglyceride metabolism on lipid storage in adipose tissue: studies using genetically engineered mouse models. Biochim Biophys Acta 2009; 1791: 479-485.

[15]   Abete I, Astrup A, Martinez JA, Thorsdottir I, Zulet M. Obesity and the metabolic syndrome: role of different dietary macronutrient distribution patterns and specific nutritional components on weight loss and maintenance. Nutr Rev 2010; 68: 214-231.

[16]   Roh C, Jung U. Screening of crude plant extracts with anti-Obesity activity. Int J Mol Sci 2012; 13: 1710-1719.

[17]   De la Garza AL, Milagro FI, Bloke N, Campion, Martinez JA. Natural inhibitors of pancreatic lipase as new players in obesity treatment. Planta Med 2011; 77(8): 733-85.

[18]   Little T, Horowitz M, Feinle-Bisset C. Modulation by high-fat diets of gastrointestinal function and hormones associated with the regulation of energy intake: implications for the pathophysiology of obesity. Am J Clin Nutr 2007; 86: 531-541.

[19]   Bays H, Blonde L, Rosenson R. Adisopathy : how do diet, exercise and weight loss drug therapies improve metabolic disease in overweight patients? Expet Rev Cardiovasc Ther 2006; 4: 871-895.

[20] Mazucotelli A, Langin D. Fatty acid mobilization and their use in adipose tissue. J Soc Biol 2006; 200: 83-91.

[21] Reeves AF, Rees JM, Schiff M, Hujoel P. Total body weight and waist circumference associated with chronic peridontitis among adolescents in the United States. Archives of Pediatrics and Adolescent Medicine 2006; 160: 894-899.

[22] Ferraro KF, Su Y, Gretebeck RJ, Black DR, and Badylak SF. Body mass index and disability in adulthood: a 20-year panel study, Am J Public Health 2002; 92(5): 834-840.

[23] Mukherjee M. Human digestive and metabolic lipase-a brief review. J Mol Catal B Enzym 2003; 22(5-6): 369-376.

[24] Rubio M, Gargallo M, Millán A, Moreno B. Drugs in the treatment of obesity: sibutramine, orlistat and rimonabant. Public Health Nutr 2007; 10: 1200-1205.

[25] Hardeman W, Griffin S, Johnston M, Kinmonth AL, Wareham NJ. Interventions to prevent weight gain: a systematic review of psychological models and behaviour change methods. Int J Obes Relat Metab Disord 2000; 24: 131-143.

[26] Rodgers RJ, Tschöp MH, Wilding JPH. Anti-obesity drugs: past, present and future. Dis Model Mech 2012; 5(5): 621-626.

[27] Cooke D, Bloom S. The obesity pipeline: current strategies in the development of anti-obesity drugs. Nat Rev Drug Discov 2006; 5: 919-931.

[28] Sargent BJ, Moore N A. New central targets for the treatment of obesity. Br J Clin Pharmacol 2009; 68: 852-860.

[29] Hasani-Ranjbar S, Nayebi N, Larijani B, Abdollahi M. A systematic review of the efficacy and safety of herbal medicines used in the treatment of obesity. World J Gastroenterol 2009; 15 (25): 3073-3085.

[30] Chaput JP, St-Pierre S, Tremblay A. Currently available drugs for the treatment of obesity: sibutramine and orlistat. Mini Rev Med Chem 2007; 7: 3-10.

[31] Mahan LK, Escott-Stump S. Krause's food, nutrition, and diet therapy. 12th ed. Philadelphia: WB Saunders and Co. 2008.

[32] Ballinger A, Peikin SR. Orlistat: its current status as an anti-obesity drug. Eur J Pharmacol 2002; 440: 109-117.

[33] Drew BS, Dixon AF, Dixon JB. Obesity management: update on orlistat. Vasc Health Risk Manag 2007; 3: 817-821.

[34] Hutton B, Fergusson D. Changes in body weight and serum lipid profile in obese patients treated with orlistat in addition to a hypocaloric diet: a systematic review of randomized clinical trials. Am J Clin Nutr 2004; 80: 1461-1468.

[35] Thurairajah PH, Syn WK, Neil DA, Stell D, Haydon G. Orlistat (xenical)-induced subacute liver failure. Eur J Gastroenterol Hepatol 2005; 17: 1437-1438.

[36] Lean ME. How does sibutramine work? Int J Obes Relat Metab Disord 2001; 4: S8-S11.

[37] Poston WS, Foreyt JP. Sibutramine and the management of obesity. Expert Opin Pharmacother 2004; 5: 633-642.

[38] Tziomalos K, Krassas GE, Tzotzas T. The use of sibutramine in the management of obesity and related disorders: an update. Vasc Health Risk Manag 2009; 5: 441-452.

[39] De Simone G, D'Addeo G. Sibutramine: balancing weight loss benefit and possible cardiovascular risk. Nutr Metab Cardiovasc Dis 2008; 18: 337-341.

[40] Slovacek L, Pavlik V, Slovackova B. The effect of sibutramine therapy on occurrence of depression symptoms among obese patients. Nutr Metab Cardiovasc Dis 2008; 18: e43-e44.

[41] Karamadoukis L, Shivashankar GH, Ludeman L, Williams AJ. An unusual complication of treatment with orlistat. Clin Nephro 2009; 71, 430-432.

[42] Halford JC. Obesity drugs in clinical development. Curr Opin Invest Drugs 2006; 7: 312-318.

[43] Melnikova I, Wages D. Anti-obesity therapies. Nat Rev Drug Discov 2006; 5, 369-370.

[44] Thompson WG, Cook DA, Clark MM, Levine JA. Treatment of obesity - concise review for clinicians. Mayo Clinic Proceedings 2007; 82: 93-103.

[45] Birari R, Bhutani K. Pancreatic lipase inhibitors from natural sources: unexplored potential. Drug Discov Today 2007; 12: 879-889.

[46] Sumantran V. Experimental approaches for studying uptake and action of herbal medicines. Phytother Res 2007; 21: 210-214

[47] Park MY, Lee KS, Sung MK. Effects of dietary mulberry, Korean red ginseng, and banaba on glucose homeostasis in relation to PPAR-a, PPAR-c, and LPL mRNA expressions. Life Sci 2005; 77: 3344–3354.

[48] Nakayama T, Suzuki S, Kudo H, Sassa S, Nomura M, Sakamoto S. Effects of three Chinese herbal medicines on plasma and liver lipids in mice fed a high fat diet. J. Ethnopharmacol 2007; 109, 236–240.

[49] Mayer MA, Hocht C, Puyo A, Taira CA. Recent advances in obesity pharmacotherapy. Curr Clin Pharmacol 2009; 4: 53–61.

[50] Moro CO, Basile G. Obesity and medicinal plants. Fitoterapia 2000; 71: S73–S82.

[51] Han LK, Kimura Y, Okuda H. Anti-obesity effects of natural products. Stud Nat Prod Chem 2005b; 30: 79-110.

[52] Rayalam S, Della-Fera MA, Baile CA. Phytochemicals and regulation of the adipocyte life cycle. J Nutr Biochem 2008; 19: 717-726.

[53] Moreno D, Ilic N, Poulev A, Brasaemle D, Fried S, Raskin I. Inhibitory effects of grape seed extract on lipases. Nutrition 2003; 19: 876-879

[54] Yoon SS, Rhee YH, Lee HJ, *et al.* Uncoupled protein 3 and p38 signal pathways are involved in anti-obesity activity of *Solanum tuberosum* L. Cv. Bora Valley. J Ethnopharmacol 2008; 118: 396-404.

[55] Kazemipoor M, Radzi CWJWM, Cordell GA, Yaze I. Safety, Efficacy and metabolism of traditional medicinal plants in the management of obesity: A Review. Inter. J of Chem Eng and Applications (IJCEA) 2012; 3(4): 288-292.

[56] Sahib NG, Saari N, Ismail A, Khatib A, Mahomoodally F, Abdul Hamid A. 2012. Plants' metabolites as potential antiobesity agents-Review Article. The Scientific World Journal; 2012: 436039; doi:10.1100/2012/436039.

[57] Tucci SA, Boyland EJ, Halford JCG. The role of lipid and carbohydrate digestive enzyme inhibitors in the management of obesity: a review of current and emerging therapeutic agents. Diabetes Metab Syndr Obes Target Ther 2010; 3: 125-143.

[58] Hadváry P, Lengsfeld H, Wolfer H. Inhibition of pancreatic lipase *in vitro* by the covalent inhibitor tetrahydrolipstatin. Biochem J 1988; 256: 357-361.

[59] Hadváry P, Sidler W, Meister W, Vetter W, Wolfer H.The lipase inhibitor tetrahydrolipstatin binds covalently to the putative active site serine of pancreatic lipase. J Biol Chem 1988; 266: 2021-2027.

[60] Bitou N, Ninomiya M, Tsujita T, Okuda H. Screening of lipase inhibitors from marine algae. Lipids 1999; 34: 441-445.

[61] Tsujita T, Takaichi H, Takaku T, Aoyama S, Hiraki J. Antiobesity action of ε-polylysine, a potent inhibitor of pancreatic lipase. J Lipid Res 2006; 47: 1852-1858.

[62] Han LK, Zheng YN, Yoshikawa M, Okuda H, Kimura Y. Anti-obesity effects of chikusetsusaponins isolated from Panax japonicus rhizomes. BMC Complement Altern Med 2005c; 5: 9.

[63] Han LK, Xu BJ, Kimura Y, Zheng Y, Okuda H. Platycodi radix affects lipid metabolism in mice with high fat diet-induced obesity. J Nutr 2000; 130: 2760-2764.

[64] Kishino E, Ito T, Fujita K, Kiuchi Y. A mixture of the *Salacia reticulata* (kotala himbutu) aqueous extract and cyclodextrin reduces the accumulation of visceral fat mass in mice and rats with high-fat diet-induced obesity. J Nutr 2006; 136: 433-439.

[65] Ono Y, Hattori E, Fukaya Y, Imai S, Ohizumi Y. Anti-obesity effect of Nelumbo nucifera leaves extract in mice and rats. J Ethnopharmacol 2006; 106: 238- 244.

[66] Slanc P, Doljak B, Mlinaric A, Strukelj B. Screening of wood damaging fungi and macrofungi for inhibitors of pancreatic lipase. Phytother Res 2004; 18: 758-762.

[67] Ahn MY, Jee SD, Lee BM. Antiobesity effects of *Isaria sinclairii* by repeated oral treatment in obese Zucker rats over a 4-month period. J Toxicol Environ Health A 2007; 70: 1395-1401.

[68] Kim HY, Kang MH. Screening of Korean medicinal plants for lipase inhibitory activity. Phytother Res 2005; 19: 359-361.

[69] Han LK, Nose R, Li W, *et al.* Reduction of fat storage in mice fed a high-fat diet long term by treatment with saponins prepared from Kochia scoparia fruit. Phytother Res 2006; 20: 877-882.

[70] Moreno DA, Ilic N, Poulev A, Raskin I. Effects of *Arachis hypogaea* nutshell extract on lipid metabolic enzymes and obesity parameters. Life Sci 2006; 8; 78 (24): 2797-803.

[71] Shimoda H, Seki E, Aitani M. Inhibitory effect of green coffee bean extract on fat accumulation and body weight gain in mice. BMC Complement Altern Med 2006; 6:9

[72] Han LK, Takaku T, Li J, Kimura Y, Okuda H. Anti-obesity action of oolong tea. Int J Obes Relat Metab Disord 1999b; 23: 98-105.

[73] Nakai M, Fukui Y, Asami S, Toyoda-Ono Y, Iwashita T, Shibata H, Mitsunaga T, Hashimoto, F, Kiso Y. Inhibitory effects of oolong tea polyphenols on pancreatic lipase *in vitro*. J Agric Food Chem 2005; 53: 4593-4598.

[74] Lin JK, Lin-Shiau SY. Mechanisms of hypolipidemic and anti-obesity effects of tea and tea polyphenols. Mol Nutr Food Res 2006; 50: 211–217.

[75] Thielecke F, Boschmann M. The potential role of green tea catechins in the prevention of the metabolic syndrome-a review. Phytochem 2009; 70: 11-24.

[76] Takao I, Fujii S, Ishii A, Han LK, Kumao T, Ozaki K. Effects of manno-oligosaccharides from coffee mannan on fat storage in mice fed a high fat diet. J Health Sci 2006; 52: 333-337.

[77] Han LK, Kimura Y, Okuda H. Reduction in fat storage during chitin-chitosan treatment in mice fed a high-fat diet. Int J Obes Relat Metab Disord 1999a; 23: 174–179.

[78] Ho SC, Tai ES, Eng PH, Tan CE, Fok AC. In the absence of dietary surveillance, chitosan does not reduce plasma lipids or obesity in hypercholesterolaemic obese Asian subjects. Singapore Med J 2001; 42: 6-10.

[79] Gallaher DD, Gallaher CM, Mahrt GJ, *et al.* A glucomannan and chitosan fiber supplement decreases plasma cholesterol and increases cholesterol excretion in overweight normocholesterolemic humans. J Am Coll Nutr 2002; 21: 428-433.

[80]   Hayashi K, Ito M. Antidiabetic action of low molecular weight chitosan in genetically obese diabetic KK-Ay mice. Biol Pharm Bull 2002; 25: 188-192.

[81]   Gades MD, Stern JS. Chitosan supplementation and fecal fat excretion in men. Obes Res 2003; 11: 683–688.

[82]   Gades MD, Stern JS. Chitosan supplementation and fat absorption in men and women. J Am Diet Assoc 2005; 105: 72-77.

[83]   Kaats GR, Michalek JE, Preuss HG. Evaluating efficacy of a chitosan product using a double-blinded, placebo-controlled protocol. J Am Coll Nutr 2006; 25: 389-394.

[84]   Sumiyoshi M, Kimura Y. Low molecular weight chitosan inhibits obesity induced by feeding a high-fat diet long-term in mice. J Pharm Pharmacol 2006; 58: 201-207.

[85]   Bondiolotti G, Bareggi SR, Frega NG, Strabioli S, Cornelli U. Activity of two different polyglucosamines, L112® and FF45®, on body weight in male rats. Eur J Pharmacol 2007; 567: 155-158.

[86]   Tomoda H, Namatame I, Omura S. Microbial metabolites with inhibitory activity against lipid metabolism. Proc Japan Acad 2002; 78: 217-240.

[87]   Liu DZ, Wang F, Liao TG, et al. Vibralactone: a lipase inhibitor with an unusual fused beta-lactone produced by cultures of the basidiomycete Boreostereum vibrans. Org Lett 2006; 8: 5749-5752.

[88]   Hopmann C, Kurz M, Mueller G, Toti L. (Aventis Pharma GMBH). Percyquinin, a process for its production and its use as pharmaceutical-European Patent Office-EPO Patent EP 1142886 (A1), Chem Abstr 2001; 287585.

[89]   Weibel EK, Hadvary P, Hochuli E, Kupfer E, Lengsfeld, H. Lipstatin, an inhibitor of pancreatic lipase, produced by *Streptomyces toxytricini*. I. Producing organism, fermentation, isolation and biological activity. J Antibiot (Tokyo) 1987; 40: 1081-1085.

[90]   Mutoh M, Nakada N, Matsukuma S, et al. Panclicins, novel pancreatic lipase inhibitors. I. Taxonomy, fermentation, isolation and biological activity. J Antibiot (Tokyo) 1994; 47: 1369-1375.

[91]   Yoshinari K, Aoki M, Ohtsuka T, et al. Panclicins, novel pancreatic lipase inhibitors. II. Structural elucidation. J Antibiot (Tokyo) 1994; 47: 1376-1384.

[92]   Kitahara M, Asano M, Naganawa H, et al. Valilactone, an inhibitor of esterase, produced by actinomycetes. J Antibiot (Tokyo) 1987; 40: 1647-1650.

[93]   Umezawa H, Aoyagi T, Uotani K, Hamada M, Takeuchi T, Takahashi S. Ebelactone, an inhibitor of esterase, produced by actinomycetes. J Antibiot (Tokyo) 1980; 33: 1594-1596.

[94]   Umezawa H, Aoyagi T, Hazato T, et al. Esterastin, an inhibitor of esterase, produced by actinomycetes. J Antibiot (Tokyo) 1978; 31: 639-641.

[95]   Celleno L, Tolaini MV, D'Amore A, Perricone NV, Preuss HG. A dietary supplement containing standardized *Phaseolus vulgaris* extract influences body composition of overweight men and women. Int J Med Sci 2007; 4: 45-52.

[96]   Bo-Linn GW, Santa-Ana CA, Morawski SG, Fordtran JS. Starch blockers-their effect on calorie absorption from a high-starch meal. N Engl J Med 1982; 307: 1413-1436.

[97]   Chantre P, Lairon D. Recent findings of green tea extract AR25 (Exolise) and its activity for the treatment of obesity. Phytomed 2002; 9: 3-8.

[98]   Halford JC, Blundell JE. Pharmacology of appetite suppression. Prog Drug Res 2000; 54: 25-58.

[99]   Wynne K, Stanley S, McGowan B, Bloom S. Appetite control. J Endocrinol 2005; 184: 291-318.

[100]   Bays HE. Current and investigational antiobesity agents and obesity therapeutic treatment targets. Obes Res 2004; 12: 1197–1211.

[101] MacLean DB, Luo LG. Increased ATP content/production in the hypothalamus may be a signal for energy-sensing of satiety: studies of the anorectic mechanism of a plant steroidal glycoside. Brain Res 2004; 1020: 1-11.

[102] Lee RA, Balick MJ. Indigenous use of *Hoodia gordonii* and appetite suppression. Explore (NY) 2007; 3: 404-406.

[103] Van Heerden FR, Marthinus Horak R, Maharaj VJ, Vleggaar R, Senabe JV, Gunning PJ. An appetite suppressant from Hoodia species. Phytochem 2007; 68: 2545-2553.

[104] Van Heerden FR. Hoodia gordonii: a natural appetite suppressant. J Ethnopharmacol 2008; 119: 434-437.

[105] Oben JE, Enyegue DM, Fomekong GI, Soukontoua YB, Agbor GA. The effect of *Cissus quadrangularis* (CQR-300) and a Cissus formulation (CORE) on obesity and obesity-induced oxidative stress. Lipids Health Dis 2007; 6: 4.

[106] Kim JH, Hahm DH, Yang DC, Kim JH, Lee HJ, Shim I. Effect of crude saponin of Korean red ginseng on high-fat diet-induced obesity in the rat. J Pharmacol Sci 2005; 97: 124-131.

[107] Kao YH, Hiipakka RA, Liao S. Modulation of endocrine systems and food intake by green tea epigallocatechin gallate. Endocrinology 2000; 141: 980-987.

[108] Nagao T, Komine Y, Soga S, *et al.* Ingestion of a tea rich in catechins leads to a reduction in body fat and malondialdehyde-modified LDL in men. Am J Clin Nutr 2005; 81: 122-129.

[109] Wolfram S, Wang Y, Thielecke F. Anti-obesity effects of green tea: from bedside to bench. Mol Nutr Food Res 2006; 50: 176-187.

[110] Moon HS, Chung CS, Lee HG, Kim TG, Choi YJ, Cho CS. Inhibitory effect of (-)-epigallocatechin-3-gallate on lipid accumulation of 3T3-L1 cells. Obesity (Silver Spring) 2007a; 15: 2571-2582.

[111] Kuriyan R, Raj T, Srinivas SK, Vaz M, Rajendran R, Kurpad AV. Effect of *Caralluma fimbriata* extract on appetite, food intake and anthropometry in adult Indian men and women. Appetite 2007; 48: 338-344.

[112] Fleming RM. The effect of ephedra and high fat dieting: a cause for concern; A case report. Angiol 2007; 58: 102-105.

[113] Klontz KC, Timbo BB, Street D. Consumption of dietary supplements containing *Citrus aurantium* (bitter orange) 2004 California behavioral risk factor surveillance survey (BRFSS). Ann Pharmacother 2006; 40 (10): 1747-1751.

[114] Baintner K, Kiss P, Pfüller U, Bardocz S, Pusztai A. Effect of orally and intraperitoneally administered plant lectins on food consumption of rats. Acta Physiol Hung 2003; 90: 97-107.

[115] Remesar X, Guijarro P, Torregrosa C, *et al.* Oral oleoyl-estrone induces the rapid loss of body fat in zucker lean rats fed a hyperlipidic diet. Int J Obes Relat Metab Disord 2000; 24: 1405-1412.

[116] Ferrer-Lorente R, Cabot C, Fernández-López JA, Alemany M. Effects of combined oleoyl-estrone and rimonabant on overweight rats. J Pharmacol Sci 2007; 104: 176-182

[117] Romero MM, Estevez M, Fernández-López JA, Alemany M. The conjugated linoleic acid ester of estrone induces the mobilisation of fat in male wistar rats. Naunyn Schmiedebergs Arch Pharmacol 2007; 375: 283-290.

[118] Salas A, Remesar X, Esteve M. Oleoyl-estrone treatment activates apoptotic mechanisms in white adipose tissue. Life Sci 2007; 80: 293-298

[119] Ohia SE, Opere CA, LeDay AM, Bagchi M, Bagchi D, Stohs SJ. Safety and mechanism of appetite suppression by a novel hydroxycitric acid extract (HCA-SX). Mol Cell Bio chem. 2002; 238: 89-103.

[120] Lane MD, Cha SH. Effect of glucose and fructose on food intake *via* malonyl-CoA signaling in the brain. Biochem Biophs Res Commun 2009; 382: 1-5.

[121] Cha SH, Wolfgang M, Tokutake Y, Chohnan S, Lane MD. Differential effects of central fructose and glucose on hypothalamic malonyl-CoA and food intake. Proc Natl Acad Sci 2008; 105: 16871-16875.

[122] Weigle DS. Pharmacological therapy of obesity: past, present, and future. J Clin Endocrinol Metab 2003; 88: 2462-2469.

[123] Avula B, Wang YH, Pawar RS, Shukla YJ, Schaneberg B, Khan IA. Determination of the appetite suppressant P57 in *Hoodia gordonii* plant extracts and dietary supplements by liquid chromatography/electrospray ionization mass spectrometry (LC-MSD-TOF) and LCUV methods. J AOAC Int 2006; 89: 606-611.

[124] Yen TT, McKee MM, Bemis KG. Ephedrine reduces weight of viable yellow obese mice (Avy/a). Life Sci 1981; 28(2): 119-128.

[125] Arch JR, Ainsworth AT, Cawthorne MA. Thermogenic and anorectic effects of ephedrine and congeners in mice and rats. Life Sci 1982; 30(21): 1817-1826.

[126] Dulloo AG, Miller DS. Thermogenic drugs for the treatment of obesity: sympathetic stimulants in animal models. Br J Nutr 1984; 52(2): 179-196.

[127] Zarrindast MR, Hosseini-Nia T, Farnoodi F. Anorectic effect of ephedrine. Gen Pharmacol 1987; 18(5): 559-561.

[128] Dulloo AG, Seydoux J, Girardier L. Potentiation of the thermogenic antiobesity effects of ephedrine by dietary methylxanthines: adenosine antagonism or phosphodiesterase inhibition? Metabolism 1992; 41(11): 1233-1241.

[129] Ramsey JJ, Colman RJ, Swick AG, Kemnitz JW. Energy expenditure, body composition, and glucose metabolism in lean and obese rhesus monkeys treated with ephedrine and caffeine. Am J Clin Nutr 1998; 68(1): 42-51.

[130] Jonderko K, Kucio C. Effect of anti-obesity drugs promoting energy expenditure, yohimbine and ephedrine, on gastric emptying in obese patients. Aliment Pharmacol Ther 1991; 5(4): 413-418.

[131] Dulloo AG, Miller DS. The thermogenic properties of ephedrine/methylxanthine mixtures: animal studies. Am J Clin Nutr 1986; 43(3): 388-394.

[132] Dulloo AG, Miller DS. Aspirin as a promoter of ephedrine-induced thermogenesis: potential use in the treatment of obesity. Am J Clin Nutr 1987a; 45(3): 564-569.

[133] Dulloo AG, Miller DS. Reversal of obesity in the genetically obese fa/fa Zucker rat with an ephedrine/methylxanthines thermogenic mixture. J Nutr 1987b; 117(2): 383-389.

[134] Astrup A, Breum L, Toubro S, Hein P, Quaade F. The effect and safety of an ephedrine caffeine compound compared to ephedrine, caffeine and placebo in obese subjects on an energy restricted diet-a doubleblind trial. Int J Obes 1992; 16: 269-77.

[135] Astrup A, Toubro S. Thermogenic, metabolic, and cardiovascular responses to ephedrine and caffeine in man. Int J Obes Relat Metab Disord 1993; 17 Suppl 1: S41-S43.

[136] Dulloo AG. Ephedrine, xanthines and prostaglandin-inhibitors: actions and interactions in the stimulation of thermogenesis. Int J Obes Relat Metab Disord 1993; 17 (Suppl 1): S35-S40.

[137] Kamphuis MM, Lejeune MP, Saris WH, Westerterp-Plantenga MS. Effect of conjugated linoleic acid supplementation after weight loss on appetite and food intake in overweight subjects. Eur J Clin Nutr 2003; 57: 1268-1274.

[138] Feltrin KL, Little TJ, Meyer JH, *et al.* Comparative effects of intraduodenal infusions of lauric and oleic acids on antropyloroduodenal motility, plasma cholecystokinin and peptide YY, appetite, and energy intake in healthy men. Am J Clin Nutr 2008; 87: 1181-1187.

[139] Sørensen LB, Cueto HT, Andersen MT, *et al.* The effect of salatrim, a low-calorie modified triacylglycerol, on appetite and energy intake. Am J Clin Nutr 2008; 87: 1163-1169.

[140] Flatt JP. Differences in basal energy expenditure and obesity. Obesity (Silver Spring) 2007; 15: 2546–2548.

[141] Redinger RN. Fat storage and the biology of energy expenditure. Transl Res 2009; 154: 52-60.

[142] Yun JW. Possible anti-obesity therapeutics from nature-A review. Phytochem 2010; 71: 1625-1641

[143] Cannon B, Nedergaard J. Brown adipose tissue: function and physiological significance. Physiol Rev 2004; 84: 277-359.

[144] Kumar MV, Sunvold GD, Scarpace PJ. Dietary vitamin a supplementation in rats: suppression of leptin and induction of UCP1 mRNA. J Lipid Res 1999; 40: 824–829.

[145] Gong DW, He Y, Karas M, Reitman M. Uncoupling protein-3 is a mediator of thermogenesis regulated by thyroid hormone, 3-adrenergic agonists, and leptin. J Biol Chem 1997; 272: 24129-24132.

[146] Cinti S. Adipocyte differentiation and trans differentiation: plasticity of the adipose organ. J Endocrinol Invest 2002; 25: 823-835.

[147] Mercader J, Ribot J, Murano I, *et al.* Remodeling of white adipose tissue after retinoic acid administration in mice. Endocrinol 2006; 14: 5325-5332.

[148] Cabrero A, Alegret M, Sanchez RM, Adzet T, Laguna JC, Vazquez M. Bezafibrate reduces mRNA levels of adipocyte markers and increases fatty acid oxidation in primary culture of adipocytes. Diabetes 2001; 50: 1883-1890.

[149] Orci L, Cook WS, Ravazzola M, *et al.* Rapid transformation of white adipocytes into fat-oxidizing machines. Proc. Natl. Acad. Sci. USA 2004; 101: 2058-2063.

[150] Flachs P, Horakova O, Brauner P, *et al.* Polyunsaturated fatty acids of marine origin upregulate mitochondrial biogenesis and induce β-oxidation in white fat. Diabetol 2005; 48: 2365–2375.

[151] Maeda H, Hosokawa M, Sashima T, Funayama K, Miyashita K. Effect of medium-chain triacylglycerols on anti-obesity effect of fucoxanthin. J Oleo Sci 2007; 56: 615-621.

[152] Racotta IS, Leblanc J, Richard D. The effect of caffeine on foodintake in rats - involvement of corticotropin-releasing factor and the sympathoadrenal system. Pharmacol Biochem Behav 1994; 48: 887-92.

[153] Kawada T, Watanabe T, Takaishi T, Tanaka T, Iwai K. Capsaicin-induced beta-adrenergic action on energy metabolism in rats: influence of capsaicin on oxygen consumption, the respiratory quotient, and substrate utilization. Proc Soc Exp Biol Med 1986; 183: 250-256.

[154] Diepvens K, Westerterp KR, Westerterp-Plantenga MS. Obesity and thermogenesis related to the consumption of caffeine, ephedrine, capsaicin, and green tea. Am J Physiol Regul Integr Comp Physiol 2007; 292: R77-R85.

[155] Borchardt RT, Huber JA. Catechol O-methyltransferase. 5. Structure–activity relationships for inhibition by flavonoids. J Med Chem 1975; 18: 120-122.

[156] Boschmann M, Thielecke F. The effects of epigallocatechin-3-gallate on thermogenesis and fat oxidation in obese men: a pilot study. J Am Coll Nutr 2007; 26: 389S-395S.

[157] Kim YJ, Shin YO, Ha YW, Lee S, Oh JK, Kim YS. Anti-obesity effect of *Pinellia ternata* extract in zucker rats. Biol Pharm Bull 2006b; 29: 1278-1281.

[158] Attele AS, Zhou YP, Xie JT, *et al.* Antidiabetic effects of Panax ginseng berry extract and the identification of an effective component. Diabetes 2002; 51, 1851-1858.

[159] Pang J, Choi Y, Park T. *Ilex paraguariensis* extract ameliorates obesity induced by high-fat diet: potential role of AMPK in the visceral adipose tissue. Arch Biochem Biophys 2008; 476, 178–185.

[160] Gregoire FM. Adipocyte differentiation: from fibroblast to endocrine cell. Exp Biol Med (Maywood) 2001; 226: 997-1002.

[161] Kim HK, Della-Fera M, Lin J, Baile, CA. Docosahexaenoic acid inhibit adipocyte differentiation and induces apoptosis in 3T3-L1 preadipocytes. J Nutr 2006a; 136: 2965–2969.

[162] Cowherd RM, Lyle RE, McGehee Jr. RE. Molecular regulation of adipocyte differentiation. Semin Cell Dev Biol 1999; 10, 3-10.

[163] Green H, Kehinde O. An established preadipose cell line and its differentiation in culture. II- Factors affecting the adipose conversion. Cell 1975; 5: 19-27.

[164] Wu Z, Puigserver P, Spiegelman BM. Transcriptional activation of adipogenesis. Curr Opin Cell Biol 1999; 11: 689-694.

[165] Lefterova MI, Lazar MA. New developments in adipogenesis. Trends Endocrin Met 2009; 20: 107-114.

[166] Lee J, Jung E, Lee J, *et al.* Isorhamnetin represses adipogenesis in 3T3-L1 cells. Obesity (Silver Spring) 2009; 17: 226-232.

[167] Okuno M, Kajiwara K, Imai S, *et al.* Perilla oil prevents the excessive growth of visceral adipose tissue in rats by down-regulating adipocyte differentiation. J Nutr 1997; 127: 1752-1757.

[168] Awad AB, Begdache, LA, Fink CS. Effect of sterols and fatty acids on growth and triglyceride accumulation in 3T3-L1 cells. J Nutr Biochem 2000; 11: 153-158.

[169] Evans M, Geigerman C, Cook J, Curtis L, Kuebler B, McIntosh M. Conjugated linoleic acid suppresses triglyceride accumulation and induces apoptosis in 3T3-L1 preadipocytes. Lipids 2000; 35: 899-910.

[170] Shimada T, Hiramatsu N, Kasai A, *et al.* Suppression of adipocyte differentiation by Cordyceps militaris through activation of the aryl hydrocarbon receptor. Am J Physiol Endocrinol Metab 2008; 295: E859-E867.

[171] Hargrave KM, Li C, Meyer BJ, Kachman *et al.* Adipose depletion and apoptosis induced by trans-10, cis-12 conjugated linoleic acid in mice. Obes Res 2002; 10: 1284-1290.

[172] Hwang JT, Park IJ, Shin JI, *et al.* Genistein, EGCG, and capsaicin inhibit adipocyte differentiation process *via* activating AMP-activated protein kinase. Biochem Biophys Res Commun 2005; 338: 694-699.

[173] Hsu CL, Yen GC. Induction of cell apoptosis in 3T3-L1 pre-adipocytes flavonoids is associated with their antioxidant activity. Mol Nutr Food Res 2006; 50: 1072-1079.

[174] Yang JY, Della-Fera MA, Hartzell DL, Nelson-Dooley C, Hausman DB, Baile CA. Esculetin induces apoptosis and inhibits adipogenesis in 3T3-L1 cells. Obesity (Silver Spring) 2006; 14: 1691-1699.

[175] Yang JY, Della-Fera MA, Baile CA. Guggulsterone inhibits adipocyte differentiation and induces apoptosis in 3T3-L1 cells. Obesity (Silver Spring) 2008; 16: 16-22.

[176] Moon HS, Lee HG, Choi YJ, Kim TG, Cho CS. Proposed mechanisms of (-) - epigallocatechin-3-gallate for anti-obesity. Chem Biol Interact 2007b; 167: 85-98.

[177] Ka SO, Kim KA, Kwon KB, Park JW, Park BH. Silibinin attenuates adipogenesis in 3T3-L1 preadipocytes through a potential upregulation of the insig pathway. Int J Mol Med 2009; 23: 633-637.

[178] Berry DC, Noy N. All-trans-retinoic acid represses obesity and insulin resistance by activatingboth peroxisome proliferation-activated receptor beta/delta and retinoic acid receptor. Mol Cell Biol 2009; 29: 3286–3296.

[179] Kong J, Li YC. Molecular mechanism of 1, 25-dihydroxyvitamin D3 inhibition of adipogenesis in 3T3-L1 cells. Am J Physiol Endocrinol Metab 2006; 290: E916-924.

[180] Hsu CL, Yen GC. Phenolic compounds: evidence for inhibitory effects against obesity and their underlying molecular signaling mechanisms. Mol Nutr Food Res 2008; 52: 53-61.

[181] Huang TH, Peng G, Li GQ, Yamahara J, Roufogalis BD, Li Y. Salacia oblonga root improves postprandial hyperlipidemia and hepatic steatosis in zucker diabetic fatty rats: activation of PPAR-α. Toxicol Appl Pharmacol 2006; 210, 225-235.

[182] Lin J, Della-Fera MA, Baile CA. Green tea polyphenol epigallocatechin gallate inhibits adipogenesis and induces apoptosis in 3T3-L1 adipocytes. Obes Res 2005; 13: 982-990.

[183] Kwon JY, Seo SG, Heo YS, *et al*. Piceatannol, natural polyphenolic stilbene, inhibits adipogenesis *via* modulation of mitotic clonal expansion and insulin receptor-dependent insulin signaling in early phase of differentiation. J Biol Chem 2012; 287(14): 11566-78.

[184] Picard F, Kurtev M, Chung N, *et al*. Sirt 1 promotes fat mobilization in white adipocytes by repressing PPAR-gamma. Nature 2004; 429: 771-776.

[185] Langin D. Adipose tissue lipolysis as a metabolic pathway to define pharmacological strategies against obesity and the metabolic syndrome. Pharmacol Res 2006; 53: 482-491.

[186] Ohkoshi E, Miyazaki H, Shindo K, Watanabe H, Yoshida A, Yajima H. Constituents from the leaves of Nelumbo nucifera stimulate lipolysis in the white adipose tissue of mice. Planta Med 2007; 73: 1255-1259.

[187] Cornelius P, MacDougald OA, Lane MD. Regulation of adipocyte development. Annu Rev Nutr 1994; 14: 99-129.

[188] Kersten S. Peroxisome proliferator activated receptors and obesity. Eur J Pharmacol 2002; 440: 223-234.

[189] Oluyemi KA, Omotuyi IO, Jimoh OR, Adesanya OA, Saalu CL, Josiah SJ. Erythropoietic and anti-obesity effects of *Garcinia cambogia* (bitter kola) in Wistar rats. Biotechnol Appl Biochem 2007; 46: 69–72.

[190] Alarcon-Aguilar FJ, Zamilpa A, Perez-Garcia MD, *et al*. Effect of *Hibiscus sabdariffa* on obesity in MSG mice. J Ethnopharmacol 2007; 114: 66-71.

[191] Lei F, Zhang XN, Wang W, *et al*. Evidence of anti-obesity effects of the pomegranate leaf extract in high-fat diet induced obese mice. Int J Obes (Lond) 2007; 31: 1023-1029.

[192] Dulloo AG, Duret C, Rohrer D, *et al*. Efficacy of a green tea extract rich in catechin polyphenols and caffeine in increasing 24-h energy expenditure and fat oxidation in humans. Am J Clin Nutr 1999; 70: 1040–1045.

[193] Kim S, Nho H. Isolation and characterization of Glucosidase inhibitor from the fungus *Ganoderma lucidum*. J Microbiol 2004; 42 (3): 223-227.

[194] Saito M, Ueno M, Ogino S, Kubo K, Nagata J, Takeuchi M. High dose of *Garcinia cambogia* is effective in suppressing fat accumulation in developing male Zucker obese rats, but highly toxic to the testis. Food ChemToxicol 2005; 43: 411-419.

[195] Li Y, Huang TH, Yamahara J. Salacia root, a unique ayurvedic medicine, meets multiple targets in diabetes and obesity. Life Sci 2008; 82: 1045–1049.

[196] Morimoto C, Satoh Y, Hara M, Inoue S, Tsujita T, Okuda H. Anti-obese action of raspberry ketone. Life Sci 2005; 77: 194-204.

[197] Park KS. Raspberry ketone increases both lipolysis and fatty acid oxidation in 3T3-L1 adipocytes. Planta med 2010; 76 (15): 1654-1658.

[198] Hu JN, Zhu XM, Han LK, *et al*. Anti-obesity effects of escins extracted from the seeds of *Aesculus turbinata* Blume (Hippocastanaceae). Chem Pharm Bull (Tokyo) 2008; 56(1): 12-6.

[199] Kimura H, Ogawa S, Sugiyama A, Jisaka M, Takeuchi T, Yokota K. Anti-obesity effects of highly polymeric proanthocyanidins from seed shells of Japanese horse chestnut (*Aesculus turbinata* Blume) Food Res Inter 2011; 44 (1), 121–126.

[200] Jongwon C, KyungTae L, WonBae K, *et al*. Effect of *Allium victorialis* var. platyphyllum leaves on triton WR-1339-induced and poloxamer-407-induced hyperlipidemic rats and on diet-induced obesity rats. Kor J Pharmacog 2005; 36: 109-115.

[201] Abidov MT, del Rio MJ, Ramazanov TZ, Klimenov AL, Dzhamize SH, Kalyuzhin OV. Effects of *Aralia mandshurica* and *Engelhardtia chrysolepis* extracts on some parameters of lipid metabolism in women with nondiabetic obesity. B Exp Biol Med 2006; 141(3): 343-6.

[202] Zhu X, Zhang W, Zhao J, Wang J, Qu W. Hypolipidaemic and hepatoprotective effects of ethanolic and aqueous extracts from *Asparagus officinalis* L. by-products in mice fed a high-fat diet. J Sci Food Agric 2010; 90 (7): 1129-1135.

[203] Chrubasik C, Maier T, Dawid C, *et al*. An observational study and quantification of the actives in a supplement with *Sambucus nigra* and *Asparagus officinalis* used for weight reduction. Phytother Res 2008; 22: 913-918.

[204] Bruno RS, Dugan CE, Smyth JA, DiNatale DA, Koo SI. Green tea extract protects leptin-deficient, spontaneously obese mice from hepatic steatosis and injury. J Nutr 2008; 138: 323-331.

[205] Oben JE, Ngondi JL, Momo CN, Agbor GA, Sobgui CS. The use of a *Cissus quadrangularis/Irvingia gabonensis* combination in the management of weight loss: a double-blind placebo-controlled study. Lipids Health Dis 2008; 7: 12.

[206] Haaz S, Fontaine KR, Cutter G, Limdi N, Perumean-Chaney S, Allison DB. Citrus aurantium and synephrine alkaloids in the treatment of overweight and obesity: An update. Obes Rev 2006; 7(1): 79-88.

[207] Sahelian R. Bitter Orange extract health benefit and side effects, review of safety, risks. [cited on 18th june 2012] Available from: http: //www.raysahelian.com/bitterorange.html

[208] Meselhy R. Inhibition of LPS-induced NO production by the oleogum resin of Commiphora wightii and its constituents. Phytochem 2003; 62(2): 213-218.

[209] Yang DJ, Chang YY, Hsu CL, *et al*. Antiobesity and Hypolipidemic Effects of Polyphenol-Rich Longan (*Dimocarpus longans* Lour.) Flower Water Extract in Hypercaloric-Dietary Rats. J Agric Food Chem 2010; 58 (3), 2020–2027.

[210] Fagotti Corrêa G, Zapparoli A. Herb Extract *Ephedra Sinica* Effect on Dipsogenesis is Dose-Dependent in Rats. Adv Stu in Biol 2012; 4 (6): 281-285.

[211] Hackman RM, Havel PJ, Schwartz HJ, *et al.* Multinutrient supplement containing ephedra and caffeine causes weight loss and improves metabolic risk factors in obese women: a randomized controlled trial. Int J Obes (Lond) 2006; 30: 1545–1556.

[212] Aoki F, Honda S, Kishida H, *et al.* Suppression by licorice flavonoids of abdominal fat accumulation and body weight gain in high-fat diet-induced obese C57BL/6J mice. Biosci Biotechnol Biochem 2007; 71: 206-214.

[213] Hioki C, Yoshimoto K, Yoshida T. Efficacy of bofu-tsusho-san, an oriental herbal medicine, in obese Japanese women with impaired glucose tolerance. Clin Exp Pharmacol Physiol 2004; 31: 614-619.

[214] Persaud SJ, Majed HA, Raman A, Jones PM. *Gymnema sylvestre* stimulates insulin release *in vitro* by increased membrane permeability. J Endocrinol 1999; 163: 207-212.

[215] Kanetkar PV, Laddha KS, Kama MY. Gymnemic acids: A molecular perspective of its action on carbohydrate metabolism. Poster presented at the 16th ICFOST meet organized by CFTRI and DFRL, Mysore, India: 2004.

[216] Pawar RS, Shukla YJ, Khan IA. New calogenin glycosides from *Hoodia gordonii*. Steroids 2007; 72: 881-891.

[217] McIntosh GH, Whyte J, McArthur R, Nestel PJ. Barley and wheat foods: influence on plasma cholesterol concentrations in hypercholesterolemic men. Am J Clin Nutr 1991; 53 (5): 1205-1209.

[218] Delaney B, Nicolosi RJ, Wilson TA, *et al.* Beta-glucan fractions from barley and oats are similarly antiatherogenic in hypercholesterolemic Syrian golden hamsters. J Nutr 2003; 133(2): 468-475.

[219] Poppitt SD. Soluble fibre oat and barley beta-glucan enriched products: can we predict cholesterol-lowering effects? Br J Nutr 2007; 97 (6): 1049-1050

[220] Lupton JR, Robinson MC, Morin JL. Cholesterol-lowering effect of barley bran flour and oil. J Am Diet Assoc 1994; 94 (1): 65-70.

[221] Dickel ML, Rates SM, Ritter MR. Plants popularly used for losing weight purposes in Porto- Alegre, South Brazil. J Ethnopharmacol 2007; 109: 60-71.

[222] Mosimann AL, Wilhelm-Filho D, da Silva EL. Aqueous extract of *Ilex paraguariensis* attenuates the progression of atherosclerosis in cholesterol-fed rabbits. Bio- factors 2006; 26: 59-70.

[223] Paganini FL, Schmidt B, Furlong EB, *et al.* Vascular responses to extractable fractions of *Ilex paraguariensis* in rats fed standard and high-cholesterol diets. Biol Res Nurs 2005; 7: 146-56.

[224] Gorzalczany S, Filip R, Alonso MR, Mino J, Ferraro GE, Acevedo C. Choleretic effect and intestinal propulsion of 'Mate' (*Ilex paraguariensis*) and its substitutes or adulterants. J Ethnopharmacol 2001; 75: 291-4.

[225] Ngondi JL, Oben JE, Minka SR. The effect of Irvingia gabonensis seeds on body weight and blood lipids of obese subjects in Cameroon. Lipids Health Dis 2005; 4: 12.

[226] Vuksan V, Jenkins DJA, Spadafora P, *et al.* Konjac-mannan (gluco- mannan) improves glycemia and other associated risk factors for coronary heart disease in type 2 diabetes. Arandomized controlled metabolic trial. Diabetes Care 1999; 22: 913-9.

[227] Arvill A, Bodin L. Effect of short-term ingestion of konjac glucomannan on serum cholesterol in healthy men. Am J Clin Nutr 1995; 61: 585-9.

[228] Yoshikawa MM, Shimada HH, Morikawa TT, *et al.* Medicinal foodstuffs. VII. On the saponin constituents with glucose and alcohol absorption-inhibitory activity from a food

garnish "Tonburi", the fruit of Japanese Kochia scoparia (L.) Schrad.: structures of scoparianosides A, B, and C. Chem Pharm Bull (Tokyo) 1997; 45(8): 1300-5.

[229] Han LK, Nose R, Li W, Gong XJ, *et al*. Reduction of fat storage in mice fed a high-fat diet long term by treatment with saponins prepared from *Kochia scoparia* fruit. Phytother Res 2006; 20 (10): 877-882.

[230] Ignjatovic V, Ogru E, Heffernan M, Libinaki R, Lim Y, Ng F. Studies on the Use of "Slimax", A Chinese herbal mixture, in the treatment of human obesity. Pharm Biol 2000; 38 (1): 30-35.

[231] Shih CC, Lin CH and Lin WL. Effects of *Momordica charantia* on insulin resistance and visceral obesity in mice on high-fat diet. Diabetes Res Clin Pract 2008; 81: 134-143.

[232] Yun SN, Moon SJ, Ko SK, Im BO, Chung SH. Wild ginseng prevents the onset of high-fat diet induced hyperglycemia and obesity in ICR mice. Arch Pharm Res 2004; 27: 790-796.

[233] Xie JT, Zhou YP, Dey L, *et al*. Ginseng berry reduces blood glucose and body weight in db/db mice. Phytomed 2002; 9: 254-258

[234] Atchibri OA, Brou KD, TH Kouakou TH, Kouadio YJ, Gnakri D. Screening for antidiabetic activity and phytochemical constituents of common bean (*Phaseolus vulgaris* L.) seeds. J Med Plant Res. (JMPR) 2010; 4(17): 1757-1761.

[235] Obiro WC, Zhang T, Jiang B. The nutraceutical role of the Phaseolus vulgaris alpha-amylase inhibitor. Br J Nutr 2008; 100 (1): 1-12.

[236] Park YS, Cha MH, Yoon YS, Ahn HS. Effects of low calorie diet and *Platycodon grandiflorum* extract on fatty acid binding protein expression in rats with diet-induced obesity. Nutritional Sciences 2006; 8: 3-9.

[237] Zheng CD, Duan YQ, Gao JM, Ruan ZG. Screening for anti-lipase properties of 37 traditional Chinese medicinal herbs. J Chin Med Assoc 2010; 73(6): 319-24.

[238] Sook PH. Effects of *Rubus coreanus* and the bioactive compounds on lipid metabolism related with adipocyte differentiation. PhD Thesis - virtues Women's University Graduate School: Department of Health Functional Advanced Materials 2011.

[239] Yoshikawa M, Shimoda H, Nishida N, Takada M, Matsuda H. *Salacia reticulata* and its polyphenolic constituents with lipase inhibitory and lipolytic activities have mild antiobesity effects in rats. J Nutr 2002; 132: 1819-1824.

[240] Gray AM, Abdel-Wahab YH and Flatt PR. The traditional plant treatment, Sambucus nigra (elder), exhibits insulin-like and insulin-releasing actions *in vitro*. J Nutr 2000; 130: 15-20.

[241] Murkovic M, Abuja PM, Bergmann AR, *et al*. Effects of elderberry juice on fasting and postprandial serum lipids and low-density lipoprotein oxidation in healthy volunteers: a randomized, double-blind, placebo-controlled study. Eur J Clin Nutr 2004; 58: 244-249.

[242] Dubey P, Jayasooriya AP, Cheema SK. Fish oil induced hyperlipidemia and oxidative stress in BioF1B hamsters is attenuated by elderberry extract. Appl. Physiol. Nutr. Metab 2012; 37 (3): 472-479.

[243] Ziauddin KS, Anwar M, Mannan A, Khan AB. Clinical efficacy of *Terminalia arjuna* Roxb. in the management of hyperlipidaemia. Hamdard Med 2004; 47: 15-18.

[244] Agoreyo FO, Agoreyo BO, Onuorah MN. Effect of aqueous extracts of *Hibiscus sabdariffa* and *Zingiber Officinale* on blood cholesterol and glucose levels of rats. Afri J of Biotech (AJB) 2008; 7 (21): 3949-3951.

[245] Fuhrman B, Rosenblat M, Hayek T, Coleman R, Aviram M. Ginger extract consumption reduces plasma cholesterol, inhibits LDL oxidation and attenuates development of atherosclerosis in atherosclerotic, apolipoprotein E-deficient mice. J Nutr 2000; 130: 1124-1131.

[246] Park MK, Jung U and Roh C. Fucoidan from marine brown algae inhibits lipid accumulation. Mar. Drugs 2011; 9: 1359-1367

[247] Maeda H, Hosokawa M, Sashima T, Murakami-Funayama K, Miyashita K. Anti-obesity and anti-diabetic effects of fucoxanthin on diet-induced obesity conditions in a murine model. Mol Med Report 2009; 2(6): 897-902.

[248] Miyashita K. The carotenoid fucoxanthin from brown seaweed affects obesity. Lipid Technolog 2009; 21 (8-9): 186-190.

[249] Hirata T, Sugahara T. Suppressive Effect of Siphonaxanthin on the Differentiation of Preadipocytes to Adipocyte. Antiobesity effects of siphoxanthin from green algae. Research Activities. SACI, Office of society Academia. Collaboration for innovation 2011. Available from: http: //www.int.icc.kyoto-u.ac.jp/?p=967.

[250] Iksoo L, Hongjin K, Ui JY, Jin PK and Byungsun M. Effect of lanostane triperpenes from the fruiting bodies of GL on Adipocyte Differentiation in 3T3 - L1 cells. Planta Med 2010; 76 (14): 1558-1563.

[251] Zhu T, Kim SH, Chen CY. A Medicinal Mushroom: *Phellinus linteus*. Curr Med Chem 2008; 15: 1330-1335.

[252] Lee JK, Jang JH, Lee JT, Lee JS. Extraction and characteristics of anti-obesity lipase inhibitor from *Phellinus linteus*. Mycobiol 2010; 38(1): 52-57

[253] Yuping L, Jing W, Weiming Z. Chemical constituents from the oil of *Sparassis crispa*. Nat Prod Res Develop 2001; 13(1): 39-41.

[254] Lee MA, Chon JW, Park JK, Kang MH, Park YK. Water-soluble extract of *Cauliflower mushroom* shows anti-obesity effects in high fat diet-induced obese mice. AKMMC J 2012; 3(2): 11-14.

[255] Tokdar P, Ranadive P, Mascarenhas M, Patil S, George S. A New Pancreatic Lipase Inhibitor Produced by a *Streptomyces* sp. MTCC 5219. International Conference on Life Science and Technology. Singapore 2011.

[256] Prashith TR, Shobha KS, Onkarappa R. Pancreatic lipase inhibitory and cytotoxic potential of a *streptomyces* species isolated from western ghat soil, Agumbe, Karnataka, India. Int J Pharmac Biolog Arch (IJPBA) 2011; 2(3): 932-937.

[257] An HM, Park SY, Lee DK, *et al*. Antiobesity and lipid-lowering effects of *Bifidobacterium* spp. in high fat diet-induced obese rats. J Ethnopharmacol 2011; 114: 66-71.

[258] Ma X, Hua J, Li Z. Probiotics improve high fat diet induced hepatic steatosis and insulin resistance by increasing hepatic NKT cells. J Hepatol 2008; 49: 821-830.

[259] Yin YN, Yu QF, Fu N, Liu XW, Lu FG. Effects of four Bifidobacteria on obesity in high fat diet induced rats. World J Gastroenterol 2010; 16: 3394-3401.

[260] Manach C, Scalbert A, Morand C, Rémésy C, Jiménez L. Polyphenols: food sources and bioavailability. Am J Clin Nutr 2004; 79 (5): 727-47.

[261] Scalbert A, Williamson G. Dietary intake and bioavailability of polyphenols. J Nutr. 2000; 130(Suppl): 2073S-85S

[262] García-Lafuente A, Guillamón E, Villares A, Rostagno M, Martínez J. Flavonoids as anti-inflammatory agents: implications in cancer and cardiovascular disease. Inflamm Res 2009; 58: 537-552.

[263] Terra X, Montagut G, Bustos M, Llopiz N, Ardvol A, Blad C. Grape-seed procyanidins prevent low-grade inflammation by modulating cytokine expression in rats fed a high-fat diet. J Nutr Biochem 2009; 20: 210-218.

[264] Ratnawati R, Indra MR, Satuman A. Epigallocatechin gallate of green tea inhibits proliferation, differentiation and TNF – α in the primary human visceral preadipocytes culture, Majalah Ilmu faal Indonesia 2007; 6 (3): 160-168.

[265] Dutt HC, Singh S, Avula B, Khan IA, Bedi YS. Pharmacological review of *Caralluma* R.Br. with special reference to appetite suppression and anti-obesity. J Med Food 2012; 15(2): 108-19.

[266] EFSA (European Food Safety Authority). Joint EFSA and ECDC report: resistant bacteria remain an important issue that can affect humans through animals and food 2011 [cited on October 3rd 2012] Available from: http: //www.efsa.europa.eu/

[267] Sparg SG, Light ME, van Staden J. Biological activities and distribution of plant saponins. J Ethnopharmacol 2004; 94: 219-243.

[268] Vincken J, Heng L, de Groot A and Gruppen H. Saponins, classification and occurrence in the plant kingdom. Phytochem 2007; 68: 275-297.

[269] Haralampidis K, Trojanowska M, Osbourn A. Biosynthesis of triterpenoid saponins in plants. Adv Biochem Eng Biotechnol 2002; 75: 31.

[270] Karu N, Reifen R, Kerem Z. Weight gain reduction in mice fed Panax ginseng saponin, a pancreatic lipase inhibitor. J Agric Food Chem 2007; 55: 2824-2828.

[271] Liu W, Zheng Y, Han L, Wang H, Saito M, Ling M. Saponins (Ginsenosides) from stems and leaves of *Panax quinquefolium* prevented high-fat diet-induced obesity in mice. Phytomed 2008; 15: 1140-1145.

[272] Lee Y, Cha B, Yamaguchi K, Choi S, Yonezawa T, Teruya T. Effects of Korean white ginseng extracts on obesity in high-fat diet-induced obese mice. Cytotechnol 2012; 62(4): 367-376.

[273] Son IS, Kim JH, Sohn HO, Son KH, Kim JS, Kwon CS. Antioxidative and hypolipidemic effects of diosgenin, a steroidal saponin of Yam (Dioscorea spp.), on high-cholesterol fed rats. Biosci Biotechnol Biochem 2007; 71(12): 3063-3071.

[274] Hu Y, Ehli EA, Kittelsrud J, *et al*. Lipid-lowering effect of berberine in human subjects and rats. Phytomed 2012; 19 (10): 861-7.

[275] Joo JI, Kim DH, Choi JW, Yun JW. Proteomic analysis for antiobesity potential of capsaicin on white adipose tissue in rats fed with a high fat diet. J Proteome Res 2010; 9 (6): 2977-87.

[276] Ninomiya K, Matsuda H, Shimoda H, *et al*. Carnosic acid, a new class of lipid absorption inhibitor from sage. Bioorg Medicinal Chem Lett 2004; 14: 1943-1946.

[277] Rau O, Wurglics M, Paulke A, *et al*. Carnosic acid and carnosol, phenolic diterpene compounds of the Labiateae herbs rosemary and sage, are activators of the human peroxisome proliferator-activated receptor gamma. Planta Med 2006; 72: 881-887.

[278] Takahashi T, Tabuchi T, Tamaki Y, Kosaka K, Takikawa Y, Satoh T. Carnosic acid and carnosol inhibit   adipocyte differentiation in mouse 3T3-Ll cells through induction of phase 2 enzymes and activation of glutathione metabolism. Biochem Biophys Res Commun 2009; 8: 549-554.

[279] Miyashita K, Maeda H, Tsukui T, Okada T, Hosokawa M. Anti-obesity effect of allene carotenoids, fucoxanthin and neoxanthin from seaweeds and vegetables. ISHS Acta Horticulturae 2007; 841: II International Symposium on Human Health Effects of Fruits and Vegetables: FAVHEALTH

[280] Maeda H, Hosokawa M, Sashima T, Funayama K, Miyashita K. Fucoxanthin from edible seaweed, *Undaria pinnatifida*, shows antiobesity effect through UCP1 expression in white adipose tissues. Biochem Biophys Res Commun 2005; 332: 392-397.

[281] Vermaak I, Viljoen AM and Hamman JH. Natural products in anti-obesity therapy. Nat. Prod. Rep., 2011; 28: 1493-1533.

[282] Soni MG, Burdock GA, Preuss HG, *et al*. Safety assessement of Hydroxy-citric acid and CitriMax,a novel calcium-Potassuim salt. Food Chem. Toxicol 2004; 42, 1513–1529.

[283] Van Heerden FR, Vleggaar R, Horak RM, Learmonth RA, Maharaj V, Whittal RD. Pharmaceutical compositions having appetite-suppressant activity. US Patent 6376657 B1; 2002

CHAPTER 4

Natural Compounds – Anti-Obesity Properties

Sara M. Reyna[1] and Jameela Banu[2,*]

[1]Department of Medicine and Medical Research Division, Edinburg Regional Academic Health Center, University of Texas Health Science Center at San Antonio, 1214, W Schunior, Edinburg, TX 78541, USA and [2]Coordinated Program in Dietetics and Department of Biology, University of Texas-Pan American, 1201, W. University Dr., Edinburg, TX 78539-2999, USA

Abstract: Obesity is a global epidemic with increasing number of individuals becoming overweight. World Health Organization (WHO) has called obesity a preventable disease mainly because most obese patients benefit by changing food habits and lifestyle. It is very well established that obesity increases the risk of several life threatening diseases like insulin resistance, diabetes, atherosclerotic vascular disease (CVD), cancer, chronic inflammation, bone disorders *etc.* Several natural products like herbs, dairy products, and products from marine organisms have been reported to have anti-obesity properties. These products reduce obesity by influencing different pathways such as decreasing intestinal absorption, fatty acid synthesis, adipocyte differentiation as well as increasing intestinal transit, beta oxidation, and metabolic rate. In this chapter, we have compiled information about the use of different natural products as anti-obesity agents and how they affect body weight.

Keywords: Adipogenesis, animal products, fat metabolism, inflammation, multi compound mixtures, natural compounds, obesity, oxidative stress, plant products, toxicity.

INTRODUCTION

Obesity is an adverse health condition that is characterized by increased accumulation of fat in the body, increasing the risk of developing severe medical problems that can lead to death. WHO declared it as a global epidemic in 1997 [1] and also considers it the most preventable disease [2]. But, there is a steady rise in

*Address correspondence to Jameela Banu: Coordinated Program in Dietetics and Department of Biology, University of Texas-Pan American, 1201, W University Dr., Edinburg, TX 78539-2999, USA; Tel: 956-665-3222; Fax: 956-665-5265; E-mail banuj@utpa.edu

Atta-ur-Rahman and M. Iqbal Choudhary (Eds)

the number of individuals that are obese and unfortunately more children are becoming obese [3]. The current total population, in the world, is about 7 billion, of which one in six adults is obese [4, 5].

CAUSES OF OBESITY

Many aspects of the disease have been studied including finding measures to prevent and reduce body weight as well as body weight gain. Living conditions and medical care have improved [6] leading to increased life expectancy around the world. In addition, more energy dense food is readily available. The downside to this is decreased physical activity and increased consumption of processed enriched food. Many reasons can be attributed to the increase in obesity including lifestyle changes, body composition, metabolic changes (endocrine, oxidative stress, activation of the sympathetic nervous system), medical conditions and genetic disorders. More recently, obesity is said to be a state of chronic low inflammation [7, 8]. There are also other non-physiological reasons for the increase in obesity including poverty and isolation [6]. Body mass index (BMI) is the main measure used to assess obesity.

Lifestyle Changes and Body Composition: Globally, we are moving to be a 'developed' society which has undoubtedly lead to 'improved living conditions' and we cannot deny the fact that global industrialization has considerably reduced physical activity both at home and at work places. Moreover, the food that is now consumed is more concentrated with high energy ingredients and imbalanced nutrients. The combination of decreased physical activity and ingestion of processed food is among the main reasons for the increase in obesity in both children as well as adults. In adults, as a process of aging, there is decreased physical activity, in addition they may have medical conditions like arthritis, depression, fractures, sarcopenia and CVD [9] which decrease physical activity. There is a strong link between mobility disorders and decreased physical activity. Apart from this, body composition and balance between lean and fat mass also changes with age [6]. The onset of decreased lean mass is around the age of 30, accelerating after 60 years of age with increase in fat mass [10]. The body fat can be either white adipose tissue (WAT) or brown adipose tissue (BAT). WAT is the primary site of storage and release of adipokines that regulate body metabolism and insulin sensitivity [6] and accumulation of fat in WAT leads to obesity. On the other hand, BAT is inversely correlated to BMI and is more of a site that involves energy expenditure [6].

***Metabolic Changes*:** In males and females, the respective dominant sex hormone levels decrease during ageing. This occurs more drastically in females during and after menopause. Decrease in estrogen is associated with increase in body weight [11]. In males, levels of testosterone secretion decreases steadily with age and the testosterone binds with sex hormone binding globulin in the plasma, contributing to further decreases in the availability of free testosterone [12, 13]. In addition to these hormones, the elderly may also face increased hypothyroidism that can lead to obesity [14].

Some of the metabolic pathways that play an important role in the development of obesity include enzymes of fatty acid digestion and absorption and fatty acid synthesis pathway. Proteins that control adipogenesis and deposition of fat in adipocytes can also cause obesity. Additionally, transcription factors, such as peroxisome proliferator-activated receptors (PPARs), CCAAT-enhancer-binding proteins (C/EBP) and uncoupling protein (UCP), are also important players in the regulation of body weight. There are three isoforms of PPARs identified and they control expression of genes that regulate cellular differentiation, development and metabolism (carbohydrate, lipid and protein) [15-18]. Increase in the expression of PPARγ results in stimulation of fat uptake and adipogenesis. Another transcription factor is C/EBP found in hepatocytes, adipocytes and several other cells and organs. There are four isoforms of C/EBP. They modulate cellular responses related to cell proliferation, growth, differentiation, metabolism and immunity. In adipocytes, C/EBP induces adipocyte differentiation, controls adipogenesis and may induce one of the PPARs (PPARγ) [19-24]. Uncoupling protein is found in the mitochondria and controls mitochondria-derived reactive oxygen species [25]. It is used to generate heat instead of adenosine triphosphate (ATP). Five isoforms have been identified so far. UCP is reported to transport fatty acids out of the mitochondrial matrix. Therefore, it may be important in maintaining the oxidative pathways in the mitochondria and protecting it from the harmful effects of fatty acids [26]. UCP seems to be modulated by triglycerides rather than free fatty acids (FFA) [27].

Other metabolic conditions such as increase in oxidative stress and inflammation can also aggravate obesity [28]. Obesity is now believed to be a state of low-grade chronic inflammation [7, 8]. As evidence of inflammation, obese individuals have elevated levels of pro-inflammatory cytokines and chemokines such as tumor necrosis factor-α (TNF-α), interleukin-1β (IL-1β), IL-6, and monocyte chemotactic protein -1 (MCP-1) [7, 8]. This is accompanied by elevated plasma levels of cholesterol, triglycerides and hormones of the rennin-angiotensin system [6]. Additionally, adipose tissue from obese individuals has chronic activation of pro-inflammatory signaling pathways, including nuclear factor κ B (NFκB) and jun N-terminal kinase (JNK) [29, 30]. The origin of these inflammatory mediators is believed to be due in large part to the obese adipose tissue. The adipocytes release these pro-inflammatory cytokines and chemokines which recruit monocytes into the adipose tissue and induce the differentiation of monocytes to M1 macrophages (pro-inflammatory) and consequently, M1 macrophages produced their own pro-inflammatory mediators [31, 32].

Nonetheless, it remains to be known as to what initiates inflammation in the adipose tissue. Indeed, evidence exists for potential sources involved in the initiation of inflammation in the adipose tissue. First, the excess of circulating FFA in obesity causes endoplasmic reticulum (ER) stress and activation of downstream signaling pathways, such as JNK, that contribute to the development of insulin resistance in obese individuals [8, 33]. Secondly, also due to the excess of nutrients, adipocytes in obesity undergo hypertrophy which eventually leads to adipocyte cell death. Subsequently, these events trigger an inflammatory response involving recruitment of macrophages to the obese adipose tissue to clear away dead cells [34, 35]. Furthermore, it is hypothesized that the high levels of FFA present in obesity can activate the cell surface receptor, Toll-like receptor 4 (TLR4) [36, 37]. The natural ligand for TLR4 is lipopolysaccharide (LPS), the Gram negative bacterial wall component which is structurally similar to FFA [36]. Indeed, obese individuals have up regulation of TLR4 in cells and tissues, including monocytes, adipose tissue, and skeletal muscle [38-40]. Therefore, a diet high in saturated FFA can activate TLR4 leading to activation of NFκB and JNK [36, 41].

Specifically, NFκB is mostly attributed to playing a central role in the development of obesity and its related complications such as insulin resistance, type 2 diabetes, and atherosclerosis [42]. NFκB proteins are a family of transcription factors that play an important role in a number of physiological processes that include cell survival, proliferation, and activation. The inhibitor of κB kinase (IKK) / inhibitor κB (IκB) / NFκB axis is activated by a wide array of exogenous and endogenous stimuli, including lipids, cytokines, hyperglycemia and reactive oxygen species (ROS) [43]. NFκB is a transcription factor that stimulates the production of several pro-inflammatory cytokines including TNF-α, IL-1, and IL-6. NFκB is a heterodimer, which usually consists of a p65 subunit and a p50 subunit. Under basal conditions, NFκB is sequestered in its inactive form in the cytoplasm by IκB. Upon activation of the IKK/IκB/NFκB axis by inflammatory stimuli, such as FFA, hyperglycemia, cytokines and oxidative stress, IKK phosphorylates IκB triggering its degradation by proteosomes. This causes the liberation of NFκB from IκB, and then NFκB translocates into the nucleus where it stimulates the transcription of number of genes involved in the production of pro-inflammatory cytokines, chemokines, and enzymes that generate mediators of inflammation, immune receptors, and adhesion molecules.

Genetic Disorders: Although there are many acquired and metabolic factors that may cause obesity, another important factor is genetic disorders. A mutation in the gene that maintains energy balance, leptin, causes obesity [44]. Leptin is secreted by the adipose and binds to its receptor (leptin receptor) in the hypothalamus. Deficiency of leptin receptor also results in obesity [44]. When leptin deficient patients are given leptin, they are no longer obese and maintain a normal body weight [45]. It is also reported that amylin, a hormone secreted from the pancreatic β cells, interacts with leptin and synergistically control body weight [44].

Other physiological conditions like loss of taste, smell, diminished sensory-specific satiety, delayed gastric emptying and food intake-related regulatory impairments for which specific mechanisms remain largely unknown [46] are also factors that can cause obesity. In addition, the elderly have less appetite and are satiated quicker [6].

Now, we can see the available therapy options for preventing and treating obesity. As mentioned there are many factors and metabolic pathways attributed to obesity. Similarly many different therapies may be developed. Certainly, life style and food habit changes can be adopted by obese individuals. In addition, they can take nutritional supplements or medications. Globally, the use of complementary and alternative medicines is common, and in the US, more than one third of the population is dependent on consumption of natural products to avoid severe side effects [47]. Some of the compounds that are available include those from 1. Plant origin; 2. Polyunsaturated fatty acids (PUFA) and 3. Other compounds isolated from natural sources. We have included products that have been shown to have direct effects on pathways that are involved in obesity or body weight changes.

In overweight and obese individuals, the major factor is increase of fat mass. Therefore, anti-obesity therapeutics should affect some of the important proteins that are for fatty acids synthesis, adipocyte proliferation, digestion and absorption of fat mass and deposition of fat globules in adipose tissue. Prevention of the expansion of WAT may be yet another way to reduce inflammation and progression of obesity [48]. Available natural compounds may modulate different pathways and result in decreased fat mass and weight gain. In the rest of the chapter, we have listed natural compounds that have shown anti-obesity properties and the pathways that they affect to prevent the development of obesity.

INFLUENCE ON FATTY ACID METABOLISM AND ENERGY MANAGEMENT

Plant Extracts and Active Ingredients of Plant Extracts

Many plant extracts or compounds have shown the ability to inhibit digestion, absorption and accumulation of fats as well as fatty acid synthesis and adipogenesis. Moreover, some others are reported to increase energy expenditure and thermogenesis (Table **1**). Different parts of plants like leaves, stem, bark, roots, flower, fruits and seeds, in addition to whole plant extracts have been tested for anti-obesity properties. Specific active ingredients of plants have also been isolated and tested.

Table 1: Anti-obesity properties of different plant extracts

Name	Mode of Action		References
	Inhibition/Reduction/Inactivation	**Activation/Increase**	
Afromomum meleguetta	Pancreatic lipase		[87]
Butea menosperma	Weight gain, triglycerides, anti-lipidemia		[76]
Camellia sinensis	Body weight, lipid absorption, visceral and hepatic fats, cholesterol, weight maintenance	Thermogenesis, expenditure energy	[49-68]
Caralluma fimbriata	Hunger, waist circumference		[94]
Cissus quadrangularis	Appetite	Muscle mass	[77-79]
Clerodendron glandulosum	LDL oxidation		[91]
Glycyrrhiza	Aabdominal fat		[120, 121]
Hibiscus sabdariffa	Body weight gain, plasma cholesterol, gastric and pancreatic lipase, accumulation of fat droplet in adipocytes, fatty acid synthetase, PPARγ, C/EBPα	Thermogenesis	[84]
Ibervillea sonorae	Weight gain, dyslipidemia		[83]
Ilex paraguariensis	Weight gain, fatty acid synthesis, IL-6, TNF-α, NFκB	UCP 2, UCP 3, AMPK phosphorylation	[116]
Irvingia gabonensis	Appetite, adipogenesis, leptin, PPARγ	Muscle mass, adiponectin	[78]
Loranthaceae (Family)	Weight reduction, appetite reduction		[75, 89]
Momordica charantia	Large adipocytes, triglyceride, mRNA of fatty acid synthase, acetyl CoA caroboxylase 1, lipoprotein lipase and adipocyte fatty acid binding protein, visceral fat accumulation, adipocyte hypertrophy		[86]
Nelumbo nucifera	α-amylase, lipase, fatty acid synthase, acetyl CoA carboxylase, HMG CoA reductase, weight gain, adipose tissue, liver triglycerides, ADD1/SREBP-1c	Expression fof UCP3	[70-73, 117, 118]
Nepata japonica	Accumulation of fat in adipocytes		[90]
Peanut shell	Fat absorption, liver triglycerols, lipoprotein lipase, pancreatic lipase		[88]
Pinella ternate	Triglycerides and free fatty acids	UCP1	[93]

Table 1: contd…

Pine needle extract	PPARγ, lipolytic activity		[123]
Populus balsamifera	Adipocyte differentiation	UCP1, hepatic fatty acid oxidation	[125]
Salacia oblonga	Hyperlipidemia, fatty liver		[80,81]
Solanun tuberosum	P38 MAPK, Leptin, serum cholesterol, triglycerides	UCP3	[74]
Spilanthes acmella	Pancreatic lipase		[87]
Taxillus chinenesis	Fatty acid synthesis		[75]
Trigonella foenum	Plasma triglyceride gain		[85]
Viscaceae (Family)	Weight reduction, appetite reduction		[75, 89]

A common beverage consumed globally is tea and many health benefits including weight loss have been associated with it. Tea is obtained from the leaves of *Camellia sinensis* and is available as green tea, oolong tea and black tea depending on how they are processed. Green tea leaves are steamed or pan-fried to inhibit polyphenol oxidase activity and has large amounts of catechins [49]. Oolong tea undergoes partial oxidation so, it retains higher levels of catechins and has unique dimeric and oligomeric polyphenols like theasinensins [50]. Black tea is further processed by crushing the leaves, which causes oxidation, a process called fermentation. This process converts most of the catechins to theaflavins and thearubigins [51]. Studies have shown that green tea is more potent than the other kinds of tea (oolong and black tea) in reducing weight in humans and animal studies. Amongst many other functions, tea also reduces lipid absorption and post prandial lipid concentrations in high fat diet fed mice [52, 53]. Interestingly, in non-obese rats, fed normal diet, tea catechins also reduces lipid metabolism [54], visceral and hepatic fat, levels of cholesterol and bile salts. The use of oolong or black tea alone is not attributed to decreased body weight [55-57]; however, there is evidence that black tea in combination with caffeine, ginger, dill weed, vitamin C, rutin, or oolong increases the metabolic rate [58-60]. Oolong tea extract decreases food intake and tea catechin reduces energy intake [61]. In humans, consumption of catechin tea results in lower body weight, total fat area, visceral fat, percent body fat, waist and hip circumference and LDL cholesterol [55, 56].

In general, weight maintenance has been better amongst tea consumers [62] may be because tea increases metabolism, thermogenesis and expenditure of energy which helps in decreasing weight gain in diet-induced obesity [63-68]. In addition, increased and prolonged interactions between polyphenols and caffeine may also control obesity [65, 69].

Several other plants are used as preventive measures for obesity. Leaf extract of the aquatic plant *Nelumbo nucifera* (lotus) inhibits the activity of α-amylase, lipase, fatty acid synthase (FAS), acetyl CoA carboxylase and HMG COA reductase [70, 71]. Mice and rats, when fed *N. nucifera* leaf extract, show decreased weight gain, adipose tissue (parametrial) and liver triglycerides [72]. In addition, it stimulates lipolysis in WAT [73]. Ethanol extraction of *Solanum* inhibits differentiation and fat accumulation of preadipocytes *in vitro* (3T3-L1 cells). It also reduces the levels of leptin, serum cholesterol and triglyceride and prevents weight gain in high fat fed diet rats [74]. Ethanolic extract of the stem of *Taxillus chinensis* inhibits fatty acid synthase [75]. A tropical tree, *Butea monosperma* (Lam), commonly called the Flame of the Forest, has several compounds including flavonoids, steroids and leucocynidin. The bark has anti-hyperlipemic properties and decreases weight gain and triglyceride levels in chemically induced obesity in rats [76]. *Cissus quadrangularis,* which is used in Ayurvedic medicine shows anti-obesity properties in humans mainly by decreasing appetite and increasing muscle mass either when used alone or in combination with another herb *Irvingia gabonensis* [77-79].

The root extract of *Salacia oblonga* attenuates hyperlipidemia and fatty liver [80, 81]. In a study with hens, it decreases plasma and muscle triglycerides [82]. In mice fed high fat diet, aqueous extract of the root of *Ibervillea sonorae* prevents weight gain and dyslipidemia [83]. The tropical flower from the genus *Hibiscus*, especially *H. sabdariffa* decreases body weight gain in chemically induced obese mice [84]. This plant compound is implicated as being antihyperglycemic, reduces plasma cholesterol levels, inhibits gastric and pancreatic lipase, stimulates thermogenesis, inhibits fat droplet accumulation in adipocytes and inhibits FAS. Another plant extract is fenugreek (*Trigonella foenum* Gracium), a common spice of South East Asia. The seed extract of fenugreek, decreases plasma triglyceride gain. In addition, the major ingredient of fenugreek extract, 4-hydroxyisoleucine, has the same effect in high fat diet fed mice [85]. Another common vegetable from the eastern part of the globe is *Momordica charantia* (bitter melon). This has been well studied and used for its anti-diabetic properties. In rats, the powder of *M.charantia* also decreases large adipocytes and triaglyceride content. It lowers the levels of mRNA of FAS, acetyl CoA carboxylase 1, lipoprotein lipase and adipocyte fatty acid binding protein. It also suppresses visceral fat accumulation and adipocyte hypertrophy [86]. Similarly, the seed extract of *I. gabonensis* also inhibits adipogenesis in adipocytes and lowers plasma leptin levels by up regulating expression of adiponectin in adipocytes [78]. The dried powder of seeds and flower buds (ethanol extracted) of two African plants *Afromomum meleguetta* (seeds) and *Spilanthes acmella* (flower bud) inhibit pancreatic lipase activity *in vitro* [87].

Moreover, peanuts are consumed widely and the shell has many health benefits. In rats, peanut inhibits fat absorption and reduces liver triglycerides, lipoprotein lipase and pancreatic lipase activity [88]. Plants from the Families Loranthaceae and Viscaceae have the properties of decreasing body weight by reducing appetite [75, 89]. *Nepata japonica* Maximowicz extract inhibits the accumulation of fat in adipocytes and may have potential anti-obesity properties [90]. Another plant extract, *Clerodendron glandulosum* Coleb prevents LDL oxidation [91] and has the potential to be used as an anti-obesity drug [92]. The *Pinellia ternate* aqueous extract lowers triglyceride and FFA levels [93]. Extract of an edible plant from India, *Caralluma fimbriata* suppresses hunger and reduces waist circumference in humans [94].

ACTIVE INGREDIENTS OF PLANTS

Specific active compounds isolated from plants and plant parts have also been tested for their anti-obesity properties (Table **2**). Many of these compounds decrease digestion and absorption of fatty acids mainly by inhibiting pancreatic lipase activity. Platycodin, a compound isolated from the root of *Platycodon grandiflorum*, a Chinese medicinal herb, inhibits pancreatic lipase activity which results in decreased body weight in diet induced obese rats [95]. It also lowers plasma lipids (total cholesterol and triglycerides), and decreases adipocyte differentiation and fat accumulation. Furthermore, it reduces subcutaneous adipose tissue weight in high fat diet fed Sprague Dawley rats by up regulating the expression of fatty acid binding protein (FBP) [96]. In another study, total chikusetsusaponins isolated from *Panax japonicum* shows prevention of body weight gain and fat storage in adipose tissue, mainly by decreasing intestinal absorption of dietary fat by inhibiting pancreatic lipase activity in high fat diet fed mice and normal rats [97]. Similarly, saponins from *Kochia scoparia* also inhibits pancreatic lipase activity *in vitro* and inhibits elevation of triglycerides, body weight and parametrial adipose tissues in high fat diet fed mice [98]. Capsinoid, isolated from peppers (genus *Capsicum),* reduces abdominal fat and increases fatty acid oxidation in humans [99]. The main ingredient in the leaves of *Acanthopanax sessiliflora* - Chiisanoside decreases plasma triglyceride levels and increases undigested triglycerides probably by inhibiting pancreatic lipase [100].

Table 2: Active ingredients of plants that show anti-obesity properties

Name of Active Ingredient	Source	Mode of Action		References
		Inhibition/Reduction/Inactivation	**Activation/Increase**	
Capsinoid	Capsicum	Abdominal fat	Fatty acid oxidation	[99]
Cathechins – EGCG	Green tea	Fatty acid, triglycerol synthesis, fat accumulation in hepatic cells, circulating lipids, PPARγ, C/EBPα, CDK2, NFκB p65, fatty acid synthase, acetyl CoA carboxylase	IL-10, energy expenditure	[69, 104, 108, 135-144]
Chiisanoside	*Acanthopanax sessiliflora*	Plasma triglycerides, pancreatic lipase		[100]
Chikusetsusaponins	*Panax japonicum*	Body weight gain, pancreatic lipase		[97]
Curcumin	*Curcuma*, Zingiber	PPARγ		[132-134]
Guabiroba		Weight gain		[103]
Theanine	Tea	Food intake		[145]
Genisten	Soy	Adipocyte formation, C/EBPβ, PPARγ		[126,127]
Lupenone	*Adenophora triphylla*	Lipid accumulation,PPARγ, C/EBPα		[146]
Oxypregnane steroidal glycoside, p57	*Hoodia*		Satiety stimulator	[130.131]

Table 2: contd…

Organosulfue (1,2DT)	*Allium sativum*	Pre-adipocyte differentiation		[48,101]
Platycodin	*Platycodon grandifloru m*	Pancreatic lipase, plasma lipid, adipocyte differentiation, fat accumulation, subcutaneous fat accumulation	Fatty acid binding protein	[95,96]
Quercetin		Adipogenesis		[128]
Resveratrol	Grapes	Adipogenesis		[129]
Saponins	*Kochia acopania*	Pancreatic lipase		[98]
Ursolic acid	Herbs and fruits	Pancreatic lipase, catabolism of triglycerides	Lipolysis	[102]

One of the most common vegetables that has been used for >5000 years as a spice and has several health benefits, including anti-obesity is garlic (*Allium sativum*). *Ex vivo* studies using human adipocytes, isolated from young women treated with garlic derived organosulfur (1,2DT) show that 1,2DT decreases pre adipocyte differentiation [48]. It is reported that organosulfur accumulates in the WAT of human and rodent adipocyte cells [48, 101]. Similarly, ursolic acid, a triterpene found in herbs and some fruits, inhibits fat absorption by inhibiting pancreatic lipase activity and enhancing lipolysis, in fat cells resulting in release of FFA and glycerol mainly by catabolism of triglycerides [102]. Another plant derivative from Brazil, Guabiroba, reduces weight gain in rats fed high fat diets [103]. The secondary metabolite in tea is catechin and the most abundant catechin in green tea is epigallocatechin gallate (EGCG). This compound has been analyzed extensively for its anti-obesity properties. EGCG (90mg) shows increased energy expenditure [69]. It also modulates several enzymes related to lipid anabolism and catabolism such as acetyl CoA carboxylase, FAS, pancreatic lipase, gastric lipase and lipooxygenase [69, 104] and has pro-oxidative and anti-oxidative properties [69, 105]. In addition, green tea can maintain weight in subjects after weight loss [106]. In humans, Monoselect *Camellia* (MonCam)(containing highly bioavailable green tea extract, GreenSelect Phytosome) when taken with a low calorie diet shows decreased total cholesterol, fasting blood sugar and total triglycerides, low density lipids, insulin and cortisol which is associated with an increase in growth hormone, high density lipids and insulin like growth factor-1 [107]. In a short term study in which overweight/obese men drank TEAVIGO which has 94% of EGCG from tea, reported in an increase in their fat oxidation [108].

MULTI COMPOUND MIXTURES

So far, we have talked about extracts and individual compounds but multi compound mixtures have also been studied and show promise as anti-obesity agents. These are readily available in the market and most are referred by their brand names. Slim339, a combination of *Garcinia cambogia*, calcium panthothenate, *Matricaria chamomilla*, *Rosa damascene*, *Lavandula officinalis*, *Cananga odorata* reduces body weight in humans [109].

Combination of bioactive compounds such as green tea extract catechins, tyrosine, anhydrous caffeine, calcium carbonate, simple or controlled release capsaicin increases the thermogenic effect, decreases fat mass and may be more useful in maintaining weight after being in a weight loss program [110]. Another study in humans has shown that plant efhedrine with caffeine, guarana, bitter orange and synephrine decreases body weight. In Japan, Bofu-Tsusho-San (traditional Japanese plant mixture of 18 crude drugs) is used against obesity and it decreases body weight and abdominal/visceral fat accumulation and total cholesterol, but has no effect on the basal metabolic rate [111].

Extracts of Non Plant Origin

A few natural products that are not plant origin have been studied and shown to have anti-obesity properties (Table **3**). A tetrahydrolipstatin (Orlistat, Xenical, Roche) isolated from *Streptomyces toxytricini* [112-114] reduces pancreatic lipase activity. Similarly, mushroom yogurt (fermented mushroom milk) decreases weight gain and triglycerides in Otsuka Long Evans Tokushima Fatty (OLETF) rats [115]. In addition to the mushroom, this preparation also has probiotic bacteria that help in the preparation of yogurt, so the effect may be from both – the compounds from mushroom as well as from the bacteria.

Table 3: Other natural products that show anti-obesity properties

Name	Source	Mode of Action		References
		Inhibition/Reduction/Inactivation	**Activation/Increase**	
Chitosan	Crustaceans	Fat absorption	Weight loss	[167]
Conjugated linoleic acids	Dairy, dairy products	Body weight, retroperitoneal fat deposits, body fat, leptin secretion, triglycerol WAT and BAT, PPARγ	Protein content, UCP-2	[158-165]
Deep sea water	<200 m sea level	C/EBPα, PPARγ	adiponectin	[169]
1-Deoxynojirimycin	Silk worm	Weight gain		[166]
Mushroon yogurt	Mushrooms	Weight gain, triglycerides		[115]
Polyunsaturated fatty acids	Fish, krill, milk, perilla, flaxseed	NFκB		[154-157]
Tetrahydrolipstatin	*Streptomyces toxytricini*	Pancreatic lipase		[112-114]

INHIBITION OF TRANSCRIPTION FACTORS INVOLVED IN ADIPOGENESIS

As mentioned earlier, certain transcription factors are also modulated by some plants. Some of them decrease the expression of PPAR-γ and C/EBP-α and UCP while others, modulate AMP activated protein kinase (AMPK) and proteins that regulate cell division and proliferation. Ethanolic extracts of the leaves from *Ilex paraguariensis* extract prevents high fat diet induced weight gain in rats by increasing the expression of coupling proteins (UCP 2 and 3) and AMPK phosphorylation which inactivates acetyl CoA carboxylase decreasing the levels of malonyl-CoA levels, thereby, decreasing fatty acid synthesis in the visceral adipose tissue [116]. Leaf extract from *Nelumbo nucifera* also increases the expression of UCP3, [117, 118] and decreases adipocyte determination and differentiation factor 1/sterol regulatory element binding protein (ADD1/SREBP-1c) in human preadipocytes [119].

Ethanolic extract of the root of *Glycyrrhiza* plant (Licorice) used in traditional medicine [120] inhibits abdominal fat lowering and hypoglycemic effects on obese diabetic mice by modulating PPAR-γ activation [121]. The flavonoid oil of licorice modulates fatty acid synthesis and oxidative pathways leading to its anti-obesity properties [122]. Ethanol extraction of the purple potato, *Solanum tuberosum,* also down regulates mitogen activated protein kinase (MAPK) p38 and activates the expression of UCP-3 in BAT and liver [74]. Furthermore, seed extract of *I. gabonensis* also down regulates PPARγ [78].

Other plant extracts like Pine needle extract (used in East Asia) suppresses the differentiation of 3T3-L1 cells in part by down regulating gene expression of PPAR-γ and also has lipolytic activity [123]. *In vitro* studies using the aqueous extract of calyx of *Hibiscus sabdariffa* show that PPAR-γ and C/EBP-α are modulated [124]. A Korean traditional treatment for removing dampness-phlegm, *Pinellia ternate,* significantly increases the expression of UCP1 mRNA in brown fat and PPARα and PGC1α mRNA expression in WAT [93]. The plant extract of *Populus balsamifera,* increases the mRNA expression of UCP1, inhibits adipocyte differentiation and decreases hepatic inflammation hepatic fatty acid oxidation [125].

Several compounds isolated from plants have shown anti-obesity properties by modulating transcription factors. For instance, genisten (soy isoflavone) inhibits adipocyte formation by decreasing the expression of C/EBPβ and PPAR-γ and also is thought to have some lipolytic activity [126, 127]. Other compounds like quercetin and resveratrol also have anti-adipogenic properties [128, 129]. A glycoside (oxypregnane steroidal glycoside, P57) from the succulent plant Genus *Hoodia* is now being developed as satiety stimulator [130, 131]. Curcumin, a polyphenol, isolated from *Curcuma* and Zingiber regulate several transcription factors like NFκB, STAT-3 and PPARγ [132]. *In vitro* studies on 3T3-L1 adipocytes have shown that curcumin inhibited PPARγ. Similarly, *in vivo* studies using high fat diet induced obese C57BL/6 mice also showed inhibition of PPARγ and reduced pro-inflammatory cytokines and c-reactive proteins [133, 134].

These studies clearly show that several plant extracts down regulates transcription factors involved in the inhibition of adipocyte differentiation and adipogenesis.

ACTIVE INGREDIENTS OF PLANTS THAT INHIBIT TRANSCRIPTION FACTORS INVOLVED IN ADIPOGENESIS

In controlled studies, the secondary metabolite of tea, catechin, decreases weight, BMI, visceral fat area, waist circumference as well as reduces CVD parameters [55,

135]. In cells (3T3-L1), catechin can also induce the phosphorylation of MAPK pathway proteins like proto-oncogene serine/threonine-protein kinase (RAF1), MAP kinase kinase (MEK) 1 and 2 and extracellular signal-regulated kinase (ERK) 1 and 2 but not JNK [136]. The mechanisms of anti-obesity properties of tea includes the reduction of adipocytogenesis and differentiation by specifically reducing the phosphorylation of MAPK, especially ERK proteins [137, 138]. In addition to this, EGCG can inhibit the activities of several enzymes related to fatty acid and triglyceride synthesis like acetyl CoA carboxylase, FAS, malic enzyme, glucose-6-phosphate dehydrogenase (G6PDH), glycerol-3-PDH and stearoyl CO A desaturase -1 resulting in decreased fat deposition in hepatocytes and adipocytes and lowering high levels of circulating lipids [53, 135, 139-142]. There is also down regulation of adipocyte marker proteins like PPAR-γ2 and C/EBPα [143]. Furthermore, green tea seed oil reduces body weight in mice fed high fat diet mainly by inhibiting PPAR-γ and CCAAT/enhancer binding protein-α and suppressing adipocyte differentiation [144]. Another compound from tea, theanine, decreases food intake and insulin levels in normal rats [145]. Similarly, the compound, lupenone, isolated from *Adenophora triphylla* var japonica decreases lipid accumulation and expression of adipogenic genes like PPAR-γ and C/EBPα in *in vitro* studies [146]

Oxidative Properties and Inflammation

Tea also has anti-oxidative properties that protects humans from oxidative damage [147, 148]. It is able to trap superoxide radical, singlet oxygen, hydroxyl radical, peroxyl radical, nitric oxide, nitrogen dioxide and peroxynitirite decreasing damage to lipid membranes proteins and nucleic acid. It appears that green tea quenches more than black tea [149]. The most active anti-oxidant in tea is EGCG. It can affect adipocyte differentiation by decreasing the activity of cyclin dependent kinase (CDK2), a kinase that is important for adipocyte proliferation [137]. AMPK can be activated by increase in ROS, and in the presence of EGCG, AMPK can be phosphorylated even more suggesting its role in anti-oxidative properties. Consistent with the general acceptance of the involvement of NFκB in metabolism and inflammation, recent studies involving natural products have targeted NFκB inhibition for the prevention of obesity. For instance, *yerba matè (Ilex paraguariensis)*, a plant consumed regularly in South Africa, has been shown to have anti-obesity properties by inhibiting NFκB activation [150, 151]. In a recent study, mice fed a high fat diet which included *yerba maté* extract exhibited a decrease in weight gain and epididymal fat compared to the animals fed a high fat diet only [151]. In addition, the use of *yerba maté* extract decreased the liver gene expression of IL-6 and TNF-α, which coincided with a reduction in the activation of NFκB in the liver.

To elucidate the effect of natural products in primary human immune cells, T_{regs}, isolated from peripheral blood of lean and obese individuals, were treated with EGCG [152]. T_{regs} are negative regulators of the immune system, producing an anti-inflammatory cytokine IL-10 and predominately express the forkhead family transcription factor 3 (Foxp3) [153]. They are important in controlling pro-inflammatory activities of T cells (Th1 and Th2) and monocytes/macrophages. Yun and colleagues demonstrated that obese individuals express less Foxp3+ T_{regs} compared to the lean group [152]. When T_{regs} from obese individuals are exposed to EGCG, there is an increase in IL-10 production without an increase in Foxp3+ T_{regs}. In addition, this was associated with a decrease in NFκB p65 activity. Therefore, this study reveals that EGCG increases Foxp3+ T_{regs} and production of the anti-inflammatory cytokine IL-10 through suppression of the NFκB signaling pathway in T cells of obese individuals.

ANIMAL PRODUCTS

Poly unsaturated fatty acids (PUFA) like docosahexaenoic acid (DHA) are anti-adipogenic by suppressing lipid accumulation and increasing basal lipolysis in 3T3-L1 adipocytes [154]. Polyphenols and PUFA have been shown to have anti-inflammatory properties and potentially a protective role against obesity (Table **3**) by decreasing the generation of pro-inflammatory cytokines, IL-6 and TNF-α [155, 156]. A recent study, examined the protective synergistic effect of polyphenols and PUFA [157]. Knowing that macrophages are key players in the development of inflammation in obesity, RAW 264.7 cells, a murine macrophage cell line, were stimulated with LPS and then exposed to a combination of polyphenols and PUFA to determine if the combination of these bioactive compounds inactivated NFκB [157]. In the presence of the polyphenol, procyanidin B3, and the PUFA, eicosapentaenoic acid (EPA), there was a decrease in NFκB p65 phosphorylation, but treatment with procyanidin B3 or

EPA alone did not induce inhibition of NFκB p65 phosphorylation. This study suggests that the combination of procyanidin B3 and EPA synergistically activate molecular mechanisms which are involved in the inactivation of the NFκB pathway.

In the last decade, the health benefits of conjugated linoleic acid (CLA) commonly found in dairy products has been established. One of the health benefits of CLA is to decrease body weight [158] (Table **3**). It is found in two isoforms of which the c9t11 isomer is formed naturally by bacteria that are found in the rumen of ruminants [159]. CLA reduces body weight by reducing WAT and serum and liver triglycerides levels [160, 161]. CLA also enhances β fatty acid oxidation in BAT and liver as well as suppresses fatty acid synthesis in the liver [59, 158, 162]. It can also reduce fat accumulation in short period of time without affecting the food intake in high fat and low fat diet fed mice [163]. This was accompanied by decreases in body weight, retroperitoneal fat deposits, body fat, leptin secretion, but with no changes in the energy intake, and an increase in protein content of the body [163]. In different studies, CLA decreases serum triglycerides in mice [164] and lipoprotein lipase activity in the adipocytes [165]. In addition, it significantly decreases both white and brown fat tissue mass in mice. The mechanism by which CLA affects fat content is by up regulating UCP-2 expression in BAT and skeletal muscles and down regulating PPARγ in cells.

Other compounds isolated from animals like silk worm and shells of invertebrates are proven to have anti-obesity properties (Table **3**). 1-Deoxynojirimycin (DNJ), an α-glucosidase inhibitor and a compound isolated from silkworms, prevents weight gain without adverse side-effects in high fat diet fed OLTEF rats [166]. Polysaccharide (chitosan) extracted from shells of invertebrates enhances weight loss and blocks fat absorption in animal studies. Humans on a diet containing chitosan for short term (60 d) lost more weight [167], but surprisingly, those individuals on a longer treatment period (180 d) did not show any significant loss of body weight [168]. Even water from the deep sea (below 200m) has been shown to decrease adipocyte differentiation by down regulating the expression of adipogenic transcription factors and adipocyte specific proteins [169] and by decreasing the C/EBPα, PPARγ, adiponectin, and fatty acid binding protein.

TOXICITY OF NATURAL COMPOUNDS

As the interest increases in the use of natural compounds to reduce body weight, there are reports of hepatotoxicity leading to chronic or even acute liver failure. Ephedra containing compounds can cause severe cardiac toxicity including myocardial infarction and arrhythmias with neuropsychiatric disorders and hepatotoxicity [170, 171]. Chronic hepatitis and hepatic necrosis is associated with ephedra consumption mainly by panacinar necrosis in severe cases and centrilobular necrosis in milder cases [172]. Trepenoids and triterpenoids, ingredient in the herbs (Tables **1** and **2**) mentioned earlier in this chapter, can increase epoxides causing hepatic necrosis, microvesicular steatosis, hepatic granulomas [173], and hepatic veno-occlusive disease [172]. In addition, they can indcue the formation of autoantibodies [172]. Toxicity of high tea consumption has been addressed, and it is mainly related to tea based dietary supplements rather than tea beverage consumption (51). Green tea extracts, especially consumption of only the active ingredients are also associated with hepatotoxicity [174-178]. In addition, mitochondrial toxicity and ROS production is attributed to excessive consumption of EGCG [179, 180]. The fatty acid CLA has been reported to induce insulin resistance and fatty liver as well as increased spleen weight [181].

Having talked about the potential toxicity, it is important to mention that individuals react to each herb differently. Some ethnic groups may react more than others which are also true for individuals in a population who may have different tolerance levels. Nevertheless, when compounds are proven to cause toxicity, they should be avoided or taken with extreme caution. Moreover, consumption of whole extracts may not cause toxicity but consumption of the active ingredients may result in severe toxicity as seen in the case of tea and EGCG. This can be explained by the fact that the active ingredient has a specific target while whole extracts may have other compounds that stabilize the overall metabolism.

Together these studies demonstrate that many pathways can be targeted to prevent and treat obesity (Fig. **1**). More recently, it is identified that inflammation may be one important pathway and specifically targeting the NFκB pathway can help in ameliorating the development of inflammation in obesity, a metabolic disorder which can eventually result to insulin resistance and type 2 diabetes mellitus. Moreover, increasing evidence has shown the clear contribution of NFκB signaling in the pathogenesis of obesity. Therefore, the critical need exists for effective and novel therapeutic strategies for blocking NFκB-induced inflammation. The use of natural products is an attractive potential intervention in the pathways linking diet, NFκB, and obesity.

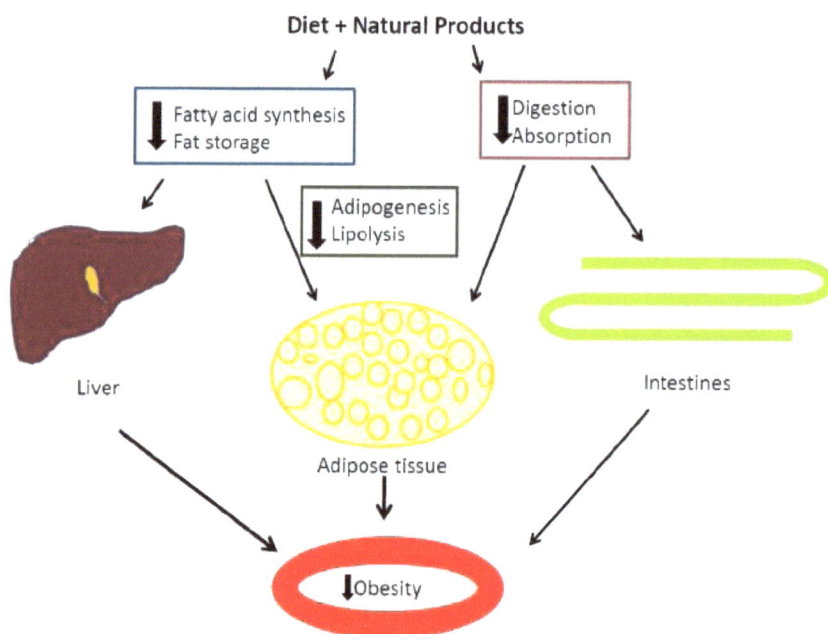

Figure 1: An outline of the effects of diet and natural compounds on obesity.

In summary, many natural products have been tested for anti-obesity properties. It has been established that different pathways can be modulated to reduce obesity using these products. Interestingly, some of the plants tested are consumed regularly in many parts of the world, while others are used in traditional medicinal practice in specific regions of the world. There is no doubt that isolated compounds should be approached with caution and in fact all of these therapies should be taken in moderation. We conclude that plant drugs having anti-obesity properties should be marketed with ample information on the potential side-effects. Additionally, consumers should approach the idea of taking anti-obesity therapy from natural products with high level of awareness and, caution by adhering to the recommended dosage and frequency.

ACKNOWLEDGEMENTS

Declared None.

CONFLICT OF INTEREST

The authors confirm that this chapter contents have no conflict of interest.

REFERENCES

[1]   Caballero B. The global epidemic of obesity: an overview. Epidemiol Rev. 2007;29:1-5.
[2]   WHO. Obesity preventing and managing the global epidemic. Report of a WHO consultation technical Report Series 894, Geneva, SwitzerSwitzerland. 2000;Switzerland.
[3]   Woodhouse R. Obesity in art: a brief overview. Front Horm Res. 2008;36:271-86.
[4]   WHO.   2008   [11/15/2012];   Available   from: www. WHO.int/mediacentre/factsheets/fs311/en/index.html.
[5]   WHO. World Health Statistics 2012: one in six adults obes, one in three hypertensive, one in 10 diabetic. 2012 [12/15/2012]; Available from: http://health.india.com/news/world-health-statistics-2012-one-in-six-adults-obese-one-inthreehypertensive/one in 10 diabetic.
[6]   Apostolopoulou M, Savopoulos C, Michalakis K, Coppack S, Dardavessis T, Hatzitolios A. Age, weight and obesity. Maturitas. 2012;71(2):115-9.
[7]   Bastard JP, Maachi M, Lagathu C, Kim MJ, Caron M, Vidal H, *et al*. Recent advances in the relationship between obesity, inflammation, and insulin resistance. Eur Cytokine Netw. 2006;17(1):4-12.
[8]   Hotamisligil GS. Inflammation and metabolic disorders. Nature. 2006;444(7121):860-7.
[9]   Wernette CM, White BD, Zizza CA. Signaling proteins that influence energy intake may affect unintentional weight loss in elderly persons. J Am Diet Assoc. 2011;111(6):864-73.
[10]   Balagopal P, Proctor D, Nair KS. Sarcopenia and hormonal changes. Endocrine. 1997;7(1):57-60.
[11]   Polotsky HN, Polotsky AJ. Metabolic implications of menopause. Semin Reprod Med. 2010;28(5):426-34.
[12]   Harman SM, Metter EJ, Tobin JD, Pearson J, Blackman MR. Longitudinal effects of aging on serum total and free testosterone levels in healthy men. Baltimore Longitudinal Study of Aging. J Clin Endocrinol Metab. 2001;86(2):724-31.
[13]   Lunenfeld B. Endocrinology of the aging male. Minerva Ginecol. 2006;58(2):153-70.
[14]   Aoki Y, Belin RM, Clickner R, Jeffries R, Phillips L, Mahaffey KR. Serum TSH and total T4 in the United States population and their association with participant characteristics: National Health and Nutrition Examination Survey (NHANES 1999-2002). Thyroid. 2007;17(12):1211-23.
[15]   Michalik L, Auwerx J, Berger JP, Chatterjee VK, Glass CK, Gonzalez FJ, *et al*. International Union of Pharmacology. LXI. Peroxisome proliferator-activated receptors. Pharmacol Rev. 2006;58(4):726-41.
[16]   Belfiore A, Genua M, Malaguarnera R. PPAR-gamma agonists and their effects on IGF-I receptor signaling: Implications for cancer. PPAR Res. 2009;2009:830501.

[17]   Berger J, Moller DE. The mechanisms of action of PPARs. Annu Rev Med. 2002;53:409-35.

[18]   Feige JN, Gelman L, Michalik L, Desvergne B, Wahli W. From molecular action to physiological outputs: peroxisome proliferator-activated receptors are nuclear receptors at the crossroads of key cellular functions. Prog Lipid Res. 2006;45(2):120-59.

[19]   Tanaka T, Yoshida N, Kishimoto T, Akira S. Defective adipocyte differentiation in mice lacking the C/EBPbeta and/or C/EBPdelta gene. EMBO J. 1997;16(24):7432-43.

[20]   Cao Z, Umek RM, McKnight SL. Regulated expression of three C/EBP isoforms during adipose conversion of 3T3-L1 cells. Genes Dev. 1991;5(9):1538-52.

[21]   Clarke SL, Robinson CE, Gimble JM. CAAT/enhancer binding proteins directly modulate transcription from the peroxisome proliferator-activated receptor gamma 2 promoter. Biochem Biophys Res Commun. 1997;240(1):99-103.

[22]   Freytag SO, Paielli DL, Gilbert JD. Ectopic expression of the CCAAT/enhancer-binding protein alpha promotes the adipogenic program in a variety of mouse fibroblastic cells. Genes Dev. 1994;8(14):1654-63.

[23]   Linhart HG, Ishimura-Oka K, DeMayo F, Kibe T, Repka D, Poindexter B, *et al.* C/EBPalpha is required for differentiation of white, but not brown, adipose tissue. Proc Natl Acad Sci U S A. 2001;98(22):12532-7.

[24]   Yeh WC, Cao Z, Classon M, McKnight SL. Cascade regulation of terminal adipocyte differentiation by three members of the C/EBP family of leucine zipper proteins. Genes Dev. 1995;9(2):168-81.

[25]   Arsenijevic D, Onuma H, Pecqueur C, Raimbault S, Manning BS, Miroux B, *et al.* Disruption of the uncoupling protein-2 gene in mice reveals a role in immunity and reactive oxygen species production. Nat Genet. 2000;26(4):435-9.

[26]   Hesselink MK, Mensink M, Schrauwen P. Human uncoupling protein-3 and obesity: an update. Obes Res. 2003;11(12):1429-43.

[27]   Mingrone G, Rosa G, Greco AV, Manco M, Vega N, Hesselink MK, *et al.* Decreased uncoupling protein expression and intramyocytic triglyceride depletion in formerly obese subjects. Obes Res. 2003;11(5):632-40.

[28]   Vincent HK, Innes KE, Vincent KR. Oxidative stress and potential interventions to reduce oxidative stress in overweight and obesity. Diabetes Obes Metab. 2007;9(6):813-39.

[29]   Olefsky JM, Glass CK. Macrophages, inflammation, and insulin resistance. Annu Rev Physiol. 2010;72:219-46.

[30]   Wellen KE, Hotamisligil GS. Inflammation, stress, and diabetes. J Clin Invest. 2005;115(5):1111-9.

[31]   Weisberg SP, McCann D, Desai M, Rosenbaum M, Leibel RL, Ferrante AW, Jr. Obesity is associated with macrophage accumulation in adipose tissue. J Clin Invest. 2003;112(12):1796-808.

[32]   Xu H, Barnes GT, Yang Q, Tan G, Yang D, Chou CJ, *et al.* Chronic inflammation in fat plays a crucial role in the development of obesity-related insulin resistance. J Clin Invest. 2003;112(12):1821-30.

[33]   Ozcan U, Cao Q, Yilmaz E, Lee AH, Iwakoshi NN, Ozdelen E, *et al.* Endoplasmic reticulum stress links obesity, insulin action, and type 2 diabetes. Science. 2004 5;306(5695):457-61.

[34]   Rutkowski JM, Davis KE, Scherer PE. Mechanisms of obesity and related pathologies: the macro- and microcirculation of adipose tissue. Febs J. 2009;276(20):5738-46.

[35]   Trayhurn P, Wood IS. Adipokines: inflammation and the pleiotropic role of white adipose tissue. Br J Nutr. 2004;92(3):347-55.

[36]   Shi H, Kokoeva MV, Inouye K, Tzameli I, Yin H, Flier JS. TLR4 links innate immunity and fatty acid-induced insulin resistance. J Clin Invest. 2006;116(11):3015-25.

[37]   Suganami T, Tanimoto-Koyama K, Nishida J, Itoh M, Yuan X, Mizuarai S, *et al*. Role of the Toll-like receptor 4/NF-kappaB pathway in saturated fatty acid-induced inflammatory changes in the interaction between adipocytes and macrophages. Arterioscler Thromb Vasc Biol. 2007;27(1):84-91.

[38]   Reyna SM, Ghosh S, Tantiwong P, Meka CS, Eagan P, Jenkinson CP, *et al*. Elevated toll-like receptor 4 expression and signaling in muscle from insulin-resistant subjects. Diabetes. 2008;57(10):2595-602.

[39]   Jialal I, Huet BA, Kaur H, Chien A, Devaraj S. Increased toll-like receptor activity in patients with metabolic syndrome. Diabetes Care. 2012;35(4):900-4.

[40]   Poulain-Godefroy O, Le Bacquer O, Plancq P, Lecoeur C, Pattou F, Fruhbeck G, *et al*. Inflammatory role of Toll-like receptors in human and murine adipose tissue. Mediators Inflamm. 2010;2010:823486.

[41]   Nguyen MT, Favelyukis S, Nguyen AK, Reichart D, Scott PA, Jenn A, *et al*. A subpopulation of macrophages infiltrates hypertrophic adipose tissue and is activated by free fatty acids *via* Toll-like receptors 2 and 4 and JNK-dependent pathways. J Biol Chem. 2007;282(48):35279-92.

[42]   Baker RG, Hayden MS, Ghosh S. NF-kappaB, inflammation, and metabolic disease. Cell Metab. 2011;13(1):11-22.

[43]   Hayden MS, Ghosh S. Shared principles in NF-kappaB signaling. Cell. 2008;132(3):344-62.

[44]   Friedman JM. Leptin and the regulation of body weigh. Keio J Med. 2011;60(1):1-9.

[45]   Dardeno TA, Chou SH, Moon HS, Chamberland JP, Fiorenza CG, Mantzoros CS. Leptin in human physiology and therapeutics. Front Neuroendocrinol. 2010;31(3):377-93.

[46]   Hays NP, Roberts SB. The anorexia of aging in humans. Physiol Behav. 2006;88(3):257-66.

[47]   Barnes PM, Bloom B, Nahin RL. Complementary and alternative medicine use among adults and children: United States, 2007. Natl Health Stat Report. 2008; 10(12):1-23.

[48]   Keophiphath M, Priem F, Jacquemond-Collet I, Clement K, Lacasa D. 1,2-vinyldithiin from garlic inhibits differentiation and inflammation of human preadipocytes. J Nutr. 2009;139(11):2055-60.

[49]   Yang CS, Maliakal P, Meng X. Inhibition of carcinogenesis by tea. Annu Rev Pharmacol Toxicol. 2002;42:25-54.

[50]   Nakai M, Fukui Y, Asami S, Toyoda-Ono Y, Iwashita T, Shibata H, *et al*. Inhibitory effects of oolong tea polyphenols on pancreatic lipase *in vitro*. J Agric Food Chem. 2005;53(11):4593-8.

[51]   Grove KA, Lambert JD. Laboratory, epidemiological, and human intervention studies show that tea (Camellia sinensis) may be useful in the prevention of obesity. J Nutr. 2010;140(3):446-53.

[52]   Bose M, Lambert JD, Ju J, Reuhl KR, Shapses SA, Yang CS. The major green tea polyphenol, (-)-epigallocatechin-3-gallate, inhibits obesity, metabolic syndrome, and fatty liver disease in high-fat-fed mice. J Nutr. 2008;138(9):1677-83.

[53] Ikeda I, Tsuda K, Suzuki Y, Kobayashi M, Unno T, Tomoyori H, *et al*. Tea catechins with a galloyl moiety suppress postprandial hypertriacylglycerolemia by delaying lymphatic transport of dietary fat in rats. J Nutr. 2005;135(2):155-9.

[54] Ito Y, Ichikawa T, Morohoshi Y, Nakamura T, Saegusa Y, Ishihara K. Effect of tea catechins on body fat accumulation in rats fed a normal diet. Biomed Res. 2008;29(1):27-32.

[55] Nagao T, Hase T, Tokimitsu I. A green tea extract high in catechins reduces body fat and cardiovascular risks in humans. Obesity (Silver Spring). 2007;15(6):1473-83.

[56] Nagao T, Komine Y, Soga S, Meguro S, Hase T, Tanaka Y, *et al*. Ingestion of a tea rich in catechins leads to a reduction in body fat and malondialdehyde-modified LDL in men. Am J Clin Nutr. 2005;81(1):122-9.

[57] Cherniack EP. Potential applications for alternative medicine to treat obesity in an aging population. Altern Med Rev. 2008;13(1):34-42.

[58] Komatsu T, Nakamori M, Komatsu K, Hosoda K, Okamura M, Toyama K, *et al*. Oolong tea increases energy metabolism in Japanese females. The journal of medical investigation : JMI. 2003;50(3-4):170-5.

[59] Roberts AT, de Jonge-Levitan L, Parker CC, Greenway F. The effect of an herbal supplement containing black tea and caffeine on metabolic parameters in humans. Altern Med Rev. 2005;10(4):321-5.

[60] Rumpler W, Seale J, Clevidence B, Judd J, Wiley E, Yamamoto S, *et al*. Oolong tea increases metabolic rate and fat oxidation in men. J Nutr. 2001;131(11):2848-52.

[61] Murase T, Nagasawa A, Suzuki J, Hase T, Tokimitsu I. Beneficial effects of tea catechins on diet-induced obesity: stimulation of lipid catabolism in the liver. Int J Obes Relat Metab Disord. 2002;26(11):1459-64.

[62] Hursel R, Viechtbauer W, Westerterp-Plantenga MS. The effects of green tea on weight loss and weight maintenance: a meta-analysis. Int J Obes (Lond). [2009;33(9):956-61.

[63] Cooper R, Morre DJ, Morre DM. Medicinal benefits of green tea: Part I. Review of noncancer health benefits. J Altern Complement Med. 2005;11(3):521-8.

[64] Diepvens K, Westerterp KR, Westerterp-Plantenga MS. Obesity and thermogenesis related to the consumption of caffeine, ephedrine, capsaicin, and green tea. American journal of physiology Regulatory, integrative and comparative physiology. 2007; 292(1):R77-85.

[65] Dulloo AG, Duret C, Rohrer D, Girardier L, Mensi N, Fathi M, *et al*. Efficacy of a green tea extract rich in catechin polyphenols and caffeine in increasing 24-h energy expenditure and fat oxidation in humans. Am J Clin Nutr. 1999;70(6):1040-5.

[66] Kao YH, Hiipakka RA, Liao S. Modulation of endocrine systems and food intake by green tea epigallocatechin gallate. Endocrinology. 2000;141(3):980-7.

[67] Shixian Q, VanCrey B, Shi J, Kakuda Y, Jiang Y. Green tea extract thermogenesis-induced weight loss by epigallocatechin gallate inhibition of catechol-O-methyltransferase. J Med Food. 2006;9(4):451-8.

[68] St-Onge MP. Dietary fats, teas, dairy, and nuts: potential functional foods for weight control? Am J Clin Nutr.2005;81(1):7-15.

[69] Dulloo AG, Seydoux J, Girardier L, Chantre P, Vandermander J. Green tea and thermogenesis: interactions between catechin-polyphenols, caffeine and sympathetic activity. Int J Obes Relat Metab Disord. 2000;24(2):252-8.

[70]   Du H, You JS, Zhao X, Park JY, Kim SH, Chang KJ. Antiobesity and hypolipidemic effects of lotus leaf hot water extract with taurine supplementation in rats fed a high fat diet. J Biomed Sci. 2010;17 Suppl 1:S42.

[71]   Wu CH, Yang MY, Chan KC, Chung PJ, Ou TT, Wang CJ. Improvement in high-fat diet-induced obesity and body fat accumulation by a Nelumbo nucifera leaf flavonoid-rich extract in mice. J Agric Food Chem. 2010;58(11):7075-81.

[72]   Ono Y, Hattori E, Fukaya Y, Imai S, Ohizumi Y. Anti-obesity effect of Nelumbo nucifera leaves extract in mice and rats. J Ethnopharmacol. 2006;106(2):238-44.

[73]   Ohkoshi E, Miyazaki H, Shindo K, Watanabe H, Yoshida A, Yajima H. Constituents from the leaves of Nelumbo nucifera stimulate lipolysis in the white adipose tissue of mice. Planta Med. 2007;73(12):1255-9.

[74]   Yoon SS, Rhee YH, Lee HJ, Lee EO, Lee MH, Ahn KS, *et al.* Uncoupled protein 3 and p38 signal pathways are involved in anti-obesity activity of Solanum tuberosum L. cv. Bora Valley. J Ethnopharmacol. 2008;118(3):396-404.

[75]   Wang Y, Deng M, Zhang SY, Zhou ZK, Tian WX. Parasitic loranthus from Loranthaceae rather than Viscaceae potently inhibits fatty acid synthase and reduces body weight in mice. J Ethnopharmacol. 2008;118(3):473-8.

[76]   Dixit P, Prakash T, Karki R, Kotresha D. Anti-obese activity of Butea monosperma (Lam) bark extract in experimentally induced obese rats. Indian J Exp Biol. 2012 Jul;50(7):476-83.

[77]   Oben JE, Enyegue DM, Fomekong GI, Soukontoua YB, Agbor GA. The effect of Cissus quadrangularis (CQR-300) and a Cissus formulation (CORE) on obesity and obesity-induced oxidative stress. Lipids Health Dis. 2007;6:4.

[78]   Oben JE, Ngondi JL, Blum K. Inhibition of Irvingia gabonensis seed extract (OB131) on adipogenesis as mediated *via* down regulation of the PPARgamma and leptin genes and up-regulation of the adiponectin gene. Lipids Health Dis. 2008;7:44.

[79]   Oben JE, Ngondi JL, Momo CN, Agbor GA, Sobgui CS. The use of a Cissus quadrangularis/Irvingia gabonensis combination in the management of weight loss: a double-blind placebo-controlled study. Lipids Health Dis. 2008;7:12.

[80]   Huang TH, He L, Qin Q, Yang Q, Peng G, Harada M, *et al.* Salacia oblonga root decreases cardiac hypertrophy in Zucker diabetic fatty rats: inhibition of cardiac expression of angiotensin II type 1 receptor. Diabetes Obes Metab. 2008;10(7):574-85.

[81]   Huang TH, Peng G, Li GQ, Yamahara J, Roufogalis BD, Li Y. Salacia oblonga root improves postprandial hyperlipidemia and hepatic steatosis in Zucker diabetic fatty rats: activation of PPAR-alpha. Toxicol Appl Pharmacol. 2006;210(3):225-35.

[82]   Wang J, Rong X, Li W, Yamahara J, Li Y. Salacia oblonga ameliorates hypertriglyceridemia and excessive ectopic fat accumulation in laying hens. J Ethnopharmacol. 2012;142(1):221-7.

[83]   Rivera-Ramirez F, Escalona-Cardoso GN, Garduno-Siciliano L, Galaviz-Hernandez C, Paniagua-Castro N. Antiobesity and hypoglycaemic effects of aqueous extract of Ibervillea sonorae in mice fed a high-fat diet with fructose. J Biomed Biotechnol. 2011;2011:968984.

[84]   Alarcon-Aguilar FJ, Zamilpa A, Perez-Garcia MD, Almanza-Perez JC, Romero-Nunez E, Campos-Sepulveda EA, *et al.* Effect of Hibiscus sabdariffa on obesity in MSG mice. J Ethnopharmacol. 2007;114(1):66-71.

[85]   Handa T, Yamaguchi K, Sono Y, Yazawa K. Effects of fenugreek seed extract in obese mice fed a high-fat diet. Biosci Biotechnol Biochem. 2005;69(6):1186-8.

[86]   Huang HL, Hong YW, Wong YH, Chen YN, Chyuan JH, Huang CJ, *et al*. Bitter melon (Momordica charantia L.) inhibits adipocyte hypertrophy and down regulates lipogenic gene expression in adipose tissue of diet-induced obese rats. Br J Nutr. 2008;99(2):230-9.

[87]   Ekanem AP, Wang M, Simon JE, Moreno DA. Antiobesity properties of two African plants (Afromomum meleguetta and Spilanthes acmella) by pancreatic lipase inhibition. Phytother Res. 2007;21(12):1253-5.

[88]   Moreno DA, Ilic N, Poulev A, Raskin I. Effects of Arachis hypogaea nutshell extract on lipid metabolic enzymes and obesity parameters. Life Sci. 2006;78(24):2797-803.

[89]   Loftus TM, Jaworsky DE, Frehywot GL, Townsend CA, Ronnett GV, Lane MD, *et al*. Reduced food intake and body weight in mice treated with fatty acid synthase inhibitors. Science. 2000;288(5475):2379-81.

[90]   Roh C, Jung U. Nepeta japonica Maximowicz extract from natural products inhibits lipid accumulation. J Sci Food Agric. 2012;92(10):2195-9.

[91]   Jadeja RN, Thounaojam MC, Devkar RV, Ramachandran AV. Clerodendron glandulosum.Coleb extract prevents *in vitro* human LDL oxidation and oxidized LDL induced apoptosis in human monocyte derived macrophages. Food Chem Toxicol. 2011;49(6):1195-202.

[92]   Jadeja RN, Thounaojam MC, Singh TB, Devkar RV, Ramachandran A. Traditional uses, phytochemistry and pharmacology of Clerodendron glandulosum Coleb--a review. Asian Pac J Trop Med. 2012;5(1):1-6.

[93]   Kim YJ, Shin YO, Ha YW, Lee S, Oh JK, Kim YS. Anti-obesity effect of Pinellia ternata extract in Zucker rats. Biol Pharm Bull. 2006;29(6):1278-81.

[94]   Kuriyan R, Raj T, Srinivas SK, Vaz M, Rajendran R, Kurpad AV. Effect of Caralluma fimbriata extract on appetite, food intake and anthropometry in adult Indian men and women. Appetite. 2007;48(3):338-44.

[95]   Zhao HL, Sim JS, Shim SH, Ha YW, Kang SS, Kim YS. Antiobese and hypolipidemic effects of platycodin saponins in diet-induced obese rats: evidences for lipase inhibition and calorie intake restriction. Int J Obes (Lond). 2005;29(8):983-90.

[96]   Park YS, Yoon Y, Ahn HS. Platycodon grandiflorum extract represses up-regulated adipocyte fatty acid binding protein triggered by a high fat feeding in obese rats. World J Gastroenterol. 2007;13(25):3493-9.

[97]   Han LK, Zheng YN, Yoshikawa M, Okuda H, Kimura Y. Anti-obesity effects of chikusetsusaponins isolated from Panax japonicus rhizomes. BMC Complement Altern Med. 2005;5:9.

[98]   Han LK, Nose R, Li W, Gong XJ, Zheng YN, Yoshikawa M, *et al*. Reduction of fat storage in mice fed a high-fat diet long term by treatment with saponins prepared from Kochia scoparia fruit. Phytother Res. 2006;20(10):877-82.

[99]   Snitker S, Fujishima Y, Shen H, Ott S, Pi-Sunyer X, Furuhata Y, *et al*. Effects of novel capsinoid treatment on fatness and energy metabolism in humans: possible pharmacogenetic implications. Am J Clin Nutr. 2009;89(1):45-50.

[100] Yoshizumi K, Murota K, Watanabe S, Tomi H, Tsuji T, Terao J. Chiisanoside is not absorbed but inhibits oil absorption in the small intestine of rodents. Biosci Biotechnol Biochem. 2008;72(4):1126-9.

[101] Egen-Schwind C, Eckard R, Jekat FW, Winterhoff H. Pharmacokinetics of vinyldithiins, transformation products of allicin. Planta Med. 1992;58(1):8-13.

[102] Kim J, Jang DS, Kim H, Kim JS. Anti-lipase and lipolytic activities of ursolic acid isolated from the roots of Actinidia arguta. Arch Pharm Res. 2009;32(7):983-7.

[103] Biavatti MW, Farias C, Curtius F, Brasil LM, Hort S, Schuster L, *et al*. Preliminary studies on Campomanesia xanthocarpa (Berg.) and Cuphea carthagenensis (Jacq.) J.F. Macbr. aqueous extract: weight control and biochemical parameters. J Ethnopharmacol. 2004;93(2-3):385-9.

[104] Safe S. Transcriptional activation of genes by 17 beta-estradiol through estrogen receptor-Sp1 interactions. Vitam Horm. 2001;62:231-52.

[105] Waltner-Law ME, Wang XL, Law BK, Hall RK, Nawano M, Granner DK. Epigallocatechin gallate, a constituent of green tea, represses hepatic glucose production. J Biol Chem. 2002;277(38):34933-40.

[106] Kovacs EM, Lejeune MP, Nijs I, Westerterp-Plantenga MS. Effects of green tea on weight maintenance after body-weight loss. Br J Nutr. 2004;91(3):431-7.

[107] Di Pierro F, Menghi AB, Barreca A, Lucarelli M, Calandrelli A. Greenselect Phytosome as an adjunct to a low-calorie diet for treatment of obesity: a clinical trial. Altern Med Rev. 2009;14(2):154-60.

[108] Boschmann M, Thielecke F. The effects of epigallocatechin-3-gallate on thermogenesis and fat oxidation in obese men: a pilot study. J Am Coll Nutr. 2007;26(4):389S-95S.

[109] Toromanyan E, Aslanyan G, Amroyan E, Gabrielyan E, Panossian A. Efficacy of Slim339 in reducing body weight of overweight and obese human subjects. Phytother Res. 2007;21(12):1177-81.

[110] Belza A, Frandsen E, Kondrup J. Body fat loss achieved by stimulation of thermogenesis by a combination of bioactive food ingredients: a placebo-controlled, double-blind 8-week intervention in obese subjects. Int J Obes (Lond). 2007;31(1):121-30.

[111] Hioki C, Yoshimoto K, Yoshida T. Efficacy of bofu-tsusho-san, an oriental herbal medicine, in obese Japanese women with impaired glucose tolerance. Clin Exp Pharmacol Physiol. 2004;31(9):614-9.

[112] Cooke D, Bloom S. The obesity pipeline: current strategies in the development of anti-obesity drugs. Nat Rev Drug Discov. 2006;5(11):919-31.

[113] Vincent RP, le Roux CW. New agents in development for the management of obesity. Int J Clin Pract. 2007;61(12):2103-12.

[114] Hadvary P, Sidler W, Meister W, Vetter W, Wolfer H. The lipase inhibitor tetrahydrolipstatin binds covalently to the putative active site serine of pancreatic lipase. J Biol Chem. 1991;266(4):2021-7.

[115] Jeon BS, Park JW, Kim BK, Kim HK, Jung TS, Hahm JR, *et al*. Fermented mushroom milk-supplemented dietary fibre prevents the onset of obesity and hypertriglyceridaemia in Otsuka Long-Evans Tokushima fatty rats. Diabetes Obes Metab. 2005;7(6):709-15.

[116] Pang J, Choi Y, Park T. Ilex paraguariensis extract ameliorates obesity induced by high-fat diet: potential role of AMPK in the visceral adipose tissue. Arch Biochem Biophys. 2008;476(2):178-85.

[117] Boss O, Samec S, Paoloni-Giacobino A, Rossier C, Dulloo A, Seydoux J, *et al*. Uncoupling protein-3: a new member of the mitochondrial carrier family with tissue-specific expression. FEBS Lett. 1997;408(1):39-42.

[118] Vidal-Puig A, Solanes G, Grujic D, Flier JS, Lowell BB. UCP3: an uncoupling protein homologue expressed preferentially and abundantly in skeletal muscle and brown adipose tissue. Biochem Biophys Res Commun. 1997;235(1):79-82.

[119] Siegner R, Heuser S, Holtzmann U, Sohle J, Schepky A, Raschke T, *et al*. Lotus leaf extract and L-carnitine influence different processes during the adipocyte life cycle. Nutr Metab (Lond). 2010;7:66.

[120] Shibata S. A drug over the millennia: pharmacognosy, chemistry, and pharmacology of licorice. Yakugaku Zasshi. 2000;120(10):849-62.

[121] Nakagawa K, Kishida H, Arai N, Nishiyama T, Mae T. Licorice flavonoids suppress abdominal fat accumulation and increase in blood glucose level in obese diabetic KK-A(y) mice. Biol Pharm Bull. 2004;27(11):1775-8.

[122] Kamisoyama H, Honda K, Tominaga Y, Yokota S, Hasegawa S. Investigation of the anti-obesity action of licorice flavonoid oil in diet-induced obese rats. Biosci Biotechnol Biochem. 2008;72(12):3225-31.

[123] Jeon JR, Kim JY. Effects of pine needle extract on differentiation of 3T3-L1 preadipocytes and obesity in high-fat diet fed rats. Biol Pharm Bull. 2006;29(10):2111-5.

[124] Kim MS, Kim JK, Kim HJ, Moon SR, Shin BC, Park KW, *et al*. Hibiscus extract inhibits the lipid droplet accumulation and adipogenic transcription factors expression of 3T3-L1 preadipocytes. J Altern Complement Med. 2003;9(4):499-504.

[125] Harbilas D, Brault A, Vallerand D, Martineau LC, Saleem A, Arnason JT, *et al*. Populus balsamifera L. (Salicaceae) mitigates the development of obesity and improves insulin sensitivity in a diet-induced obese mouse model. J Ethnopharmacol. 2012;141(3):1012-20.

[126] Harmon AW, Harp JB. Differential effects of flavonoids on 3T3-L1 adipogenesis and lipolysis. Am J Physiol Cell Physiol. 2001;280(4):C807-13.

[127] Harmon AW, Patel YM, Harp JB. Genistein inhibits CCAAT/enhancer-binding protein beta (C/EBPbeta) activity and 3T3-L1 adipogenesis by increasing C/EBP homologous protein expression. Biochem J. 2002;367(Pt 1):203-8.

[128] Park HJ, Della-Fera MA, Hausman DB, Rayalam S, Ambati S, Baile CA. Genistein inhibits differentiation of primary human adipocytes. J Nutr Biochem. 2009;20(2):140-8.

[129] Park HJ, Yang JY, Ambati S, Della-Fera MA, Hausman DB, Rayalam S, *et al*. Combined effects of genistein, quercetin, and resveratrol in human and 3T3-L1 adipocytes. J Med Food. 2008;11(4):773-83.

[130] van Heerden FR. Hoodia gordonii: a natural appetite suppressant. J Ethnopharmacol. 2008;119(3):434-7.

[131] van Heerden FR, Marthinus Horak R, Maharaj VJ, Vleggaar R, Senabe JV, Gunning PJ. An appetite suppressant from Hoodia species. Phytochemistry. 2007;68(20):2545-53.

[132] Zhou H, Beevers CS, Huang S. The targets of curcumin. Curr Drug Targets. 2010 Mar 1;12(3):332-47.

[133] Alappat L, Awad AB. Curcumin and obesity: evidence and mechanisms. Nutr Rev. 2010;68(12):729-38.

[134] Ejaz A, Wu D, Kwan P, Meydani M. Curcumin inhibits adipogenesis in 3T3-L1 adipocytes and angiogenesis and obesity in C57/BL mice. J Nutr. 2009;139(5):919-25.

[135] Wang H, Wen Y, Du Y, Yan X, Guo H, Rycroft JA, *et al*. Effects of catechin enriched green tea on body composition. Obesity (Silver Spring). 2009;18(4):773-9.

[136] Ku HC, Chang HH, Liu HC, Hsiao CH, Lee MJ, Hu YJ, *et al*. Green tea (-)-epigallocatechin gallate inhibits insulin stimulation of 3T3-L1 preadipocyte mitogenesis *via* the 67-kDa laminin receptor pathway. Am J Physiol Cell Physiol. 2009;297(1):C121-32.

[137] Hung PF, Wu BT, Chen HC, Chen YH, Chen CL, Wu MH, *et al*. Antimitogenic effect of green tea (-)-epigallocatechin gallate on 3T3-L1 preadipocytes depends on the ERK and Cdk2 pathways. Am J Physiol Cell Physiol. 2005 288(5):C1094-108.

[138] Levites Y, Amit T, Youdim MB, Mandel S. Involvement of protein kinase C activation and cell survival/ cell cycle genes in green tea polyphenol (-)-epigallocatechin 3-gallate neuroprotective action. J Biol Chem. 2002;277(34):30574-80.

[139] Ahmad N, Mukhtar H. Green tea polyphenols and cancer: biologic mechanisms and practical implications. Nutr Rev. 1999;57(3):78-83.

[140] Kao YH, Chang HH, Lee MJ, Chen CL. Tea, obesity, and diabetes. Mol Nutr Food Res. 2006;50(2):188-210.

[141] Lin JK, Liang YC, Lin-Shiau SY. Cancer chemoprevention by tea polyphenols through mitotic signal transduction blockade. Biochem Pharmacol. 1999;58(6):911-5.

[142] Lin JK, Lin-Shiau SY. Mechanisms of hypolipidemic and anti-obesity effects of tea and tea polyphenols. Mol Nutr Food Res. 2006;50(2):211-7.

[143] Yang CS, Wang ZY. Tea and cancer. J Natl Cancer Inst. 1993;85(13):1038-49.

[144] Kim NH, Choi SK, Kim SJ, Moon PD, Lim HS, Choi IY, *et al*. Green tea seed oil reduces weight gain in C57BL/6J mice and influences adipocyte differentiation by suppressing peroxisome proliferator-activated receptor-gamma. Pflugers Arch. 2008;457(2):293-302.

[145] Yamada T, Nishimura Y, Sakurai T, Terashima T, Okubo T, Juneja LR, *et al*. Administration of theanine, a unique amino acid in tea leaves, changed feeding-relating components in serum and feeding behavior in rats. Biosci Biotechnol Biochem. 2008;72(5):1352-5.

[146] Ahn EK, Oh JS. Lupenone Isolated from Adenophora triphylla var. japonica Extract Inhibits Adipogenic Differentiation through the Downregulation of PPARgamma in 3T3-L1 Cells. Phytother Res. 2012; 27:761-6.

[147] Mukhtar H, Ahmad N. Tea polyphenols: prevention of cancer and optimizing health. Am J Clin Nutr. [Review]. 2000;71(6 Suppl):1698S-702S; discussion 703S-4S.

[148] Erba D, Riso P, Bordoni A, Foti P, Biagi PL, Testolin G. Effectiveness of moderate green tea consumption on antioxidative status and plasma lipid profile in humans. J Nutr Biochem. 2005;16(3):144-9.

[149] Khan N, Mukhtar H. Tea polyphenols for health promotion. Life Sci. 2007;81(7):519-33.

[150] Oliveira DM, Freitas HS, Souza MF, Arcari DP, Ribeiro ML, Carvalho PO, *et al*. Yerba Mate (Ilex paraguariensis) aqueous extract decreases intestinal SGLT1 gene expression but does not affect other biochemical parameters in alloxan-diabetic Wistar rats. J Agric Food Chem. 2008;56(22):10527-32.

[151] Arcari DP, Bartchewsky W, Jr., dos Santos TW, Oliveira KA, DeOliveira CC, Gotardo EM, *et al*. Anti-inflammatory effects of yerba mate extract (Ilex paraguariensis) ameliorate insulin resistance in mice with high fat diet-induced obesity. Mol Cell Endocrinol. 2011;335(2):110-5.

[152] Yun JM, Jialal I, Devaraj S. Effects of epigallocatechin gallate on regulatory T cell number and function in obese v. lean volunteers. Br J Nutr. 2010;103(12):1771-7.

[153] O'Garra A, Vieira P. Regulatory T cells and mechanisms of immune system control. Nat Med. 2004 Aug;10(8):801-5.

[154] Kim HK, Della-Fera M, Lin J, Baile CA. Docosahexaenoic acid inhibits adipocyte differentiation and induces apoptosis in 3T3-L1 preadipocytes. J Nutr. 2006;136(12):2965-9.

[155] Rahman I, Biswas SK, Kirkham PA. Regulation of inflammation and redox signaling by dietary polyphenols. Biochem Pharmacol. 2006;72(11):1439-52.

[156] Calder PC. Polyunsaturated fatty acids and inflammation. Biochem Soc Trans. 2005;33(Pt 2):423-7.

[157] Pallares V, Calay D, Cedo L, Castell-Auvi A, Raes M, Pinent M, *et al*. Additive, antagonistic, and synergistic effects of procyanidins and polyunsaturated fatty acids over inflammation in RAW 264.7 macrophages activated by lipopolysaccharide. Nutrition. 2012;28(4):447-57.

[158] Nagao K, Yanagita T. Conjugated fatty acids in food and their health benefits. Journal of bioscience and bioengineering. [Review]. 2005 Aug;100(2):152-7.

[159] Kepler CR, Hirons KP, McNeill JJ, Tove SB. Intermediates and products of the biohydrogenation of linoleic acid by Butyrinvibrio fibrisolvens. J Biol Chem. [*In Vitro*]. 1966;241(6):1350-4.

[160] Teachey MK, Taylor ZC, Maier T, Saengsirisuwan V, Sloniger JA, Jacob S, *et al*. Interactions of conjugated linoleic acid and lipoic acid on insulin action in the obese Zucker rat. Metabolism. 2003;52(9):1167-74.

[161] Wang YM, Nagao K, Inoue N, Ujino Y, Shimada Y, Nagao T, *et al*. Isomer-specific anti-obese and hypolipidemic properties of conjugated linoleic acid in obese OLETF rats. Biosci Biotechnol Biochem. 2006;70(2):355-62.

[162] Rahman SM, Wang Y, Yotsumoto H, Cha J, Han S, Inoue S, *et al*. Effects of conjugated linoleic acid on serum leptin concentration, body-fat accumulation, and beta-oxidation of fatty acid in OLETF rats. Nutrition. 2001;17(5):385-90.

[163] DeLany JP, Blohm F, Truett AA, Scimeca JA, West DB. Conjugated linoleic acid rapidly reduces body fat content in mice without affecting energy intake. Am J Physiol. 1999;276(4 Pt 2):R1172-9.

[164] Takahashi Y, Kushiro M, Shinohara K, Ide T. Dietary conjugated linoleic acid reduces body fat mass and affects gene expression of proteins regulating energy metabolism in mice. Comparative biochemistry and physiology Part B, Biochemistry & molecular biology. 2002;133(3):395-404.

[165] Park Y, Albright KJ, Storkson JM, Liu W, Cook ME, Pariza MW. Changes in body composition in mice during feeding and withdrawal of conjugated linoleic acid. Lipids. 1999;34(3):243-8.

[166] Kong WH, Oh SH, Ahn YR, Kim KW, Kim JH, Seo SW. Antiobesity effects and improvement of insulin sensitivity by 1-deoxynojirimycin in animal models. J Agric Food Chem. 2008;56(8):2613-9.

[167] Kaats GR, Michalek JE, Preuss HG. Evaluating efficacy of a chitosan product using a double-blinded, placebo-controlled protocol. J Am Coll Nutr. 2006;25(5):389-94.

[168] Mhurchu CN, Poppitt SD, McGill AT, Leahy FE, Bennett DA, Lin RB, *et al*. The effect of the dietary supplement, Chitosan, on body weight: a randomised controlled trial in 250 overweight and obese adults. Int J Obes Relat Metab Disord. 2004;28(9):1149-56.

[169] Hwang HS, Kim SH, Yoo YG, Chu YS, Shon YH, Nam KS, *et al*. Inhibitory effect of deep-sea water on differentiation of 3T3-L1 adipocytes. Marine biotechnology. 2009;11(2):161-8.

[170] Bajaj J, Knox JF, Komorowski R, Saeian K. The irony of herbal hepatitis: Ma-Huang-induced hepatotoxicity associated with compound heterozygosity for hereditary hemochromatosis. Digestive diseases and sciences. 2003;48(10):1925-8.

[171] Nadir A, Agrawal S, King PD, Marshall JB. Acute hepatitis associated with the use of a Chinese herbal product, ma-huang. The American journal of gastroenterology. 1996;91(7):1436-8.

[172] Chitturi S, Farrell GC. Herbal hepatotoxicity: an expanding but poorly defined problem. Journal of gastroenterology and hepatology. 2000;15(10):1093-9.

[173] Jorge OA, Jorge AD. Hepatotoxicity associated with the ingestion of Centella asiatica. Revista espanola de enfermedades digestivas : organo oficial de la Sociedad Espanola de Patologia Digestiva. 2005;97(2):115-24.

[174] Gloro R, Hourmand-Ollivier I, Mosquet B, Mosquet L, Rousselot P, Salame E, *et al*. Fulminant hepatitis during self-medication with hydroalcoholic extract of green tea. European journal of gastroenterology & hepatology. 2005;17(10):1135-7.

[175] Molinari M, Watt KD, Kruszyna T, Nelson R, Walsh M, Huang WY, *et al*. Acute liver failure induced by green tea extracts: case report and review of the literature. Liver transplantation : official publication of the American Association for the Study of Liver Diseases and the International Liver Transplantation Society. 2006;12(12):1892-5.

[176] Pedros C, Cereza G, Garcia N, Laporte JR. [Liver toxicity of Camellia sinensis dried etanolic extract]. Medicina clinica. 2003;121(15):598-9.

[177] Thiolet C, Mennecier D, Bredin C, Moulin O, Rimlinger H, Nizou C, *et al*. [Acute cytolysis induced by Chinese tea]. Gastroenterologie clinique et biologique. 2002;26(10):939-40.

[178] Vial T, Bernard G, Lewden B, Dumortier J, Descotes J. [Acute hepatitis due to Exolise, a Camellia sinensis-derived drug]. Gastroenterologie clinique et biologique. 2003;27(12):1166-7.

[179] Galati G, Lin A, Sultan AM, O'Brien PJ. Cellular and *in vivo* hepatotoxicity caused by green tea phenolic acids and catechins. Free Radic Biol Med. 2006;40(4):570-80.

[180] Schmidt M, Schmitz HJ, Baumgart A, Guedon D, Netsch MI, Kreuter MH, *et al*. Toxicity of green tea extracts and their constituents in rat hepatocytes in primary culture. Food Chem Toxicol. 2005;43(2):307-14.

[181] Li JJ, Huang CJ, Xie D. Anti-obesity effects of conjugated linoleic acid, docosahexaenoic acid, and eicosapentaenoic acid. Mol Nutr Food Res. 2008;52(6):631-45.

Send Orders for Reprints to reprints@benthamscience.net

CHAPTER 5

Sphingolipid Turnover Inhibitors as Modulators of Cellular Metabolism and Obesity

Nataliya A. Babenko*

Department of Physiology of Ontogenesis, Institute of Biology, Kharkov Karazin National University, 4 Svobody pl., 61077 Kharkov, Ukraine

Abstract: Sphingolipids are important structural components of cellular membranes which are involved in the regulation of cell growth and death. Sphingolipids metabolites have profound effects on energy production, nutrient utilization and cellular metabolism. Ceramide-induced metabolic impairments contribute to the tissue malfunction associated with obesity. Ceramides are the key intermediates in the biosynthesis of all complex sphingolipids, located in the membranes, where they participate in raft formation and are accumulated in the cells in response to the stress stimuli. Ceramide accumulation in blood serum, liver, adipose tissue, and muscle are associated with the obesity and metabolic disease. Sphingomyelin hydrolysis, *de novo* synthesis and the salvage pathway are three major pathways for ceramide production and the key enzymes of ceramide metabolism can be the useful targets for cellular lipid modulation. The inhibition of ceramide production results in reduced weight, prevented the diet-induced obesity and a variety of obesity-induced metabolic disorders, too. This chapter will be focused on the role of sphingolipid metabolites in the regulation of lipid storage in cells and tissues. Much attention will be given to the role of ceramide in lipogenesis deregulation. The metabolic benefits of sphingolipid turnover inhibition in obese rodents will be analyzed.

Keywords: Cellular metabolism regulation, ceramidase, ceramide synthase, ceramides, dihydroceramide desaturase, glucosylceramide synthase, inhibitors of sphingolipid turnover, obesity, serine palmitoyltransferase, sphingomyelinases.

INTRODUCTION

Obesity and associated disorders are the major public health problems. Recent evidence suggests that sphingolipids have been implicated in the obesity and

*Address Correspondence to Nataliya A. Babenko: Department of Physiology of Ontogenesis, Institute of Biology, Kharkov Karazin National University, 4 Svobody pl., 61077 Kharkov, Ukraine; Tel: 38(057) 7062148; Fax: 38(057) 3352923; Email: babenko@univer.kharkov.ua

metabolism violation [1-4]. Sphingolipids are components of biological membranes and important regulators of various stress responses and growth mechanisms. Such sphingolipids as ceramide, sphingosine and sphingosine 1-phosphate are a novel class of molecules of bio-effectors involved in the regulation of different signaling pathways. Ceramides are the key intermediates in the biosynthesis of all complex sphingolipids, located in the membranes where they participate in raft formation and are accumulated in the cell in response to the stress stimuli [5-9]. There are three major pathways for the ceramide production in the cells. *De novo* ceramide synthesis is the best known pathway which starts with the transfer of serine residue onto a fatty acyl-CoA to form 3-keto-sphinganine (3KSn). This reaction is catalyzed with the rate-limiting enzyme serine palmitoyltransferase. Subsequent activation of 3KSn reductase, (dihydro)ceramide synthase, and dihydroceramide desaturase converts this intermediate into ceramide. Sphingomyelin hydrolysis is the second ceramide-generating pathway. Different sphingomyelinases, distinguished by their pH optima and subcellular location, hydrolyze sphingomyelin to form the ceramide. Taking into account that sphingomyelin is the most abundant sphingolipid in mammalian cells, it becomes evident that sphingomyelinase-dependent pathway plays the important role in ceramide accumulation in the cells. However, other complex sphingolipids can be the source of ceramide, as well. An increase in cellular concentration of ceramide can come from glucosylceramide and ceramide-1-phosphate and from the reacylation of sphingosine, too.

Factors that alter sphingolipids metabolism and ceramide production increase risk and progression of the pathogenesis of obesity, diabetes and atherosclerosis [10]. Nearly all stress factors induce sphingolipid synthesis, ceramide and ceramide metabolites accumulation in different tissues. Glucocorticoid-, saturated fat-, and obesity-induced insulin resistance is associated with increased ceramide synthesis [11]. However, inhibition of ceramide synthesis markedly improves glucose tolerance and prevents diabetes development in obese rodents. The high-fat diet increased the ceramide as well as triacylglycerol production in the liver [12]. The palmitate flux through ceramide and triacylglycerol synthetic pathways is regulated in the liver in a competitive fashion. The capacity of liver to handle excess dietary fat and to accumulate triacylglycerol is an important factor in the regulation of overall glucose homeostasis. Elevation of sphingolipid synthesis activates the major transcription factors of lipid metabolism, the sterol-regulatory element binding proteins (SREBPs), that regulate genes of fatty acids, cholesterol, and phospholipids synthetic enzymes [2]. Moreover, significant increase of the newly synthesized fatty acids, ceramide and sphingosine levels in the liver, muscles, hippocampus and brain cortex has been defined in aged rats, chronically maintained on calorie high saturated fat-enriched diet [13]. Ceramide and free fatty acids accumulation in brain structures were associated with farther decline in cognitive function and development of central insulin resistance of old animals as compared with the age-matched normal control [13, 14].

Recent studies have demonstrated that high-fat diet increased expression and activity of acid sphingomyelinase and ceramide level in the adipose tissues and plasma isolated from C57BL/6J mice [15, 16]. Ceramide accumulation was associated with increased body weight and glomerular injury [16]. Neutral and acid sphingomyelinases were elevated in the adipose tissues of obese rodents, while absence of acid enzyme in humans with type-1 Niemann-Pick disease was followed by the weight loss [17, 18]. Chronic calorie uptake reduction-induced weight loss was accompanied by a decrease in neutral sphingomyelinase, ceramide synthase activities, ceramides, hexosylceramides and lactosylceramides contents in kidney, liver and brain cortex [19-21]. These findings provide definitive evidence of changing the key enzymes of sphingolipid turnover in obese and calorie-restricted rodents. Ceramide is a key molecule involved in the development of the obesity-related pathology. The inhibition of ceramide production in obese rodents delays or prevents disease onset [22-24].

MECHANISM OF CERAMIDE ACTION ON THE LIPOGENESIS AND WHOLE-BODY METABOLISM

Lipid biosynthesis is essential for the cellular homeostasis. The newly synthesized lipids are used as an energy source/reserve, precursors of cellular glycerolphospholipids, sphingolipids and cholesterol, and signaling molecules. Energy homeostasis depends on the ability to control the balance between lipid synthesis, storage and lipid mobilization [25, 26]. Stored fat is deposited as triacylglycerols in intracellular lipid droplets [27], which are accumulated in adipose and other body tissues. Different defects of lipid metabolism contribute to the development of many pathological states, including obesity, insulin resistance, type 2 diabetes, non-alcoholic fatty liver disease, and cancer.

Recent studies performed on obese humans and animals revealed an important role of sphingolipids in regulation of *de novo* lipogenesis and lipid storage. Sphingolipids and their numerous metabolites participate in the regulation of variety of cellular processes. Different ceramides (C2-and NBD-ceramides) have been demonstrated to be effective in lipogenesis regulation in HL60 cells (a human leukocytic line) and baby-hamster kidney (BHK) fibroblasts [28]. Addition of ceramides to the culture media significantly reduced contents of newly synthesized phosphatidylcholine, sphingomyelin and glucosylceramide and increased diacylglycerol and triacylglycerol levels in the cells. Treatment of [^{14}C]acetate-labeled BHK fibroblasts with B. cereus sphingomyelinase increased significantly [^{14}C]ceramide, [^{14}C]diacylglycerol and [^{14}C]triacylglycerol contents, and had no effect on phosphatidylcholine synthesis. It can be concluded that ceramide directly affecting lipids synthesis *de novo* causes diacylglycerol and triacylglycerol accumulation. However, the direct mechanisms of lipid synthesis regulation by sphingolipids are currently unknown.

Increased triacylglycerol synthesis and lipid droplets accumulation have been determined in the etoposide-treated cells of different lines (HCT116, EL4, DU145, and C4-2b) [29]. Etoposide is a widely used drug for apoptosis induction in cancer cells. Ceramide accumulation *via* sphingolipid synthesis enhancement precedes the drug-induced cell death [30, 31]. Etoposide-induced triacylglycerol synthesis results from the inhibition of mitochondrial fatty acid β-oxidation and is associated with increased acyl-CoA synthetase activity [29]. Thus, the drug targets fatty acids away from oxidation pathway to neutral lipids synthesis.

Recently, the schlank gene has been identified as a major regulator of lipid homeostasis in Drosophila [32]. Schlank encodes a conserved member of the Lass/CerS family of ceramide synthases, containing a catalytic Lag1 motif and a homeobox transcription factor domain. Gene mutant shows the reduced levels of sphingolipids and depleted fat stores as a result of upregulation of triacylglycerol lipases and a downregulation of SREBP-dependent fatty acid synthesis. It is worth-noticing that members of the conserved Lass/CerS family also influence on lipid homeostasis in mammals [33]. The results obtained suggest a novel role of ceramide synthases in regulating the body fat metabolism.

Ceramide synthesized *de novo* or derived from the sphingomyelin regulates mature SREBP levels [34, 35]. Ceramide synthesis elevation due to exogenous sphingosine addition or sphingosine kinase inhibition led to the sterol-regulatory elements-mediated gene transcription and mature SREBP levels increase in the CHO (Chinese hamster ovary) cells [35].

The central role of ceramide in body weight regulation, energy metabolism, and the metabolic syndrome has been determined [16, 36, 37]. Inhibition of ceramide synthesis or acid sphingomyelinase in high-fat-induced or genetic obese mice has been found to significantly improve the features of metabolic syndrome. However, a high-fat diet does not cause triacylglycerol accumulation in the liver of acid sphingomyelinase-deficient mice [12]. The acid sphingomyelinase inhibitor, desipramine, attenuates the palmitic acid-induced triacylglycerol accumulation in HepG2 cells. The overexpression of acid sphingomyelinase in the liver improves glucose tolerance in wild-type and diabetic *db/db* mice and induces lipid accumulation in hepatocytes *via* sphingosine-1-phosphate formation [38].

Other target of ceramide derived from sphingomyelin is the leptin. A close link between plasma leptin, obesity and insulin resistance has been reported [39-44].

Hyperleptinemia, increased food intake, and decreased metabolism are the prime consequences of leptin resistance [44-46]. Content of circulating leptin increases with increasing calorie intake. However, leptin failed to change feeding behavior, to prevent weight rise and to modify gluconeogenesis in overfed animals. High-fat diet increased significantly the leptin level in the plasma [16]. The administration of inhibitor of acid sphingomyelinase, amitriptiline, to animals, treated with a high-fat diet, reduced ceramide levels in the plasma and adipose tissue and leptin concentration in the plasma, too. Hypothalamic arcuate nucleus (Arc) pretreatment with a cell-penetrating analog of natural ceramide C2-ceramide blocked the leptin-induced anorectic effect [47]. Arc myriocin administration, which effectively inhibited the serine palmitoyltransferase and reduced ceramide level in the hypothalamus, lowered food uptake and weight gain.

Chronic treatment of obese (*ob/ob*) or high-fat-induced obese mice with an inhibitor of *de novo* ceramide synthesis, myriocin, decreased C16-and C18-ceramide molecular species, and total ceramide content in the blood plasma [36]. The decrease in the ceramide level was followed by weight loss, hepatic steatosis decrease, glucose homeostasis improvement, expression of suppressor of cytokine signaling-3 (SOCS-3) and induced adipose uncoupling protein-3 (UCP3) decrease. Taking into account that ceramide could directly induce SOCS-3 and inhibit UCP3 mRNA in cultured adipocytes, a reasonable assumption might be made that ceramide plays a key role in metabolism regulation *via* direct effects on genes involved in energy metabolism and expenditure [36]. However, finding that in *db/db* mice the muscle ceramide levels did not elevate, but inhibition of *de novo* ceramide synthesis with myriocin still prevented the insulin resistance development, it was assumed that such ceramide metabolite as glucosylceramide is more important in mediating the skeletal muscle insulin resistance than the ceramide itself [37]. Furthermore, a specific inhibitor of glucosylceramide synthase, N-(5'-adamantane-1'-yl-methoxy)-pentyl-1-deoxynojirimycin, enhanced the insulin sensitivity *via* lowering of glucosylceramide and ganglioside contents, without significant reduction of ceramide level in the tissues of *ob/ob* mice as well as in the high-fat-fed and Zucker diabetic *fa/fa* rats [48]. Moreover, it has been demonstrated that not only the ceramide but also the sphingosine-1-phosphate are involved in glucose and lipid metabolism regulation [38, 49, 50].

The above results provide a convincing proof of an important role of sphingolipids in lipogenesis regulation and obesity development. Ceramide is the key but not a single molecule contributing into the lipogenesis deregulation. The key enzymes of ceramide production and turnover modulation can be chosen as a strategy for obesity and obesity-related symptoms treatment.

INHIBITION OF SPHINGOLIPID SYNTHESIS AND TURNOVER AS A STRATEGY FOR IMPROVEMENT OF CELLULAR METABOLISM

It is well documented that lipotoxic sphingolipid metabolites accumulation in adipose tissues and tissues not suited for lipid storage is a feature of obese individuals with an elevated risk of insulin-resistance, diabetes and cardiovascular disease. Among the numerous sphingolipid species, stored in these tissues, ceramide is the most toxic one. However, recent studies have shown that the alteration in cellular and whole-body metabolism is a direct consequence of ceramide accumulation [3, 16, 32, 33, 36, 37, 50]. Taking into consideration that ceramide synthesis *de novo*, sphingomyelin hydrolysis, and salvage pathway altered in obese animal models and obese individuals, attention will be focused on the inhibitors of these three major pathways.

Ceramide Synthesis *De Novo*

Serine palmitoyltransferase activation initiates the process of sphingolipid synthesis *de novo* (Fig. **1**). The enzyme is highly selective for fatty acyl-CoA with 16 ± 1 carbon atoms and the presence of both the serine and palmitoyl-CoA are necessary for the activation of this step in sphingolipid synthesis. Other fatty acids can inhibit the synthesis by competing for the CoA pool [51, 52]. Serine palmitoyltransferase is inhibited by a number of synthetic and natural products. The inhibition of the first enzyme of sphingolipid synthesis is followed by a decrease in the ceramide and sphingosine or sphingomyelin levels in the cells. Among the potent and specific inhibitors of serine palmitoyltransferase are beta-chloroalanine, L-cycloserine and the inhibitors isolated from microorganisms (sphingofungins, lipoxamycins, and ISP1/myriocin) [53, 54] (Fig. **1**). Myriocin is widely used to clarify the serine palmitoyltransferase impact on ceramide accumulation in adipose and muscle tissues, blood plasma and liver under fatty acids oversupply. Myriocin treatment (4-8-week-long) of *ob/ob* obese mice or animals maintained on a high-fat diet abolished ceramide accumulation in blood plasma [36] and skeletal muscle [37]. Besides, myriocin reduced body weight and fat mass. Drug-induced inhibition of ceramide synthesis was associated with a reduction in adipocytes diameter, abdominal subcutaneous and epididymal fat pad weights, and body weight [36]. Myriocin did not change the food intake and respiratory exchange ratio while increased the V_{02} and CO_2 output and horizontal activity.

Moreover, myriocin reduced the leptin gene expression in epididymal fat pads and liver of obese mice, liver triacylglycerol level and ameliorated hepatic steatosis, the most common liver abnormality in obese rodents and humans, which contributes to hepatic insulin resistance.

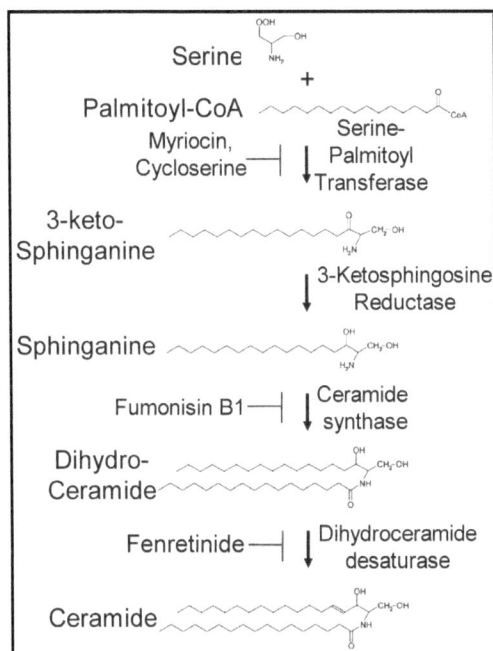

Figure 1: Inhibition of ceramide synthesis *de novo* pathway.

Experiments conducted on isolated hepatocytes have demonstrated that age-dependent and palmitic acid- or C2-ceramide-induced insulin resistance can be improved by myriocin [55]. Short-term cells pretreatment with myriocin reduced significantly the ceramide level which is elevated in the old and palmitic acid/C2-ceramide-treated hepatocytes. Myriocin increased induction of glucose uptake, glycogen synthesis and phospholipase D by insulin in insulin-resistant liver cells. However, short-term action of myriocin on primary hepatocytes did not completely restore glucose metabolism in insulin-resistant cells. Myriocin administered orally or intraperitonealy significantly reduced liver, soleus muscle and serum ceramide levels as well as triacylglycerol content in the blood serum, improved glucose homeostasis in Zucker diabetic fatty rats and prevented diabetes development [11]. Beneficial effects of myriocin could be seen after the first, second and third weeks of treatment. But the short-term soleus muscle strips pretreatment with myriocin or another serine palmitoyltransferase inhibitor, cycloserine, prevented palmitate-induced ceramide accumulation, abolished the antagonistic effect of palmitic acid on insulin-stimulated glucose uptake and did not affect on the diacylglycerol content.

Myriocin or cycloserine nullified palmitic acid-induced ceramide accumulation and inhibitory effect of palmitic acid on Akt/protein kinase B (PKB) and glycogen synthase kinase 3β (GSK3β) phosphorylation in the C2C12 myoblasts and L6 myotubes [56-58]. In contrast, the long-term (7-day-long) treatment of muscle cells with myriocin did not ameliorate the palmitate-induced loss of PKB activation and glucose uptake, but significantly reduced the serine palmitoyltransferase activity and palmitate-induced ceramide accumulation in the L6 miotubes [57]. Sustained chronic serine palmitoyltransferase inhibition imitated enzyme silencing effects not changing the enzyme expression. However, a stable loss of serine palmitoyltransferase activity *via* shRNA-mediated silencing of the enzyme or its pharmacological inhibition led to increased diacylglycerol content in L6 cells. Diacylglycerol is a well known activator of novel and conventional protein kinases (PKC), implicated in lipid-induced insulin resistance [59]. With increase in fatty acyl-CoA and diacylglycerol contents, a novel PKC, PKCθ, activity increased that led to negative regulation of insulin signaling in muscle cells [59-62]. The excess of the *de novo* synthesized diacylglycerol activated PKC, phosphorylation of insulin receptor substrate-1 (IRS-1), thus suppressing the IRS-1 tyrosine phosphorylation and diminishing phosphatidylinositol 3-kinase activation and blocking the insulin signaling in the target cells [63-68]. The results obtained allow to make a conclusion that the chronically reduced serine palmitoyltransferase activity and elevated *de novo* diacylglycerol synthesis define the defective insulin-stimulated glucose transport in the muscle cells.

Besides inhibitors of serine palmitoyltransferase, ceramide synthesis could be inhibited by reduction of the (dihydro)ceramide synthase [69] (Fig. **1**). The (dihydro)ceramide synthase is the target of Fumonisin B_1 and other fungal inhibitors [70-72]. Fumonisin B_1 is used to study the biological role of ceramide and complex sphingolipids in different cells and tissues. Drug exposure results in decrease of sphingomyelin, other sphingolipids and diacylglycerol contents in different cells and tissues [73-75]. The long-term culturing of NIH/3T3 fibroblasts in the presence of Fumonisin B_1 decreased sphingolipids and glycosylsphingolipids contents, increased glycosyltransferases in the pathway of globotraosylceramide (Gb3) synthesis and did not change the ganglioside 3

(GM3) and sphingomyelin synthase activities [76]. Using the CHOs cells, stable transfectants for an SRE-reporter gene, treated with Fumonisin B_1 or other ceramide synthesis inhibitors (myriocin, cycloserine) for 8 hours demonstrated that decreased ceramide synthesis was correlated with diminished SRE-mediated gene transcription and mature SREBP [35]. Pretreatment (16 hours-long) of C2C12 myotubes with Fumonisin B_1 as well as with myriocin prevented palmitate-induced ceramide accumulation and insulin signaling disruption [55]. Fumonisin B_1, like myriocin and cycloserine, revoked palmitate effect on Akt/PKB and GSK3β, and did not prevent the Akt/PKB phosphorylation inhibition by synthetic C2-ceramide. The long-term daily mice treatment with Fumonisin B_1 significantly increased the sphinganine and sphingosine contents in the liver of both wild-type mice and mice with deleted NOS-2 gene, as well as levels of sphingosine 1-phosphate and sphinganine 1-phosphate in wild-type animals [77]. The administration of the Fumonisin B_1 to mice increased the gene expression of two subunits of serine palmitoyltransferase (LCB1 and LCB2) and sphingosine kinase 1 [77].

Fumonisin B_1 effect is specific and adapts cells to chronic reduction of ceramide synthesis. It is quite possible that increased activity of acid sphingomyelinase, which has a house keeping function in cells, can adapt cells to a reduced ceramide level by producing ceramide *via* sphingomyelin hydrolysis. Indeed, 5 day-long injection of Fumonisin B_1 did not change the ceramide level in liver, kidney, and brain [78].

It is worth noting that the mycotoxins are extremely toxic and carcinogenic substances [78-81]. Fumonisin B_1-induced ceramide synthesis inhibition results in disruption of different pathways of sphingolipid metabolism and turnover. Thus, it should be remembered that Fumonisin B_1 is not appropriate in all cases.

The promising results have been obtained in recent experiments with the dihydroceramide desaturase inhibitor, fenretinide (Fig. **1**) [82]. The long-term treatment of obese mice with fenretinide markedly reduced adiposity and hyperleptinemia and did not have any effect on energy expenditure, food intake, physical activity or stool lipid content [83]. Fenretinide improved insulin action on glucose uptake and glycogen levels in muscle and reduced hepatic steatosis.

Sphingomyelin Hydrolysis

Sphingomyelin is the most abundant sphingolipid and its hydrolysis under the action of sphingomyelinases is the important pathway of ceramide generation in cells. The pathway is activated by oxidative stress and inflammatory signals. A new role of sphingomyelinases in regulation of metabolism and obesity has been demonstrated [12, 38]. Chronic treatment of adult rats with dietetic saturated fat significantly increased the ceramide/sphingomyelin ratio in the liver and brain cortex with respect to control ones [14]. If it is recalled that the altered ceramide/sphingomyelin ratio may itself be a result of the elevated sphingomyelinase activity, our findings suggest that the saturated fat, chronically added to the diet of rats, can enchance the sphingomyelinase activity in the liver and brain. The long-term feeding of mice with the saturated fat led to the pronounced increase of sphingomyelinases expression and activity in liver and epididymal and subcutaneous fat pads [15, 84]. However, a high fat diet affected the expression of both neutral and acid sphingomyelinases in the fat tissues [15], enhanced activity of neutral sphingomyelinase in liver and liver cell nuclei [85] and activated the acid sphingomyelinase, but not the neutral sphingomyelinase in the colon [86]. From these results it is evident that dietetic saturated fat-induced expression of sphingomyelinases mRNA can be an important reason of chronic sustained ceramide accumulation in the different tissues.

Acid sphingomyelinase inhibitors (Fig. **2**) are widely used to protect cells from the stress-induced and receptor-mediated apoptosis and to promote the cell proliferation [87, 88]. Using acid sphingomyelinase inhibitor made it possible to determine the enzyme role in lipid metabolism regulation. Acid sphingomyelinase inhibitor, amitriptyline, attenuated obesity and obesity-associated renal injury induced with the high-fat-diet treatment [16]. Inhibition of acid sphingomyelinase by desipramine significantly reduced triacylglycerol synthesis and content and increased the (dihidro)ceramide synthesis in the HepG2 cells, cultured in the presence of exogenous palmitic acid of high concentration [12]. Addition of ceramide synthesis inhibitors (myriocin or Fumonisin B_1) to the culture media containing the desipramine-treated liver cells attenuated the desipramine effect on ceramide synthesis. Similar results were obtained for acid sphingomyelinase-deficient mice fed with saturated fat enriched-diet. They provide direct evidence that acid sphingomyelinase regulates the partitioning of increased palmitic acid supply mainly to sphingolipid synthesis. In contrast, the overexpression of acid sphingomyelinase in the diabetic *db/db* mice is associated with glucose and lipid metabolism improvement [38]. Acid sphingomyelinase inhibition with imipramine results in decrease of glucose uptake by liver cells and glycogen and lipid deposition in hepatocytes that clearly demonstrates the important role of enzyme inhibitors in determination of acid sphingomyelinase in glucose and lipid metabolisms regulation.

Desipramine and imipramine are tricyclic antidepressants, which efficiently supress the acid sphingomyelinase activity in cells (Fig. **2**) [87, 88] and in different tissues [89] as experiments *in vitro* and *in vivo* have shown, respectively. These drugs are able to enter the lysosomes and after accumulation they stimulate the proteolytic enzyme degradation. However, the desipramine has been found to inhibit the acid ceramidase in addition to acid sphingomyelinase in the human prostate cancer cell line DU145, bladder cancer cell line 5637, and Hela cervical cancer cells [90], though this drug has no effect on a majority of other lisosomal enzymes [88]. As the tricyclic antidepressants are minimally toxic and licensed for medical use in humans, this group of sphingomyelinase inhibitors can be potentially used in treatment of acid sphingomyelinase-dependent metabolic dysfunctions. The effects of other inhibitors of sphingomyelinase activity on cellular metabolism remain to be established. Besides classical sphingomyelinase inhibitors, the other approaches exist. As the recent studies have shown, the long-term feeding of rats with the fish oil-enriched diet reduced the elevated ceramide production and increased the reduced phosphatidylserine and sphingomyelin levels in the brain structure of old animals [91]. This dietetic effect could be mimicked by the exogenous phosphatidylserine. The phosphatidylserine administration to old rats reduced significantly the neutral sphingomyelinase activity in brain.

Since the *n-3* PUFA (polyunsaturated fatty acids) as well as phosphatidylserine have anti-inflammatory effects [92] and reduced content of known stimulator of neutral sphingomyelinase, interleikin-1β [93], a reasonable assumption has been made that in old animals *n-3* PUFA preventes the ceramide accumulation *via*

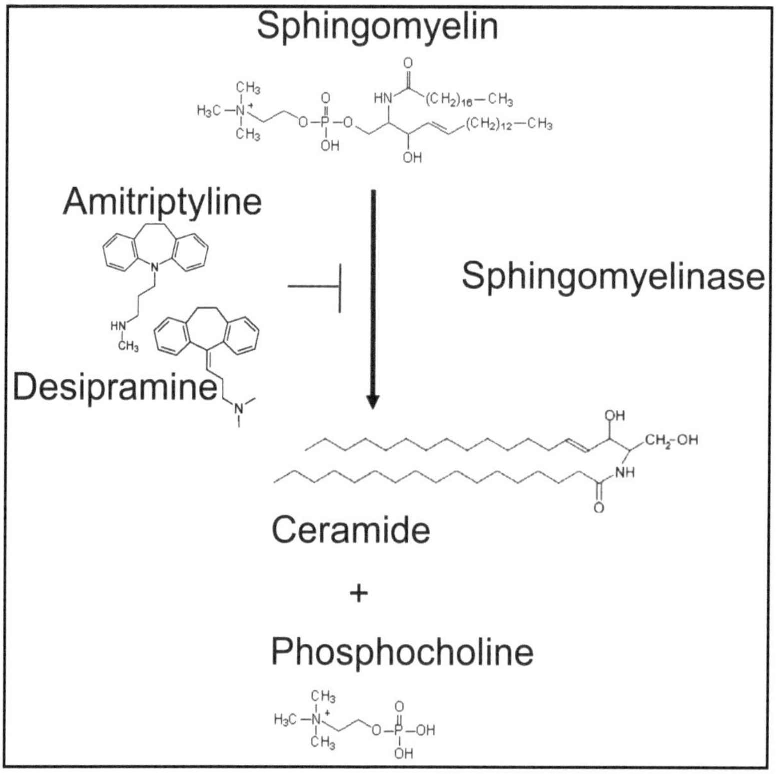

Figure 2: Acid sphingomielinase inhibitors.

phosphatidylserine-mediated cytokine-induced sphingomyelinase inhibition. Other indirect inhibitors of sphingomyelinase activity have also been determined [87]. Among the natural sphingomyelinase inhibitors, the plant-derived flavonoids are worth consideration. The administration of Chamomilla recutita flavonoids (apigenin, luteolin, apigenin-7-glucoside (AP7Glu), luteolin-7-glucoside (LU7Glu), isorhamnetin and quercetin) to old rats decreased the elevated neutral and acid sphingomyelinases activities and ceramide mass and did not affect the ceramide conversion to the sphingosine or sphingomyelin [94]. These data suggest a key role of sphingomyelinases in the flavonoid-induced decrease of ceramide levels in the liver of old rats. Because of their antioxidant properties, the flavonoids were able to reduce the damage of hepatocytes induced by chemicals *in vitro* and *in vivo*. The intragastric administration of the mixture of Chamomilla recutita flavonoid isomers (such as apigenin, luteolin, AP7Glu, LU7Glu, isorhamnetin and quercetin (chamiloflan)) to adult rats nullified the CCl_4-induced increase of serum alanine aminotransferase, aspartate aminotransferase and gamma-glutamile transpeptidase activities in blood serum and prevented the hepatocellular fatty degeneration [95, 96]. The flavonoids completely restored the triacylglycerol, free fatty acids and ceramide levels and decreased the elevated ceramide/sphingomyelin ratio in the damaged liver of CCl_4-treated animals or isolated hepatocytes [97]. The administration of flavonoids to rats normalized the elevated ceramide content in the damaged liver *via* neutral sphingomyelinase inhibition and ceramidase activation. Effects of flavonoids on sphingomyelin turnover can be imitated by α-tocopherol. Both compounds, flavonoids and α-tocopherol, increased the level of negative regulator of the neutral sphingomyelinase, glutathione in cells and thus supressed the enzyme activity [98]. Both the long- and short-term effects of α-tocopherol on sphingolipid turnover have been determined. α-Tocopherol could ameliorate the palmitate-induced ceramide accumulation in the hepatocytes of young animals *via* the inhibition of sphingolipid synthesis. By using the α-tocopherol, the intracellular accumulation of ceramides can be prevented by inhibition of the acid and neutral sphingomyelinase, as well as ceramide synthesis *de novo*.

Other Pathways of Ceramide Turnover

A growing body of evidence implicates glycosphingolipids in the pathogenesis of insulin resistance and metabolism deregulation. Inhibiting glycosphingolipids synthesis (Fig. **3**) in *ob/ob* mice with Genz-123346, a specific inhibitor of glucosylceramide synthase, the initial enzyme implicated in the synthesis of glycosphingolipids, lowered glucose and hemoglobin A1c (HbA1c) levels, as well as the liver/body weight ratio, the accumulation of triglycerides, liver glucosylceramide and improved the several markers of liver pathology [99].

Similar results were obtained for other inhibitor (Genz-112638), which is currently being evaluated clinically for a lysosomal storage disorder (Gaucher disease) treatment [100]. Drug treatment also reduced the expression of several genes associated with hepatic steatosis involved in lipogenesis, gluconeogenesis, and inflammation. Drug-induced inhibition of glycosphingolipids synthesis in obese mice prevented the development of steatosis. Using a highly specific inhibitor (iminosugar derivative *N*-(5′-adamantane-1′-yl-methoxy)pentyl-1-

deoxynoijrimycin (AMP-DNM)) of glucosylceramide synthase, the improvement of insulin signaling in cultured 3T3-L1 adipocytes has been demonstrated [47].

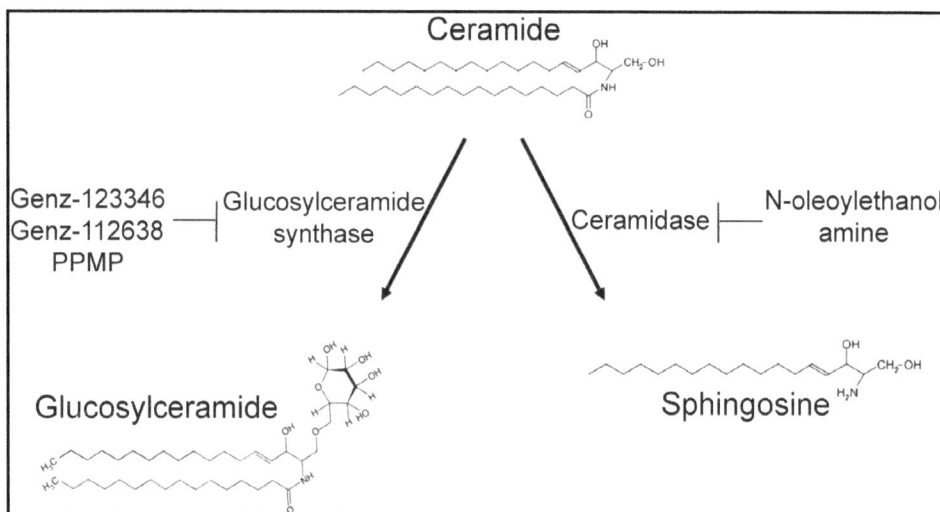

Figure 3: Inhibitors of ceramide utilization.

Treatment of *ob/ob* mice with AMP-DNM normalized the elevated tissues glucosylceramide levels, markedly lowered plasma glucose levels, improved oral glucose tolerance, and insulin sensitivity in muscle and liver.

Similarly beneficial metabolic effects of the inhibitor were seen in high-fat–fed mice and diabetic rats. These findings provide further evidence that inhibition of glycosphingolipid biosynthesis might present a novel approach to prevent the insulin resistance and associated metabolic disorders.

To increase ceramide levels in the treated cells, the other group of glucosylceramide synthase inhibitors was used. For example, treatment of SHO cells with DL-treo-1-Phenyl-2palmitoylamino-3morpholino-1-propanol-HCl (PPMP), an inhibitor of glucosylceramide synthase, increased the intracellular ceramide level, decreased the ceramide synthesis *de novo*, as measured by [^{3}H]serine incorporation, and also decreased the SRE-mediated gene transcription [35]. The glucosylceramide synthase inhibitor, N-Butyldeoxynojirimycin-HCl (NB-DNJ), which had no effect on the ceramide content and synthesis in the cells, did not change the SRE-mediated gene transcription. Addition of PPMP, as well as ceramidase inhibitor, *N*-oleoylethanolamine (Fig. **3**), to the culture media of C2C12 miotubes farther increased the ceramide accumulation and markedly inhibited the insulin-stimulated Akt/PKB phosphorylation [55]. Administration of *N*-oleoylethanolamine caused weight loss due to increased fatty acid metabolism and oxidation [101-104]. In adipocytes and hepatocytes the *N*-oleoylethanolamine inhibited mitogenic and metabolic signaling by the insulin receptor and produced glucose intolerance. The role of *N*-oleoylethanolamine as antiobesity drug and its role in metabolic control are discussed.

CONCLUDING REMARKS

Sphingolipids are the source of bioactive metabolites which are involved in the regulation of cellular metabolism and thereby cell functions, its growth and death. Different defects in sphingolipid synthesis or turnover contribute to the development of many pathological states and depend on deregulation of key enzymes of sphingolipid metabolism. Overexpression of serine palmitoyltransferase, ceramide synthase and sphingomyelinase in the tissues of obese rodents is the main reason of ceramide accumulation in the tissues of obese and diabetic rodents. Nevertheless, contribution of other enzymes of ceramide turnover, such as glucosylceramide synthase, ceramidases and sphingosine kinases can not be ruled out in ceramide deregulation. Inhibitors of sphingolipid metabolism are able to block or enhance the ceramide production and accumulation within the cells and are useful tools for investigation of ceramide role in cell pathology. Inhibitors of sphingolipid metabolism and turnover are used not only *in vitro*, but in long-term experiments *in vivo*, too. Late approach allows to answer the question how altered sphingolipid metabolism can regulate the whole body weight and metabolism and to determine the central role of ceramide in metabolic syndrome development. However, the beneficial clinical effect of sphingolipid metabolism inhibitors remains to be studied.

ACKNOWLEDGEMENTS

Declared none

CONFLICT OF INTEREST

The author confirms that this chapter contents have no conflict of interest.

REFERENCES

[1]   Worgall TS. Sphingolipids: major regulators of lipid metabolism. Curr Opin Clin Nutr Metab Care 2007; 10(2): 149-55.

[2]   Worgall TS. Sphingolipid synthetic pathways are major regulators of lipid homeostasis. Adv Exp Med Biol 2011; 721: 139-48.

[3]   Bikman BT, Summers SA. Ceramides as modulators of cellular and whole-body metabolism. J Clin Invest 2011; 121(11): 4222-30.

[4]   Chavez JA, Summers SA. A ceramide-centric view of insulin resistance. Cell Metab 2012; 15: 585-94.

[5]   Hannun YA, Obeid LM. Principles of bioactive lipid signalling: lessons from sphingolipids. Nat Rev Mol Cell Biol. 2008; 9(2): 139-50.

[6]   Gault CR, Obeid LM, Hannun YA. An overview of sphingolipid metabolism: from synthesis to breakdown. Adv Exp Med Biol. 2010; 688:1-23.

[7]   Hannun YA, Obeid LM. The ceramide-centric universe of lipid-mediated cell regulation: stress encounters of the lipid kind. J Biol Chem 2002; 277(29): 25847-50.

[8]   Sawai H, Hannun YA. Ceramide and sphyngomyelinases in the regulation of stress responses. Chem Phys Lipids 1999; 102 (1-2): 141-7.

[9]   Hannun YA, Luberto C. Ceramide in the eukaryotic stress response. Trends Cell Biol 2000; 10(2): 73-80.

[10]   Cutler RG, Mattson MP. Sphingomyelin and ceramide as regulators of development and lifespan. Mech Ageing Dev 2001; 122: 895–908.

[11]   Holland WL, Brozinick JT, Wang L-P, *et al.* Inhibition of ceramide synthesis ameliorates glucocorticoid-, saturated-fat-, and obesity-induced insulin resistance. Cell Metab 2007; 5: 167-79.

[12]   Deevska GM, Rozenova KA, Giltiay NV, *et al.* Acid sphingomyelinase deficiency prevents diet-induced hepatic triacylglycerol accumulation and hyperglycemia in mice. J Biol Chem 2009; 284(13): 8359-69.

[13]   Babenko NA, Semenova YaA, Kharchenko *VS.* Effects of fat-enriched diet on the content of sphingolipids in the brain and on cognitive functions in old rats. Neurophysiol 2009; 41: 258-63.

[14]   Babenko NA. Effects of short-and long-term saturated fat-enriched diet on the ceramide and neutral lipids accumulation in the insulin responsive tissues of rats. In: Langella JP. Saturated Fats: Metabolism, Disease Risks and Public Awareness. New York; Nova Science Publishers 2012; pp. 71-97.

[15]   Shah C, Yang G, Lee I, *et al.* Protection from high fat diet-induced increase in ceramide in mice lacking plasminogen activator inhibitor. J Biol Chem 2008; 283: 13538-48.

[16]   Boini KM, Zhang Ch, Xia M, Poklis JL, Li P-L. Role of sphingolipid mediator ceramide in obesity and renal injury in mice fed a high-fat diet. J Pharm Exp Ther 2010; 334(3): 839-46.

[17]   Samad F, Hester KD, Yang G, Hannun YA, Bielawski J. Altered adipose and plasma sphingolipid metabolism in obesity. A potential mechanism for cardiovascular and metabolic risk. Diabetes 2006; 55: 2579-87.

[18]   Crocker AC, Farber S. Niemann-Pick disease: a review of eighteen patients. Medicine (Baltimore) 1958; 34(1): 1-95.

[19] Hernandez-Corbacho MJ, Jenkins RW, Clarke ChJ, *et al*. Accumulation of long-chain glycosphingolipids during aging is prevented by caloric restriction. PLoS ONE 2011; 6(6): 1-9.

[20] Rutkute K, Asmis RH, and Nikolova-Karakashian MN. Regulation of neutral sphingomyelinase-2 by GSH: a new insight to the role of oxidative stress in agind-associated inflammation. J Lipid Res 2007; 48: 2443-52.

[21] Costantini C, Weindruch R, Valle GD, Puglielli L. A TrkA-to-p75[NTR] molecular switch activates amyloid β-peptide generation during aging. Biochem J 2005; 391: 59-67.

[22] Quan-Jiang Zhang Q-J, Holland WL, Wilson L, *et al*. Ceramide mediates vascular dysfunction in diet-induced obesity by PP2A-mediated dephosphorylation of the eNOS-Akt complex. Diabetes 2012; 61: 1848–59.

[23] Ussher JR, Folmes CDL, Keung W, *et al*. Inhibition of serine palmitoyl transferase I reduces cardiac ceramide levels and increases glycolysis rates following diet-induced insulin resistance. PLoS ONE 2012; 7(5): e37703.

[24] Schiffmann S, Ferreiros N, Birod K, *et al*. Ceramide synthase 6 plays a critical role in the development of experimental autoimmune encephalomyelitis. J Immunol 1103109 2012; doi: 10.4049/jimmunol.1103109

[25] Hay N, Sonenberg N. Upstream and downstream of mTOR. Genes Dev 2008; 18: 1926–45.

[26] Zechner R, Strauss JG, Haemmerle G, Lass A, Zimmermann R. Lipolysis: pathway under construction. Curr Opin Lipidol 2005; 16: 333–40.

[27] Martin S, Parton RG. Lipid droplets: a unified view of a dynamic organelle. Nat Rev Mol Cell Biol 2006; 7: 373–378.

[28] Allan D. Lipid metabolic changes caused by short-chain ceramides and the connection with apoptosis. Biochem J 2000; 345: 603-10.

[29] Boren J, Brindle KM. Apoptosis-induced mitochondrial dysfunction causes cytoplasmic lipid droplet formation. Cell death and differentiation 2012; doi:10.1038/odd.2012.34.

[30] Perry DK, Carton J, Shah AK, *et al*. Serine palmitoyltransferase regulates *de novo* ceramide generation during etoposide-induced apoptosis. J Biol Chem 2000; 275(12): 9078-84.

[31] Sawada M, Nakashima S, Banno Y, *et al*. Ordering of ceramide formation, caspase activation, and Bax/Bcl-2 expression during etoposide-induced apoptosis in C6 glioma cells. Cell Death Differ 2000; 7(9): 761-72.

[32] Bauer R, Voelzmann A, Breiden B, *et al*. Schlank, a member of the ceramide synthase family controls growth and body fat in Drosophila. EMBO J 2009; 28: 3706-16.

[33] Pewzner-Jung Y, Park H, Lavid EL, *et al*. A critical role for ceramide synthase 2 in liver metabolic pathways. J Biol Chem 2010; 285: 10902-10.

[34] Worgall TS, Johnson RA, Seo T, Gierens H, Deckelbaum RJ. Unsaturated fatty acid-mediated decreases in sterol regulatory element-mediated gene transcription are linked to cellular sphingolipid metabolism. J Biol Chem 2002; 277: 3878-85.

[35] Worgall TS, Juliano RA, Seo T, Deckelbaum RJ. Ceramide synthesis correlates with the posttranscriptional regulation of the sterol-regulatory element-binding protein. Arterioscler Thromb Vasc Biol 2004; 24: 943-8.

[36] Yang G, Badeanlou L, Bielawski J, Roberts AJ, Hannun YA. Central role of ceramide biosynthesis in body weight regulation, energy metabolism, and the metabolic syndrome. Am J Physiol Endocrinol Metab 2009; 297: E211-E224.

[37] Ussher JR, Koves TR, Cadete VJJ, *et al*. Inhibition of *de novo* ceramide synthesis reverses diet-induced insulin resistance and enhances whole-body oxygen consumption. Diabetes 2010; 59: 2453-64.

[38]   Osawa Y, Seki E, Kodama Y, *et al*. Acid sphingomyelinase regulates glucose and lipid metabolism in hepatocytes through AKT activation and AMP-activated protein kinase suppression. FASEB J 2011; 25: 1133-44.

[39]   Dobrian AD, Davies MJ, Schriver SD, Lauterio TJ, Prewitt RL. Oxidative stress in a rat model of obesity-induced hypertension. Hypertension 2011; 37: 554–60.

[40]   Abdullah AR, Hasan HA, Raigangar VL. Analysis of the relationship of leptin, high-sensitivity C-reactive protein, adiponectin, insulin, and uric acid to metabolic syndrome in lean, overweight, and obese young females. Metab Syndr Relat Disord 2009; 7(1): 17-22.

[41]   Pehlivanov B, Mitkov M. Serum leptin levels correlate with clinical and biochemical indices of insulin resistance in women with polycystic ovary syndrome. Eur J Contracept Reprod Health Care 2009; 14(2): 153-9.

[42]   Miesel A, Müller H, Thermann M, Heidbreder M, Dominiak P, Raasch W. Overfeeding-induced obesity in spontaneously hypertensive rats: an animal model of the human metabolic syndrome. Ann Nutr Metab. 2010; 56(2): 127-42.

[43]   Knight SF, Quigley JE, Yuan J, Roy SS, Elmarakby A, Imig JD. Endothelial dysfunction and the development of renal injury in spontaneously hypertensive rats fed a high-fat diet. Hypertension 2008; 51: 352–9.

[44]   Wang J, Obici S, Morgan K, Barzilai N, Feng Z, Rossetti L. Overfeeding rapidly induces leptin and insulin resistance. Diabetes. 2001; 50(12): 2786-91.

[45]   Friedman JM, Halaas JL. Leptin and the regulation of body weight in mammals. Nature 1998; 395: 763–70.

[46]   Gao S, Zhu G, Gao X, *et al*. Important roles of brain-specific carnitine palmitoyltraansferase and ceramide metabolism in leptin hypothalamic control of feeding. PNAS 2011; 108(23): 9691-96.

[47]   Aerts JM, Ottenhoff R, Powlson AS, *et al*. Pharmacological inhibition of glucosylceramide synthase enhances insulin sensitivity. Diabetes 2007; 56: 1341-9.

[48]   Ma MM, Chen JL, Wang GC, *et al*. Sphingosine kinase 1 participates in insulin signaling and regulates glucose metabolism and homeostasis in KK/Ay diabetic mice. Diabetologia 2007; 50(4): 891-900.

[49]   Rapizzi E, Taddei ML, Fiaschi T, *et al*. Sphingosine-1-phosphate increases glucose uptake through trans-activation of insulin receptor. Cell Mol Life Sci 2009; 66(19): 3207-18.

[50]   Guenther GG, Edinger AL. A new take on ceramide. Starving cells by cutting off the nutrient supply. Cell cycle 2009; 8(8): 1122-6.

[51]   Merrill AH Jr, Wang E, Mullins RE. Kinetics of long-chain (sphingoid) base biosynthesis in intact LM cells: effects of varying the extracellular concentrations of serine and fatty acid precursors of this pathway. Biochemistry 1988; 27 (1): 340-5.

[52]   Miyake Y, Kozutsumi Y, Nakamura S, Fujita T, Kawasaki T. Serine palmitoyltransferase is the primary target of a sphingosine-like immunosuppressant, ISP-1/myriocin. Biochem Biophys Res Commun 1994; 211: 396-403.

[53]   Mandala SM, Harris GH. Isolation and characterization of novel inhibitors of sphingolipid synthesis: australifungin, viridiofungins, rustmicin, and khafrefungin. Methods Enzymol 2000; 311: 335-48.

[54]   Babenko NA, Kharchenko *VS*. Ceramides inhibit phospholipase D-dependent insulin signaling in liver cells of old rats. Biochemistry (Moscow) 2012; 77: 180-6.

[55]   Chavez JA, Knotts TA, Wang L-P, *et al*. A role for ceramide, but not diacylglycerol, in the antagonism of insulin signal transduction by saturated fatty acids. J Biol Chem 2003; 278(12): 10297-303.

[56]   Powell DJ, Turban S, Gray A, Hajduch E, Hundal HS. Intracellular ceramide synthesis and protein kinase Cζ activation play an essential role in palmitate-induced insulin resistance in rat L6 skeletal muscle cells. Biochem J 2004; 382: 619-29.

[57]   Watson ML, Coghlan M, Hundal HS. Modulating serine palmitoyl transferase (SPT) expression and activity unveils a crucial role in lipid-induced insulin resistance in rat skeletal muscle cells. Biochem J 2009; 417: 791-801.

[58]   Erion DM, Shulman GI. Diacylglycerol-mediated insulin resistance.Nature Medicine2010; 16: 400–2.Haasch D, Berg C, Clampit JE, *et al*. PKCθ is a key player in the development of insulin resistance. Biochem Biophys Res Commun 2006; 343: 361-68.

[59]   Qu X, Seale JP, Donnelly R. Tissue and isoform-selective activation of protein kinase C in insulin-resistant obese Zucker rats: effects of feeding. J Endocrinol 1999; 162: 207-14.

[60]   Griffin ME, Marcucci MJ, Cline GW, *et al*. Free fatty acid-induced insulin resistance is associated with activation of protein kinase Cθ and alterations in the insulin signaling cascade. Diabetes 1999; 48: 1270-4.

[61]   Itani SI, Hou Q, Pories WJ, Macdonald KG, Dohm GL. Involvment of protein kinase C in human skeletal muscle insulin resistance and obesity. Diabetes 2000; 49: 1353-8.

[62]   Jornayvaz FR, Birkenfeld AL, Jurczak MJ, *et al*. Hepatic insulin resistance in mice with hepatic overexpression of diacylglycerol acyltransferase 2. Proc Natl Acad Sci USA 2011; 108(14): 5748-52.

[63]   Zhang L, Ussher JR, Oka T, *et al*. Cardiac diacylglycerol accumulation in high fat-fed mice is associated with impaired insulin-stimulated glucose oxidation. Cardiovascular Research 2011; 89: 148–56.

[64]   Neschen SK, Morino LE, Hammond D, *et al*. Prevention of hepatic steatosis and hepatic insulin resistance in mitochondrial acyl-CoA:glycerol-sn-3-phosphate acyltransferase 1 knockout mice. Cell Metab 2005; 2: 55–65.

[65]   Nagle CA, An J, Shiota M, *et al*. Hepatic overexpression of glycerol-sn-3-phosphate acyltransferase 1 in rats causes insulin resistance. J Biol Chem 2007; 282: 14807–15.

[66]   Boden G, She P, Mozzoli M, *et al*. Free fatty acids produce insulin resistance and activate the proinflammatory nuclear factor-κB pathway in rat liver. Diabetes 2005; 54(12): 3458-65.

[67]   Benoit SC, Kemp CJ, Elias CF, *et al*. Palmitic acid mediates hypothalamic insulin resistance by altering PKC-theta subcellular localization in rodents. J Clin Invest 2009; 119: 2577-89.

[68]   Merrill AH Jr. *De novo* sphingolipid biosynthesis: a necessary, but dangerous, pathway. J Biol Chem 2002; 277(29): 25843-46.

[69]   Vesper H, Schmelz E-M, Nikolova-Karakashian MN, *et al*. Sphingolipids in food and the emerging importance of sphingolipids to nutrition. J Nutr 1999; 129(7): 1239-50.

[70]   Mandala SM, Thornton RA, Frommer Br, *et al*. The discovery of australifungin, a novel inhibitor of sphinganine N-acyltransferase from Sporomiella australis. Producing organism, fermentation, isolation, and biological activity. J Antibiot (Tokyo) 1995; 48(5): 349-56.

[71]   Humpf HU, Schmelz EM, Meredith FI, *et al*. Acylation of naturally occurring and synthetic 1-deoxysphinganines by ceramide synthase. Formation of N-palmitoyl-aminopentol

produces a toxic metabolite of hydrolyzed fumonisin, AP1, and a new category of ceramide synthase inhibitor. J Biol Chem 1998; 273(30): 19060-4.

[72] Wu WI, McDonough VM, Nickels JT Jr, Ko J, Fischl AS, Vales TR, Merrill AH Jr, Carman GM. Regulation of lipid biosynthesis in Saccharomyces cerevisiae by fumonisin B1. J Biol Chem 1995; 270: 13171–8.

[73] Yoo HS, Norred WP, Showker J, Riley RT. Elevated sphingoid bases and complex sphingolipid depletion as contributing factors in fumonisin-induced cytotoxicity. Toxicol Appl Pharmacol 1996; 138: 211–8.

[74] He Q, Suzuki H, Sharma N, Sharma RP. Ceramide synthase inhibition by Fumonisin B1 treatment activates sphingolipid-metabolizing systems in mouse liver. Toxicol Sci 2006; 94(2): 388–97.

[75] Meivar-Levy I, Futerman AH. Up-regulation of neutral glycosphingolipid synthesis upon long term inhibition of ceramide synthesis by fumonisin b1. J Biol Chem 1999; 274: 4607–12

[76] Suzuki H, Riley RT, Sharma RP. Inducible nitric oxide has protective effect on fumonisin B_1 hepatotoxicity in mice *via* modulation of sphingosine kinase. Toxicology 2007; 229(1-2): 42–53.

[77] Tsunoda M, Sharma RP, Riley RT. Early fumonisin B1 toxicity in relation to disrupted sphingolipid metabolism in male BALB/c mice. J Biochem Mol Toxicol 1998; 12(5): 281-9.

[78] Gelderblom WC, Kriek NP, Marasas WF, Thiel PG. Toxicity and carcinogenicity of the Fusarium moniliforme metabolite, fumonisin B1, in rats. Carcinogenesis 1991; 12 (7): 1247-51.

[79] Harrison LR, Colvin BM, Greene JT, Newman LE, Cole JR Jr. Pulmonary edema and hydrothorax in swine produced by fumonisin B1, a toxic metabolite of Fusarium moliniforme. J Vet Diagn Invest 1990; 2(3): 217-21.

[80] Dugyala RR, Sharma RP, Tsunoda M, Riley RT. Tumor necrosis factor-alpha as a contributor in fumonisin B1 toxicity. J Pharmacol Exp Ther 1998; 285(1): 317-24.

[81] Bikman BT, Guan Y, Shui G, *et al*. Fenretinide prevents lipid-induced insulin resistance by blocking ceramide biosynthesis. J Biol Chem 2012; 287: 17426-37.

[82] Preitner F, Mody N, Graham TE, Peroni OD, Kahn BB. Long-term fenretinide treatment prevents high-fat diet-induced obesity, insulin resistance, and hepatic steatosis. Am J Physiol Endocrinol Metab 2009; 297(6): E1420-E1429.

[83] Lyn-Cook LE Jr, Lawton M, Tong M, *et al*. Hepatic ceramide may mediate brain insulin resistance and neurodegeneration in type 2 diabetes and non-alcoholic steatohepatitis. J Alzheimer Dis 2009; 16: 715-29.

[84] Chocian G, Chabowski A, Zendzian-Piotrowska M, *et al*. High fat diet induces ceramide and sphingomyelin formation in rat's liver nuclei. Mol Cell Biochem 2010; 340; 125-31.

[85] Cheng Y, Ohlsson L, Duan R-D. Psyllium and fat in diets diferentially affect the activities and expressions of colonic sphingomyelinases and caspase in mice. Br J Nutr 2004; 91: 715-23.

[86] Arenz C. Small molecule inhibitors of acid sphingomyelinase. Cell Physiol Biochem 2010; 26: 1-8.

[87] Kornhuber J, Tripal Ph, Reichel M, *et al*. Functional inhibitors of acid sphingomyelinase (FIASMAs): a novel pharmacological group of drugs with broad clinical applications. Cell Physiol Biochem 2010; 26: 9-20.

[88]   Garkavenko VV, Storozhenko GV, Krasnikova ON, Babenko NA. Correction of age-related disorders of sphingolipid content in rat tissues by acid sphingomyelinase inhibition. Int J Physiol Pathophysiol. 2012; 3(3): 281-286.

[89]   Elojeimy S, Holman DH, Liu X, *et al*. New insights on the use of desipramine as an inhibitor for acid ceramidase. FEBS Letters 2006; 580: 4751-6.

[90]   Babenko NA, Semenova YaA. Effects of long-term fish oil-enriched diet on the sphingolipid metabolism in brain of old rats. Exp Gerontol 2010; 45: 375-80.

[91]   Calder PC. N-3 polyunsaturated fatty acids, inflammation, and inflammatory diseases. Am J Clin Nutr 2006; 83: 1505S–19S.

[92]   O'Donnell E, Vereker E, Lynch MA. Age-related impairment in LTP is accompanied by enhanced activity of stress-activated protein kinases: analysis of underlying mechanisms. Eur J Neurosci 2000; 12: 345–52.

[93]   Babenko N, Shakhova E. Effects of Chamomilla recutita flavonoids on age-related liver sphingolipid turnover in rats. Exp Gerontol 2006; 41(1): 32-9.

[94]   Babenko N, Shachova E. Effects of flavonoids on carbon tetrachloride induced accumulation of lipids in the liver. Annales Universitatis Mariae Curie-Sklodowska (Lublin-Polonia) 2004; 17: 173-5.

[95]   Babenko NA, Shachova EG. Effects of flavonoids on CCl$_4$-induced ceramide and diacylglycerol accumulation in the liver. Ukrainian Biochem J 2005; 77(2): 94.

[96]   Babenko N, Shachova E. Effects of flavonoids on sphingolipid turnover in the toxin-damaged liver and liver cells. Lipids Health Disease 2008; 7: 1

[97]   Babenko NA, Hassouneh LKhM, Kharchenko VS, Garkavenko VV. Vitamin E prevents the age-dependent and palmitate-induced disturbances of sphingolipid turnover in liver cells. Age 2012; 34: 905-15.

[98]   Zhao H, Przybylska M, Wu IH, *et al*. Inhibiting glycosphingolipid synthesis ameolirates hepatic steatosis in obese mice. Hepatology 2009; 50(1): 85-93.

[99]   Yew NS, Zhao H, Hong E-G, *et al*. Increased Hepatic Insulin Action in Diet-Induced Obese Mice Following Inhibition of Glucosylceramide Synthase. PLoS ONE 2010; 5(6): e11239. Available from: doi:10.1371/journal.pone.0011239

[100]   Overton HA, Babbs AJ, Doel SM, *et al*. Deorphanization of a G protein-coupled receptor for oleoylethanolamide and its use in the discovery of small-molecule hypophagic agents. Cell Metab 2006; 3: 167–75.

[101]   Lo Verme J, Gaetani S, Fu J, Oveisi F, Burton K, Piomelli D. Regulation of food intake by oleoylethanolamide. Cell Mol Life Sci 2005; 62: 708–16.

[102]   Guzman M, Lo Verme J, Fu J, Oveisi F, Blazquez C, Piomelli D. Oleoylethanolamide stimulates lipolysis by activating the nuclear receptor peroxisome proliferator-activated receptor alpha (PPAR-alpha) J Biol Chem 2004; 279: 27849–54.

[103]   Fu J, Gaetani S, Oveisi F, Lo Verme J, Serrano A, Rodriguez De Fonseca F, *et al*. Oleoylethanolamine regulates feeding and body weight through activation of the nuclear receptor PPAR-alpha. Nature 2003; 425: 90–3.

[104]   Wang J, Ueda N. Role of the endocannabinoid system in metabolic control. Curr Opin Nephrol Hypertens 2008; 17(1): 1-10.

Anti-Obesity Drug Discovery and Development, Vol. 2, 2014, 264-286

Index

A

Abdominal obesity   11, 14, 16, 58, 105, 112
Absorption   44, 133, 180, 213, 216, 220
Absorption inhibitors   135
Acetyl CoA carboxylase (ACC)   142, 217, 219-22, 226
Acid
  eicosapentaenoic (EPA)   227
  hydroxyl citric (HCA)   140, 158, 192
  palmitic   249-50
      sphingomyelinase   242, 244, 246, 251-3, 255
  carnosic   188-9
  conjugated linoleic   140, 144-5, 224, 228
  phenolic   181
      poly unsaturated fatty (PUFA)   144, 216, 227
Actinobacteria   179-80
Actinomycetales   179
Activity
  antiobesity   147
  lipolytic   218, 225
  lipoprotein lipase   53, 228
  serine palmitoyltransferase   250
Adenosine monophosphate protein kinase (AMPK)   20, 140, 142, 224, 226
Adipocyte   10, 19-21, 23, 26-30, 37, 53, 95-6, 98, 142-8, 188-9, 211, 213-14, 216-22, 224-8, 247-8, 256-7
  central   95-6
  large   217, 220
  inhibition of   130, 225
mature   143, 145
Adipocyte hypertrophy   29-30, 217, 220
Adipocyte life-cycle   135, 142-3, 145-6
Adipocyte proliferation   143, 216, 226
Adipocytokines   20, 90, 95

M

Macrophage inflammatory protein (MIP)   26

Macrophage inhibitory factor (MIF)   28

Macrophages   26-8, 37, 62, 214, 227

Magnetic resonance imaging (MRI)   100

Malignancies   86-8, 90, 97, 99-101, 103, 107, 113-14, 116

Mature SREBP levels   246

MCP-1   23, 28, 42, 214

Mediterranean diet (MD)   42-3

Melanin-concentrating hormone (MCH)   139

Menopausal transition   105-6

Menopause   87, 89, 92, 94, 96, 98, 100-1, 105-6, 110, 116, 213

Metabolic   21, 26, 32, 43, 48, 57-8, 61, 86-7, 89, 94, 96, 102-3

Metabolic changes   9, 60, 62, 212-13

Metabolic disease   19, 21, 29-30, 53, 144, 242

Metabolic inflexibility   3, 30, 38, 57-8

Metabolic IR   40-1

Metabolic processes   48, 86

Metabolic syndrome (MetS)   3, 8, 11-18, 20-1, 23-7, 30, 38, 42, 48, 58, 86-8, 90-4, 101, 111, 246

Metabolism   10, 15, 35, 95, 142, 163, 189, 213, 219, 226, 229, 252, 257

Metabolites   9, 136, 140, 176, 245

  microbial   137, 180, 190

  secondary   185, 190-1, 222, 225

Metabolomics   180-1

Metaflammation   8, 26, 31

MetS components   18, 23

Micro-organisms   131, 179

Microbial sources   130, 135, 139, 147, 190-1

Migraine   51, 58-60

Mitochondria   213

Monocytes   23, 28, 214

Mortality   42, 88-9, 106, 114, 131

mRNA expression   23, 225

Peptide YY (PYY) 7, 9, 134

Peptides 20, 23, 194

Peripheral nervous system 55

Pernatural 177-8

Peroxisome 35, 144-6, 188, 213

Peroxisome proliferator-activated receptors, (PPAR) 20, 144, 146, 148, 171, 188, 213, 217-18, 221, 224-6, 228

PGC-1 35

Phenolics 144, 157, 173, 181

Phentermine 3, 8, 45-6, 50, 55-6, 133

Phosphodiesterase 142

Phosphorylation 97, 144, 226-8, 250

Phyllum 179-80

Physical activity 3, 6, 42, 44, 107, 109-11, 133, 141, 212, 251

  decreased 131, 212

  reduced 107, 132, 212

  regular 109

Physical exercise 10, 35, 41-2, 56, 98, 109, 130

Phytochemicals 131, 136

Phytoestrogens 98-9, 108

PL inhibitors 136, 148, 179-81, 193

PL inhibitory effects 136-7

Plant extracts 139, 192, 216-17, 219-20, 225

Plant origin 216, 223

Plant products 211

Plants 131, 134-6, 139-40, 158, 185-6, 189, 193, 216, 219-22, 224-6, 230

  medicinal 134, 180-1, 194

Plasma 154, 162, 174, 186, 213, 219, 244, 246

Plasma lipids 220, 222

Plasma triglyceride gain 218-19

Platycodin 220, 222

Polycystic ovarian syndrome 41, 93, 103, 110-11

Polyphenols 130, 136-7, 140, 181, 219, 225, 227

Postprandial state 19, 29-30